Praise for Using Insulin

"This book is a tremendous resource for all patients and medical personnel who deal with diabetes. Comprehensive, easily un... all ages and both Type 1 and Type 2 diabetes. I highl

— Ken Cathcart, D.O., F.A.C.E.
Adult and pediatric endocrinologist, Spok

"A great mix of vast information, guidance, and conversational tone with tables, quizzes, sidebars and humor. I now realize how much I have taken insulin for granted all these years and how narrow my scope has been."

— Judith Ambrosini
Author and chef extraordinaire at the Diabetes Cyber Kitchen
www.diabetesnet.com/cyber_kitchen/

"A great resource-book packed full of up-to-date and useful information for those who have diabetes and the health professionals who care for them. Step-by-step guidelines are clarified by creative charts, case studies and chapter summaries. Thank you for all the hard work that makes my job easier."

— JoAnne Scott, R.N., C.D.E.
Diabetes educator and person with diabetes, Spokane, Washington

"Congratulations on this invaluable contribution to diabetes treatment! A book that is comprehensive, well-researched, yet very readable."

— George Dailey III, M.D., endocrinologist at the Diabetes and Endocrinology Division, Scripps Clinical Research Foundation, La Jolla, California

"An essential and comprehensive guide for anyone who uses insulin – even I learned new things!"

— Sheri R. Colberg, Ph.D., Author of **The Diabetic Athlete**
Professor of exercise physiology at Old Dominion University, Type 1 diabetes for over 35 years, Norfolk, Virginia

"**Using Insulin** is an excellent resource for persons using insulin to control their diabetes and for the professionals who participate in their care. A Great Book."

— Jo-Ann Shartel, R.N., C.D.E.
Diabetes educator and insulin user, San Diego, California

Using INSULIN

Everything You Need For Success With Insulin

by John Walsh, P.A., C.D.E.,
Ruth Roberts, M.A.,
Chandrasekhar Varma, M.D., F.A.C.P., F.A.C.E.,
and Timothy Bailey, M.D., F.A.C.P., F.A.C.E.

Torrey Pines Press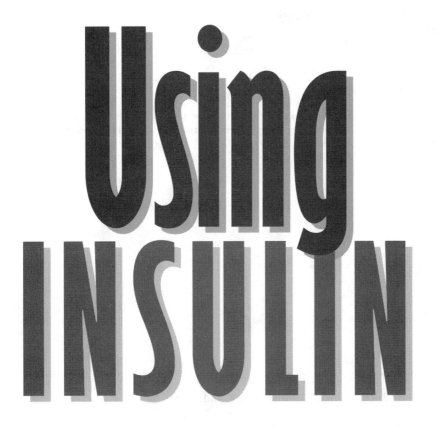
San Diego

Torrey Pines Press
1030 West Upas Street
San Diego, California 92103-3821
1-619-497-0900

Library of Congress Cataloging in Publication Data
Walsh, John; Roberts, Ruth; Varma, Chandrasekhar; and Bailey, Timothy
Using Insulin
    Everything you need for success with insulin
    by John Walsh, P.A., C.D.E., Ruth Roberts, M.A., Chandrasekhar Varma, M.D., F.A.C.P., F.A.C.E., Timothy Bailey, M.D., F.A.C.P., F.A.C.E.

p. cm.
Includes bibliographical references.
Includes index.
1. Diabetes Popular Books
2. Diabetes Insulin
3. Diabetes Insulin-dependent diabetes
4. Diabetes Research
5. Insulin Therapeutic use
I. Title

Library of Congress Control Number: 2003097719
ISBN 1-884804-85-3 $23.95 Paperback

Printed in the United States of America

10 9 8 7 6 5 4 3 2

About the Authors

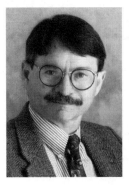

John Walsh, P.A., C.D.E., is a Physician Assistant and Diabetes Clinical Specialist, working for the last ten years at North County Endocrine in Escondido, CA. He has provided clinical care to thousands of people with diabetes in various clinical settings, including 10 years in the Endocrine Division of a large HMO in San Diego. He has over 30 years of personal experience with multiple injections and over 20 years with pumps.

Mr. Walsh is a popular speaker on diabetes topics to physicians, health professionals and people with diabetes, as well as a guest on radio and TV programs as an authority on intensive diabetes management. He is President of Diabetes Services, Inc., and has served on the Board of Directors for both corporate and nonprofit corporations. He is author or coauthor of hundreds of diabetes articles and books, and a consultant for several medical corporations. He specializes in identifying and providing clinical care to those at risk of developing diabetes complications, stabilizing and reversing these complications, and enhancing blood sugar control through innovative methods.

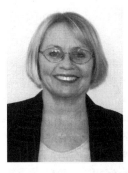

Ruth Roberts, M.A., is CEO of The Diabetes Mall and a medical writer. She has served as a corporate training administrator, technical writer, and instructional designer for 15 years in San Diego. She has been involved in diabetes support groups for over 20 years, and has coauthored several books on diabetes.

Ruth is a professional member of the American Diabetes Association, has served on the Board of Directors for the International Diabetes Athletes Association, and is editor and frequent contributor to "Diabetes This Week", a weekly internet newsletter on the forefront of covering the latest developments in diabetes research and business. She has been a guest on "Living With Diabetes", and is an educational consultant on intensive self-management.

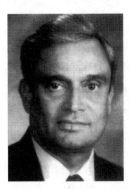

Chandrasekhar Varma M.D., F.A.C.E., F.A.C.P., provides clinical care as a Board Certified Endocrinologist at North County Endocrine and provides rapidly evolving technology to treat common and rare endocrine disorders. Dr. Varma received his medical degree in his native country of India and completed his internship at Drake Memorial Hospital in Cincinnati, his residency at the V.A. Hospital, Brooklyn, New York, and his fellowship at Nassau County Medical Center, New York.

Dr. Varma is clinical assistant professor at the UCSD School of Medicine. He is a Fellow of the American College of Physicians and the American College of Endocrinology.

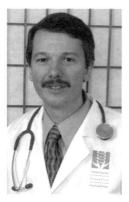

Timothy Bailey M.D., F.A.C.E., F.A.C.P., is Board-Certified in Endocrinology, Metabolism and Internal Medicine. He specializes in the treatment of diabetes, osteoporosis, thyroid diseases, and lipid disorders at North County Endocrine. He is in full-time clinical practice.

Dr. Bailey received his medical degree from Mount Sinai Medical School, New York. He completed his residency at St. Luke's - Roosevelt Hospital, New York and his fellowship in Endocrinology was completed at Downstate Medical Center of New York.

He is a fellow of the American Association of Clinical Endocrinologists, and the American College of Physicians. He is also a member of the American Medical Association, American Diabetes Association, and the Endocrine Society.

In 1994, he founded MetaMedix Inc., a company that developed diabetes and nutrition management software. He led the company to profitability and a successful acquisition by iMetrikus Inc. in August of 2000. He continues to consult for a number of biomedical and pharmaceutical firms.

As a clinical assistant professor at the UCSD School of Medicine, he is active in the education of Endocrinology fellows. He is a frequent speaker to both physician and patient groups.

Contributing Author for Chapter 25, Kids And Teens

Shannon I. Brow, R.N., B.S., C.D.E. is a pediatric diabetes nurse educator and consultant in Houston, Texas. She has developed many patient education materials for use with children, their families, and adults in a variety of inpatient, outpatient, and clinic settings. She also teaches in local colleges of nursing.

Shannon has had diabetes since adolescence and is jokingly referred to as a "Peripatetic Diabetic" because of her love of travel. She "packs her diabetes in her suitcase" and travels around the world 1-2 times a year.

Shannon donates her summers as a medical staff volunteer to several day, weekend, and residential camping programs for children and young adults with diabetes. She is a member of the American Association of Diabetes Educators, and has served as an officer in the South Texas Association of Diabetes Educators. She is a volunteer for the American Diabetes Association and Juvenile Diabetes Foundation.

Other books by John Walsh, P.A., C.D.E. and Ruth Roberts, M.A.:

Pumping Insulin, *third edition, Torrey Pines Press, 2000*

Second edition, 1994; First edition, 1989

STOP the Rollercoaster, *Torrey Pines Press, 1996*

Pocket Pancreas, *Torrey Pines Press, 1995, 1998*

Insulin Pump Therapy Handbook, *1990*

Diabetes Advanced Workbook, *1988*

Acknowledgments

Using Insulin is the product of years of personal and professional experience with diabetes. Many major contributions have been made by our patients, friends, family members, colleagues and fellow travelers.

We especially want to thank the following individuals who graciously and critically reviewed and improved upon this book:

- Helen Oswalt, support group leader and editor, par excellence, of San Diego, CA

- Sheri Colberg, Ph.D., Professor of exercise physiology at Old Dominion University in Norfolk, VA, and has lived with Type 1 diabetes for over 35 years

- Ken Cathcart, D.O., F.A.C.E., adult and pediatric endocrinologist in Spokane, WA

- George Dailey III, M.D., at the Diabetes and Endocrinology Division at Scripps Clinical Research Foundation in La Jolla, CA

- Jeff Hitchcock, Director and Founder of the massive Children With Diabetes website at www.childrenwithdiabetes.com, father of a daughter with Type1

- JoAnne Scott, R.N., C.D.E. Diabetes Educator and insulin user in Spokane, WA

- Rick Mendosa, who has Type 2 diabetes and is the author and webmaster at a comprehensive diabetes site at www.mendosa.com

- Nancy J.V. Bohannon, M.D., F.A.C.E., board-certified endocrinologist, San Francisco, CA

- Diane R. Krieger, M.D., board-certified endocrinologist, Medical Director of the South Miami Hospital Diabetes Care Center, Miami, FL

- Judith Ambrosini, diabetes writer, organizer, and Chief Chef of the Diabetes Cyber Kitchen at www.diabetesnet.com/cyber_kitchen/, Type 1

- Steven V. Edelman, M.D., Prof. of Medicine, U.C.S.D School of Medicine, Founder and Director of Taking Control of Your Diabetes, www.tcoyd.org

- Cindy Onufer, R.N., M.A., Bc-A.D.M., C.D.E., Diabetes Nurse Specialist

- Jean Betschart-Roemer, M.S.N., C.P.N.P., C.D.E., author of numerous books for and about children with diabetes

- Scott King, Publisher of *Diabetes Interview*, Type 1 diabetes, San Francisco, CA

- Carol Wysham, M.D., Rockwood Clinic, Spokane, WA

- Joe Largay, P.A.C., C.D.E., Clinical Instructor, U.N.C. Diabetes Care Center of Raleigh, NC

– Paul C. Davidson, M.D., F.A.C.E., board-certified endocrinologist, Atlanta, GA

– Sara Hohn, R.N., M.S., D.C.N.S., C.D.E., Diabetes Education Coordinator of the OHSU Diabetes Center, Portland, OR

Our special thanks to Richard Morris, III, an independent graphics artist of San Diego, for the cover design, chapter headings, and all the wonderful tables and figures. His work allows us to send this information across in a clear, crisp way.

We and everyone with diabetes are indebted to:

The American Diabetes Association, the Juvenile Diabetes Foundation, the National Institute of Health, and other national agencies that generously support diabetes education and research, as well as the many researchers and clinicians who dedicate their lives to improving health for others.

Table Of Contents

Tables

Graphs

Go Figures

Important Note

    Using Insulin has been developed as a guide to using insulin for diabetes control. Graphs, charts, figures, examples, situations, and tips provide basic as well as advanced information related to the basal/bolus approach for diabetes management. Insulin requirements and treatment protocols differ significantly from one person to the next. The information included in this book should be used only as a guide. It is not a substitute for the sound medical advice of your personal physician or health care team.

    Specific treatment plans, insulin dosages, and other aspects of health care for a person with diabetes, must be based on individualized treatment protocols under the guidance of your physician or health care team. The information in this book is provided to enhance your understanding of diabetes and insulin use so that you can manage the daily challenges you face. It can never be relied upon as a sole source for your personal diabetes regimen.

    While every reasonable precaution has been taken in the preparation of this information, the authors and publishers assume no responsibility for errors or omissions, nor for the uses made of the materials contained herein and the decisions based on such use. No warranties are made, expressed, or implied, with regard to the contents of this work or to its applicability to specific individuals. The authors and publishers shall not be liable for direct, indirect, special, incidental, or consequential damages arising out of the use of or inability to use the contents of this book.

Read This!

    Never use this book on your own! Any suggestion made in this book for improving blood sugar control should only be followed with the approval and under the guidance of your personal physician. We have provided the best information and tools available for you to use your insulin to do its job of normalizing your blood sugars.

    However, this book is not enough. We have worked with individuals who have used this information together with guidance from their physician, and they have excelled. We have also seen others who get themselves into trouble by a selective use of this or other material, and by ignoring or not seeking excellent medical advice.

    Always seek the advice and guidance of your physician and health care team. No book can ever help you as much as they will. They have the benefit of objectivity and experience gained from working with many others on insulin. Your own participation in the process of good control is essential, but never minimize the importance of good professional advice and support. Teams win where individuals fail, and teamwork takes trust and communication from everyone.

We wish all users of this book good health and great control using insulin.

Diabetes Terms Used

Basal/Bolus Approach

A method of managing diabetes that matches insulin to need to best mimic a normal pancreas.

Basal/Bolus Balance

The balance between basal and bolus insulin doses during the day. Generally, the total basal doses and bolus doses during a day will be approximately 50% each for optimal control.

Basal Insulin Dose

An around the clock delivery of insulin that matches background need. When background or basal doses of a long-acting insulin are correctly set, the blood sugar does not rise or fall during periods in which the person does not eat.

Carb Bolus

An injection of rapid insulin delivered to match carbohydrates in an upcoming meal or snack. Most people on injections use between 1 unit of Humalog or Novolog for each 5 grams to 1 unit for each 25 grams.

Correction Bolus

An injection of rapid insulin delivered to bring a high blood sugar back to normal. Usually combined with a carb bolus before a meal. For most people, a correction bolus will lower the blood sugar from 10 to 100 mg/dl per unit of Humalog or Novolog over four hours.

mg/dl

Milligrams per deciliter is the unit of measurement for glucose concentration in the blood that is used in the United States. Millimoles or mmol is how glucose is measured in Europe, Canada, and many other countries. To convert mg/dl to mmol, divide mg/dl by 18, and to convert mmol to mg/dl, multiply mmol by 18.

TDD or Total Daily Dose of Insulin

This is the total units of insulin used per day and is obtained by adding up all the basal doses, carb boluses, and correction boluses for the day.

Additional terms can be found in the Glossary that starts on page 327.

Introduction

If you are considering using insulin, beginning insulin use, or been on it for a while but would like to improve your control, the answers to your questions are here. This book gives the information and in-depth detail you need for success using insulin. It can help anyone who uses insulin, whether Type 1, Type 1.5, or Type 2, and anyone who assists people in their insulin use.

Using Insulin is for:

- Everyone considering or beginning to use insulin
- Current insulin users who want to improve their control
- Physicians, nurses, dieticians, physician assistants, nurse practitioners, diabetes educators, and others who assist people with insulin use
- Everyone who wants to end blood sugar highs and lows
- Everyone who wants to match insulin need with insulin delivery

Using Insulin tells you:

- What insulin is and how it works
- How to chart and analyze your blood sugars
- How to count carbohydrates and match them to insulin
- How to test, set and regulate basal rates and boluses for better control
- How to manage low blood sugars and high blood sugars
- How to analyze and solve problem blood sugar patterns
- How to feel better and live a healthier life
- When to seek help

This book provides step-by-step directions for setting and testing your insulin doses, checklists for improving control, and specific examples of blood sugar management techniques. Included are advanced blood sugar charting methods, carbohydrate counting instructions, approaches to exercise and pregnancy, specific directions for children and teens on insulin, and information on how to avoid complications.

Fast Forward

Seeking specific information relevant to your diabetes challenges? This will help you find where to go.

Benefits Of Blood Sugar Control

The number of people with diabetes is impressive. Over 11 million people in the U.S. know they have diabetes and another seven million have it but are unaware of it. Several million more have an early stage called prediabetes. As part of their treatment, five million people use insulin, including 1.4 million with Type 1 and 4 million with Type 2 diabetes. Many others with Type 2 diabetes who are not currently on insulin would benefit if it were being used.

Many people on insulin, however, face up and down readings on a daily basis. Rarely at peace with their control, they may wonder, "Will I ever be able to use insulin effectively and have optimal control?"

Success with diabetes comes through trial and error, learning, and applying that learning. For those of us with diabetes, the benefits of taking on this task and learning how to use insulin are tremendous, namely a more productive life today and a healthier and longer life in the future.

Today's developments in insulin analogs, insulin delivery, blood sugar testing, and pattern recognition have enabled many to mimic the action of their pancreas and achieve desirable readings. These advances have made diabetes control easier for those who learn to apply this technology. This book is designed to make these recent advances more useful and provide the tools needed to achieve more normal blood sugars while using insulin.

This chapter presents:

- The goal – optimal control
- Why high blood sugars are destructive
- The benefits of better control

What Is Optimal Control?

People without diabetes typically have blood sugars in the 70 to 140 mg/dl* (3.6 to 7.8 mmol) range, depending on how soon after eating a test is taken, as shown in Figure 1.1. Most people with diabetes who control their blood sugar well with insulin and have excellent A1c test results will have some readings that are outside an ideal range every day. When you have diabetes, it is not possible to

---

* Values are all plasma glucose unless otherwise indicated. See Table 1.7 for information.

1.1 Normal Blood Sugars

Normal blood sugars in plasma go from 70 to 110 mg/dl (3.9 to 6.1 mmol) before meals and no higher than 140 mg/dl (7.8 mmol) one to two hours after a meal. The graph shows normal daily readings with the rise seen after meals.

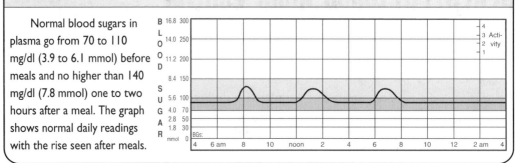

maintain ideal blood sugars 24 hours a day. No health professional expects that kind of control, even though the handouts they give you suggest that ideals can be met with every blood sugar test.

Those who have diabetes vary greatly in their ideas about optimal control. For some, no matter how great their readings are, they are not satisfied because their readings do not stay between 70 and 120 (3.9 and 6.7 mmol) before meals. Some may have nightmares about complications if they occasionally have a premeal blood sugar over 120 mg/dl (6.7 mmol). Others go to the opposite extreme and don't even blink at readings above 200 mg/dl (11 mmol), because that's what their blood sugars have always read since they began to check them.

So how do you tell if your blood sugar is adequately controlled? An excellent way to measure your overall control is with an A1c test which measures your average blood sugar for the last six weeks. Ask your doctor for this important test. See Textbox 1.3 about the A1c test.

1.2 The Diagnosis Of Diabetes Mellitus

The plasma glucose values below show readings for those without diabetes, those who have impaired glucose tolerance or prediabetes, and those with diabetes. Any value in the last column must be found on two different days to diagnose diabetes.

	Normal	Prediabetes	Diabetes Mellitus
FPG	< 110 mg/dl	110 mg/dl to 126 mg/dl	≥ 126 mg/dl
2 hr OGTT	< 140 mg/dl	140 mg/dl to 200 mg/dl	≥ 200 mg/dl
Or			Diabetes symptoms + random PG ≥ 200 mg/dl

FPG = Fasting plasma glucose, OGTT = Oral glucose tolerance test, PG = plasma glucose

Most people want their A1c value to stay below 6.5% to 7%, or no higher than 1% above a lab's upper range for those without diabetes, which is 4% to 6% at most labs.

Although the A1c test is based on your average blood sugar reading, it does not indicate how stable your blood sugar is. You could have numerous up and down swings in your readings and still achieve an A1c which shows your control is "excellent."

Testing before meals, two hours after meals, occasionally at 2:00 a.m., and whenever you think your blood sugar may be high or low will reveal your true readings and the patterns within those readings. With frequent testing, you do not have to wait for the A1c test results and you have a better guide to making insulin dose adjustments each day. If you use a continuous monitor, blood sugar patterns quickly become apparent because of how frequently readings are done. This level of detail shows how close to normal your blood sugars really are.

Most meters display an average of your readings and how many tests were actually done over the last 14 and 30 days. This is another tool you can use to gradually lower your average blood sugar until it eventually comes down to 150 mg/dl (8.3 mmol) or less for combined pre and postmeal readings. Circumstances such as having a history of hypoglycemia unawareness or living alone will dictate a higher target, while pregnancy will lower it.

> ## 1.3 The A1c Or HbA1c Test
>
> The hemoglobin A1c test can be ordered by your physician or can be done at home with new tests.
>
> Hemoglobin is the protein in red cells which carries oxygen. The A1c test measures the percentage of hemoglobin which has become glycosylated over the past eight weeks. The more glucose in the blood during this time, the more glucose that will permanently bond or glycosylate to hemoglobin.
>
> Glycosylation of proteins damages their structure. The A1c test measures the current average blood sugar and also provides a picture of how much damage is occurring to proteins in the body, such as enzymes, collagen, and other structural proteins in blood vessels and cell walls.

The Price Of High Blood Sugars

High blood sugars that occur frequently can cause internal damage and lead over time to complications such as kidney damage, retinopathy, nerve damage and heart disease. In contrast, relatively normal blood sugars can minimize complications or prevent them altogether.

Damage from high readings is gradual, remains hidden for years, and lulls people into thinking their control is adequate. *"It is not at all uncommon for the careless person who has diabetes and lacks the initiative to self-manage to come abruptly to the recognition that a major complication has occurred without any detectable early warning. Diabetes can be silent for decades."* says William M. Bortz, II, M.D. People eventually develop symptoms they can no longer ignore, only to realize that their organs now have advanced damage and their overall health has been greatly diminished.

Damage begins at a submicroscopic level due to unwanted interactions between excess glucose and nearby structural proteins and enzymes. High blood sugars impair the normal flow of energy that enzymes depend on to do their work. Damage gradually spreads, affecting structures such as blood vessels, eyes, kidneys, and nerves, while other organs, like the liver, muscles and lungs show little effect from high blood sugars. The liver may accumulate fatty deposits and the lungs undergo a reduction in air flow, but these changes usually do not have a significant effect on function.

Why are some organs damaged while others are not? Different cells have different mechanisms by which they access glucose. Although all cells depend on a supply of energy that comes largely from glucose and free fatty acids circulating in the blood, some cells require insulin to open specific paths in their outer wall for the glucose to enter. The cells that depend on insulin for glucose to enter do not become flooded by glucose when glucose levels are high in the blood because insulin levels at this time are low. Organs and tissues with cells that depend on insulin, such as those in muscle, liver and fat, stay relatively protected when blood sugars go high.

Other cells, like those in nerves, blood vessels, eyes, and kidneys, require a steady source of glucose all the time. They have evolved so they do not require

---

1.4 Complication Risk In Type 1 Diabetes

These percentages indicate average risk for developing each complication in someone with Type 1 diabetes whose A1c is about 9.7%. These values reflect data obtained prior to the DCCT Trial completed in 1993.

Organ	Lifetime Risk (unless noted)
Eyes	
Cataract	25-35%
Cataract removal	3-5%
Retinopathy	
any degree	90%
proliferative retinopathy	50% (15 yrs)
laser treatment	40-50%
blindness	3-5% (30 yrs)
Frozen Shoulder	10%
Trigger finger (DuPuytren's)	10%
Kidneys	
End stage renal disease	35%
Nerves	
Gastroparesis symptoms	1-5%
Peripheral neuropathy	54%
Autonomic neuropathy	
Bladder dysfunction	1-5%
Impotence	25%
Diarrhea	1%

For each 10% reduction in A1c, the risk of eye and kidney problems drops about 35% and may be similar for other complications.

Adapted from D.M. Nathan, Chap 5 in Atlas of Clinical Endocrinology Vol. 2: Management and Prevention of Complications in Type 1 Diabetes. Ed: C.R. Kahn, Current Medicine, Inc., Philadelphia, 2000

	1.5 Early Detection And Intervention Prevents Damage			
Organ	**Early Detection**	**Prevents**	**Overt Symptoms**	**Show Up**
Eyes	regular eye exams	blindness	loss of vision, a "spider web", or blurred vision*	late
Kidneys	urine test for microalbumin	kidney failure, requiring dialysis or transplant	excess bubbles in urine, tiredness	very late
Heart	cholesterol levels, BP, C-reactive protein	heart attack or stroke	angina, CHF, heart attack	early to late
Nerves	testing feet with a monofilament	amputation	numbness, tingling, shooting pain in feet	early to late

* Many newly-diagnosed people experience blurred vision shortly after starting on insulin. This occurs in both eyes, is caused by a sudden drop in blood sugar levels, and gradually resolves over about a month. When blurring occurs in one eye or without a dramatic change in blood sugar, it should be checked immediately by an ophthalmologist.

insulin which means they will absorb any excess glucose from the blood. When glucose levels are high, they become flooded with glucose. These organs are susceptible to damage when the blood sugar remains high for more than a few hours.

Do high blood sugars always lead to complications? Not always. Occasionally, someone escapes serious health problems despite a long history of poor control. It is rare, however, to find no damage at all when blood sugars have remained high over several years. Although cholesterol levels, genetics, nutrition, exercise, blood pressure, smoking, alcohol intake, hormone levels, vitamin and mineral balance, and stress all play a role in determining the extent of damage, the vast majority of people with poor control eventually develop one or more of the complications typical of diabetes.

The world contains an excellent control group of several billion individuals whose blood sugars stay normal because they do not have diabetes. Having normal blood sugars, they do not develop diabetes complications. Keeping blood sugars close to normal is the key factor for staying healthy with diabetes and avoiding complications. Blood sugar control becomes easier, more systematic, and more understandable once you learn how to use insulin.

Benefits of Better Blood Sugar Control

Most people find that improvement in their day-to-day quality of life provides better motivation than prevention of long-range problems. When insulin is given in the right amount at the right time, they no longer have frightening low blood sugars, the fluctuations of "brittle diabetes," an inability to tell when the blood sugar is low, nor high morning blood sugars that wreck the rest of the day. They discover they can have variety in their exercise and eating schedules without losing control.

People say: "For the first time in years, I can eat when I want to," or "I can really control my blood sugars now, and I feel better, too." They have a greater sense of security with a better quality of life each day, and they are preventing complications in the future. Let's look at these benefits.

Less Hypoglycemia

Hypoglycemia or low blood sugars can be frightening and exhausting. Some people will do anything to avoid them, including running the blood sugar high or giving up entirely on their control because of fear.

Cells in the brain and the nervous system depend exclusively on glucose for fuel. Deprived of glucose, they have trouble performing normal functions like thought and coordination. Luckily, the blood sugar has to be extremely low for many hours before permanent brain damage is seen, and this usually occurs only after repeated episodes of unconsciousness or grand mal seizure activity. Nonetheless, lows do affect a person's sense of self-control and temporarily weaken the body.

Lows occur when there is more insulin circulating in the blood than is required for the body's needs at that time.

Common causes of lows include:

- Too much rapid insulin has been injected for some reason
- Insulin is taken for a meal that is miscalculated, delayed, or missed
- The amount or the timing of long-acting insulin is misjudged
- Insulin absorption is increased, as when exercise or heat increases blood flow

For most people, the best way to deliver insulin is with frequent, precise doses that are being matched to an individual's needs: basal insulin to cover background need and bolus insulin to cover carbohydrates or to bring down high blood sugars. Precise dosing is critical for those who are sensitive to insulin, usually people who require less than 40 units a day. Precise dosing is important for people who have Type 1 diabetes because they make no insulin of their own and cannot raise or lower their own insulin production to compensate for an insulin dose that is miscalculated.

Some people with Type 1 diabetes end up with insulin doses set too high. This can lead to overeating to avoid lows or, even worse, to frequent and severe hypoglycemia. A major benefit of improving control is that less insulin is usually required. Correct doses lower insulin need, improve control, and can help with weight loss.

The DCCT or Diabetes Control and Complications Trial clearly showed that one drawback in regulating blood sugar control closely was an increased risk of low

1.6 What Are Your Goals?					
How important are these for you?					
	not very				very
A freer lifestyle	1	2	3	4	5
Feeling better	1	2	3	4	5
Fewer reactions	1	2	3	4	5
Stop/reverse complications	1	2	3	4	5
A lower A1c	1	2	3	4	5
A healthy life	1	2	3	4	5
A healthy pregnancy	1	2	3	4	5
Other _____	1	2	3	4	5

blood sugars. Severe hypoglycemia, requiring the assistance of another person, was three times as frequent in the intensive control group as in the control group.[1] Some participants had several episodes, while others had none at all, indicating

1.7 Normal Plasma Versus Whole Blood Glucose			
	Normal glucose values for:		
	interstitial fluid	whole blood	plasma
before meals	90 mg/dl or less (5 mmol)	100 mg/dl or less (5.6 mmol)	110 mg/dl or less (6.1 mmol)
2 hrs after meals	120 mg/dl or less (6.3 mmol)	130 mg/dl or less (6.9 mmol)	140 mg/dl or less (7.8 mmol)

Plasma readings are similar to lab values. Whole blood readings are about 10% lower than plasma values, while interstitial values read by many continuous monitors are about 20% lower than plasma. Know which value your meter is giving you.   2003 Diabetes Services, Inc.

that matching insulin to need is more critical in some people than in others.

In the DCCT study, severe hypoglycemia occurred once every year and a half, on average, in the intensive group, compared to only once every five years in the control group. More severe lows with unconsciousness or seizure activity occurred once every six years in the intensive group compared to once every 20 years in the control group. However, the overall benefit of lower risks for eye, kidney, and nerve damage clearly outweighed the increased risk for hypoglycemia.

This risk-to-benefit ratio may need to be reevaluated if the person lives alone and has no one available to help treat a serious low. In some circumstances, it may be better to focus on safe dosages despite the higher risk for complications.

Proper insulin dosing reduces the risk of hypoglycemia. One benefit of frequent, smaller insulin doses is that when a low blood sugar does occur, it will be less severe and shorter in duration. When insulin doses match need, blood sugars drop more slowly, allowing symptoms to be recognized and treatment to begin.

No More "Brittle Diabetes"

Some people believe they have been cursed with "brittle diabetes" because their blood sugars rise and fall more than is typical of other people, leaving them frequently out of control. Wide fluctuations like this are unnecessary. Fluctuating blood sugars indicate that insulin doses are not matched to need. "Brittle diabetes" can be eliminated by taking advantage of the equipment and knowledge available today and taking the time to learn how to adjust insulin doses.

By learning how to control blood sugars, highs and lows can be avoided. Many clinicians believe that when blood sugars often swing from high to low and back they may create organ damage even though the average blood sugar, as measured by the A1c test, appears to be close to normal. Whether these swings are damaging is uncertain, but the misery they cause can be avoided with appropriate use of insulin. A steady lifestyle can help, of course. One teenager acknowledged this by saying, "Why do I live wildly, when it just makes me feel bad?"

Many people have simply not learned how to use insulin well. When injected insulin is better matched to need, insulin doses become more appropriate and results more predictable. Covering carbs and correcting high blood sugars becomes simpler to do as each insulin fulfills a specific role. "Brittle diabetes" disappears as insulin is matched to need.

Regain Hypoglycemia Awareness

When someone has a low blood sugar but doesn't recognize it, he or she has hypoglycemia unawareness. When this person has a low blood sugar, it may be recognized only when someone else realizes what is happening. Hypoglycemia unawareness can be dangerous if no one else is around to help or if the person with the low is convinced he or she has no problem, becomes stubborn, and refuses treatment.

Hypoglycemia unawareness is more common when someone has had diabetes for many years, when insulin doses are excessive, and especially following a series of mild lows. Hypoglycemia unawareness becomes less likely and can be reversed as the total number of lows is reduced or lows are avoided altogether. Avoiding lows allows depleted counter-regulatory hormones to be replenished so that a person can once more recognize the warning signals needed to treat their lows. Better insulin dosing allows additional time to recognize that a low blood sugar is underway before it becomes severe. New continuous monitoring devices are designed to sound an alarm if a low is likely based on the current trend in the blood sugar. This enables the person to treat an approaching low before it occurs.

Bring Down High Morning Readings

The first blood sugar of the day is usually the most important one for controlling the entire day's readings. "If I wake up high, my whole day is shot!" is a typical complaint. Early morning highs are more difficult to bring down and often require several correction boluses through the morning and early afternoon hours.

Some 50% to 70% of people with Type 1 diabetes find they need more background insulin in the early morning hours to offset a rise in their blood sugar at that time.[2] This rise, called the Dawn Phenomenon, results from a normal increase in growth hormone levels, as well as cortisol and epinephrine levels, during the early morning hours.[3] When these hormones are produced, but no additional insulin is available to counteract them, the liver begins to produce more glucose. If the insulin level goes up slightly around 2 a.m., the liver does not produce glucose and the blood sugar does not rise as daylight approaches. Insulin delivery for someone with a Dawn Phenomenon requires that slightly more insulin be delivered during the early morning hours to keep the blood sugar from rising.

Controlling the morning blood sugar is also difficult for a large percentage of people with Type 2 diabetes who have excess fat cells in the abdomen. At night, this abdominal fat is released into the portal vein which goes directly to the liver. More fat makes the liver less sensitive to insulin. With its sensitivity reduced, the liver interprets a normal or elevated insulin level as low, which means glucose should also be low, although it is not. The liver proceeds to make unneeded glucose. A precisely timed increase in the nighttime insulin level reduces excess glucose production by the liver, improves the uptake of glucose by muscle cells, and reduces excess fat release so that a person can wake up with normal blood sugars.

Allow Variety In Your Life

One way to match insulin to need is to live a regulated lifestyle and take set doses of insulin. Though this works for some, for many others a life with variety is more desirable, even if it requires learning to adjust daily insulin doses to match their lifestyle. Diabetes specialist Alan Marcus, M.D., summarizes it this way: "A basic tenet of diabetes care is that the degree of lifestyle flexibility that can be achieved is directly related to the number of daily insulin injections." [4]

For most of us, work hours can vary, meetings and events pop up, meals are delayed or missed, and eating may be on the run. Weekends are meant for rising earlier or later, changing the exercise schedule, enjoying a large family meal, or dining late after a movie. By learning how to match insulin to these changes in routine, people open up a new and delightful freedom.

Convenience sometimes leads people to try getting by with one or two injections a day. However, this convenience leads to the inconvenience of solving serious control problems. After a blood sugar becomes high or low, the person cannot determine which insulin dose was poorly matched to need. "My blood sugar's high. I don't know if I didn't cover dinner with enough Humalog or if I need to raise my breakfast NPH," becomes a typical and common dilemma.

High and low blood sugars in your logbook or meter are a clear sign that your insulin doses are not the ones you need. The best way to set up one's insulin doses is to give each insulin injection a specific purpose. Each insulin then can be individually tested and adjusted when a control problem arises. With insulin matched to need, life can be safer and at the same time more spontaneous. Setting up effective insulin doses begins by matching long-acting insulin to background need. Once basal insulin is correctly set, meals can be eaten late or skipped entirely without having the blood sugar fall. It will be possible to go all day with perhaps only an occasional snack to maintain normal blood sugars.

Rapid insulin is given to match the carbohydrate count and to correct the current blood sugar before any meals or snacks. If basal doses have been correctly set, these boluses can be matched to carbohydrate intake, and control takes far less effort.

There is more flexibility for leisure activities with less concern about low or high blood sugars. If the sugar becomes high, a bolus can be given just for that purpose.

One person expressed the new freedom allowed by this basal/bolus approach by saying: "I don't have to eat at a certain time. I can wait until I feel hungry. I had forgotten what hunger feels like." Another person commented, "Just recently I began taking a more aggressive approach toward my diabetes, though it was diagnosed over 17 years ago when I was 10. After many failed attempts to monitor my blood sugars, I feel like I'm on the right track this time. I actually want to know what my blood sugars are. I started four shots a day a few months ago and love it. I have a new freedom."

Prevent And Control Complications

People with diabetes rightly worry about what may be going on inside, even though they see nothing wrong outside. Changes in kidney function, nerve conduction, and many other unwanted physical changes have no outer symptoms until 10 or more years of high blood sugars have passed. Only special tests, such as a urine test for microalbumin to detect kidney disease, will give an early indication of a specific diabetes complication. However, high blood sugars always show up when testing is done regularly, long before complications develop. High readings should be the warning on which action is taken before a problem has a chance to develop.

In the Diabetes Control and Complications Trial or DCCT, which started in the mid-1980s, 1,441 people participated to see whether tight control would reduce complications. Half of the group received conventional treatment and started the trial using urine testing and one or two injections a day. The other half received intensive treatment, with monitoring done several times a day and use of multiple injections or an insulin pump. Frequent feedback via telephone and clinic visits assisted them in adjusting their insulin doses as needed. By 1993, when the study ended, the intensive control group had better A1c values and were experiencing far fewer complications than the conventional control group.

Preventing complications at an early stage is an important reason to match insulin delivery to need. All of the complications associated with diabetes – neuropathy, nephropathy, retinopathy, and some heart problems – develop in the presence of high blood sugars. Most complications do not have apparent symptoms until they have become quite severe, and then careful control can only delay further damage at best. Reversal of damage may be possible if a problem is caught early, but prevention pays healthier rewards.

Control of blood sugars effectively reduces the risk of developing complications if it is done early enough. These risks are not minor. Each year in the U.S., 5,000 new cases of blindness are caused by proliferative retinopathy (new vessel growth in the retina), 56,000 cases of blurred or impaired vision are caused by macular edema, and 55,000 amputations occur in people with diabetes. Most of this could be avoided.

Controlling risk factors other than high blood sugars also is important. Reducing fat and protein intake to the amount needed nutritionally, lowering elevated

1.9 Millions Have Undiagnosed Type 2 Diabetes

Some 18 million people in the U.S. have diabetes, but only 11 million know it. Data from the Center for Disease Control suggests that 7 million people are not yet aware they have diabetes. Another 16 million are expected to develop diabetes in the U.S. in the next 10 years. The health problems that accompany this exploding population are beginning to place an enormous burden on the U.S. economy.

Symptoms of Type 2 diabetes are often minimal for several years before diagnosis. High blood sugars may be discovered only after a routine physical or a doctor visit for another problem. Everyone with a family history of diabetes or who suspects they may have diabetes should request that a glucose test be done.

A family member or friend may have a blood sugar meter available and this can be used to check at home for suspected diabetes. Doing a test on a home meter may uncover diabetes and lead to earlier treatment. Early diagnosis is critical in Type 2 diabetes because 20% have kidney disease and more have some form of heart disease by the time they are diagnosed with diabetes.

Short of a fasting blood glucose at your doctor's office, the best way to find out if someone has diabetes is to test the blood sugar an hour or two after a large carb breakfast (pancakes, or cereal and fruit). At this point, the blood sugar would normally be no higher than 140 mg/dl. Anything higher should raise suspicion and generate a doctor visit.

blood pressure, exercising, improving the diet in general, avoiding smoking, and controlling cholesterol levels have all shown benefits in reducing complications. It is estimated that improving blood sugar control to the 7.2% A1c levels achieved in the DCCT trial would save $624 million spent on eye damage each year. It would increase vision by 174,000 person years.[5,6] Using a combination of better control and better care, over 90% of vision loss is believed to be preventable.[7,8]

Now reconsider the value of matching insulin to the body's true needs. Can it help slow or reverse complications? In most cases the answer is yes, especially when damage is caught early.

Do Not Overdo It

Be aware that for some people, a strict adherence to tight control creates its own problems. For those who want near-perfect blood sugar readings or have other unrealistic expectations for control, intensive care can be overdone. A lower A1c value may look impressive but not if it comes at the price of unconsciousness or grand mal seizures. Lows may impair coordination and thinking, create personality changes such as temper tantrums or a self-destructive attitude, or lead to a car accident and even death. An excessive focus on avoiding complications can become counterproductive.

Health care providers who recognize these tendencies in overly-conscientious patients will advise them to set goals that are safer for them to achieve. This may mean a premeal target of 100 to 150 mg/dl (5.5 to 8.3 mmol) and avoidance of all blood sugars below 70 mg/dl (3.9 mmol). Reasonable goals encourage safer insulin use and often result in more consistent readings with little or no rise in the A1c value. The person will feel safer driving or be able to live alone with far more confidence.

Summary

When people with diabetes use insulin well, they begin to feel better, live more freely, and are far less likely to have diabetes-related health problems. They are confident that their blood sugar will remain stable because they are meeting their need for insulin with the right dose at the right time.

Once people become competent in using insulin, they say things like, "Why didn't I do this before?" or "It wasn't as hard as I thought it would be once I paid attention to my records and got some professional help." One person expressed it this way: "The insecurity is gone. I feel so much more hopeful and positive about life now that my insulin is set up right. My control was OK in the past according to my A1c, but my blood sugars jumped around unpredictably and I couldn't avoid overnight or daytime lows that stressed me day after day. For the first time I am in charge of my body again."

Will a picture of improved health and happiness be enough to make you take on the challenge of blood sugar control? We hope so. Not only will tomorrow's health look rosier, but you start feeling better physically and emotionally as soon as you begin to master your blood sugars. This improved sense of well-being and the higher quality of life that can come from stable and normal blood sugars motivates many people with diabetes to optimize their control.

If you often feel tired, have trouble thinking clearly, remembering names or events, taking tests at school, feel numbness creeping into your feet, or are fed up with family and friends being overly-concerned about your well-being and diabetes management, you are ready to use this book to improve your blood sugar readings.

A normal blood sugar is important to health, so understanding how to make this happen pays tremendous benefits. This book will assist you in becoming a pro at using insulin. It helps you set and achieve reasonable blood sugar goals, and guides you in how to use the tools that are available to achieve them. With awareness and experience, you can improve control, reduce blood sugar swings, feel better, and prevent or reverse complications. You can stop the highs and lows that give you so many problems as you become a master over your diabetes.

Control usually improves when insulin is given more often in smaller doses.

"Make your own recovery the first priority in your life."
Robin Norwood

Normal Insulin Delivery
— Your Best Guide

2

Using Insulin shows you how to stay within your target range more often while using insulin. Optimal control is the result of insulin delivered in a way that mimics the normal pancreas.

This chapter defines and develops:

- The basal/bolus method for delivering insulin to mimic the pancreas
- How many injections are needed a day to do this
- How this book will help

A certain amount of insulin must always be present in the blood and near cell surfaces. The insulin level in the blood has to remain at the right level to facilitate the transport of glucose into fat, liver and muscle cells for fuel. Background or basal insulin levels may rise at times to counterbalance a rise in stress hormones, growth hormone, and other regulatory hormones. They may also fall during periods of the day when activity is increased.

When eating occurs, the second need for insulin appears. In contrast to a slow, steady release of insulin for background metabolism, insulin release for food occurs rapidly in proportion to the amount of carbohydrate ingested. Healthy beta cells release a short burst or bolus of insulin to match the amount of carbohydrate in each meal or snack.

Figure 2.1 depicts normal insulin release into the blood after a meal. The darker band at the bottom of the figure represents the relatively constant, 24-hour release of basal insulin. Basal insulin need varies from person to person and may vary slightly from day to day in the same person based on activity and stress levels. Basal insulin makes up about half of the day's total insulin production.

When food is eaten, stores of insulin are released rapidly in the first 15 minutes, as shown in the figure. This first phase insulin release comes from stores in the beta cells of the pancreas. This phase is followed by a more gradual second phase over the next hour and a half to three hours as the production of insulin by the beta cells rises to match a rising blood glucose as carbohydrates are digested.

Unlike the steadier basal insulin pattern, bolus insulin release varies greatly from meal to meal depending on how much carbohydrate is eaten. If someone eats a big stack of pancakes, the release of bolus insulin will be quite large, but a leafy salad results in only a slight release.

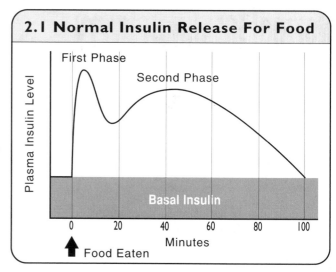

2.1 Normal Insulin Release For Food

Other circumstances can quickly change how much insulin is needed, such as having an infection (more insulin) or engaging in exercise (less insulin). If someone engages in moderate or strenuous physical activity for several hours, less basal and bolus insulin is needed for the next 24 to 48 hours.

The beta cells form part of the body's system of checks and balances to keep the blood sugar within a relatively narrow range. The liver senses insulin, not glucose, and begins to produce glucose when the insulin level goes low. The counter-regulatory hormones – epinephrine, growth hormone, and cortisol – mobilize stored glucose from liver and muscle cells into the blood stream when the blood sugar begins to fall.

The beauty of normal beta cells is that they deliver the exact amount of insulin required to move glucose from the blood into fat, muscle, and liver cells for normal metabolism, yet they leave enough glucose behind in the blood to avoid hypoglycemia. The brain and nervous system depend on having just the right amount of glucose in the blood at all times to fuel their vital functions.

How To Mimic Normal Insulin Delivery With Injections

The best way to use insulin to control blood sugars is to imitate the pancreas and use the same basal/bolus approach. This approach allows effective basal insulin and carb bolus coverage to be set up and tested when a problem arises.

Improving your control comes from matching these two needs:

- The first need for background or basal insulin is met by one to three injections of a long-acting insulin, such as NPH, Lente, Ultralente, Lantus (glargine) or the newest basal insulin, called Detemir. Insulin need may vary slightly through the day, such as having a higher need during the early morning hours when the production of growth hormone and cortisol may increase.
- The second need for food coverage is provided by an injection or bolus of a rapid insulin, such as Humalog (lispro), Novolog (aspart), or Regular, to match the amount of carbohydrate that will be eaten in a meal.

When these two needs are not handled in diabetes, a third need also arises. Additional boluses of insulin may be needed to lower high blood sugars that occur because of illness, a basal insulin dose set too low, a carb bolus that is too small, or other miscalculations. The correction dose is calculated so it returns a high blood sugar to normal.

The beauty of matching insulin doses to these three needs is that each need can be covered independently. Each need can be evaluated separately to ensure proper matching for each aspect of the control process. These three insulin needs are easier to quantify than most people imagine, and once this is done, do not usually vary greatly.

The old style of insulin delivery where fixed doses are given once or twice a day will rarely provide adequate control. An advisory panel from the Joslin Diabetes Center in Boston looked at data from the DCCT trial and decided that to optimize blood sugar control "three or more injections a day or use of an insulin pump should be recommended, unless clearly contraindicated." [9]

Testing and setting an individual's basal insulin doses, insulin-to-carb ratio, and correction factor can usually be completed within a four to six week period. Once basal doses are set, they may occasionally need to be adjusted for changes in weight or activity, or when blood sugar control is no longer optimal. Basal or bolus doses may be adjusted for better control at times, so it is important to watch the balance between basal and bolus totals within the total daily dose. When changes are made, retesting can usually be completed over a few days to regain control. It is important to start out with appropriate doses and to change them when the need arises.

How Many Injections A Day?

How many injections a day are enough to mimic normal insulin responses? The answer is "as many as it takes to achieve control." People with Type 2 diabetes who still produce considerable amounts of their own insulin will be able to achieve control using fewer injections than those with Type 1 who produce no insulin at all. Everyone would prefer fewer injections for convenience sake, but giving smaller, more frequent injections through the day has major advantages.

Advantages Of Frequent Injections

• Blood sugars are easier to control because each dose is matched to a particular need.[10, 11]

• Reduced doses lessen the risk of weight gain. Smaller meals can be matched with smaller boluses. Fewer low blood sugars occur and fewer carbs are needed to regain control.

• Blood sugar control is smoother, with less spiking after meals and steadier control through the night.

• Better control after meals directly lowers A1c values in both Type 1 and Type 2 diabetes to lessen the risk of complications.

• Better after meal readings lower triglyceride levels which can be dangerously high in Type 2 diabetes.

- Fewer swings in the blood sugar also mean a more stable personality, eliminating the emotional swings often seen with lows and highs.

Do not focus on how many injections you have to take for great control. Focus instead on how to deliver your insulin in the best way to meet your specific needs. For most people on insulin, at least three injections a day provides the best way to achieve control.

Where Using Insulin Takes You

This book is for people who are ready to control their blood sugars by using insulin in a way that mimics the normal pancreas. It is ideal for those with Type 1 diabetes who make little or no insulin of their own and those with Type 2 diabetes after the pancreas no longer produces sufficient insulin. Readers who still retain much of their insulin production can learn the benefits of flexible insulin use.

Taking set doses of insulin without matching insulin to daily needs will not control your diabetes. The process involved in this book is based on first calculating the total daily dose of insulin or TDD which is then used to determine accurate basal and bolus doses.

To match insulin to need, the blood sugar must be tested from four to eight times a day. Test results are compared to target ranges set for premeal, postmeal and

---

2.2 Mimic The Pancreas – Match Your Insulin Doses To Your Needs

- Take 3 or more injections of insulin a day.
- Test your blood sugars at least four to eight times a day or use a continuous monitor for excellent control in Type 1 diabetes. In Type 2, testing frequency depends on your residual insulin production and how good your current control is.
- Calculate food effects on your blood sugar by learning carb counting and use of a carb factor.
- Record your blood sugars, insulin doses and carbs in a way that helps you recognize blood sugar patterns.
- Analyze patterns in your readings so you can modify your treatment and improve control.
- Adjust insulin doses and carbs to get rid of unwanted patterns.
    - Set basal doses so that they keep your blood sugars flat when you do not eat.
    - Use carb boluses to balance the carbs you eat in each meal or snack.
    - Use correction boluses to lower the highs that can result from miscalculation.
- As insulin needs change with exercise, menses, or stress, readjust your doses and other factors such as eating until you regain control
- Consult with your physician and health care personnel when you cannot correct a blood sugar problem on your own. Keep detailed records. These can be used to quickly spot patterns and problem areas.

bedtime values. It helps to keep a record of insulin doses, carbs eaten, exercise, stress and other factors, and blood sugar tests on a one page graph or enhanced logbook to determine the interplay of these factors with your blood sugar.

Problem patterns are revealed by reviewing this data every 7 to 10 days. Problem patterns can be matched to examples shown later in the book where solutions are also suggested. Unwanted patterns can be corrected by adjusting the TDD, basal doses, carb and correction boluses, the timing, quantity and glycemic index of carbs, exercise, stress, or anything else that affects the blood sugar.

Basal insulin doses are the least likely to need adjustment. Once correctly set, basal doses need only be changed when a major change in activity is planned or insulin sensitivity or insulin production changes significantly.

Most insulin adjustments are made with carbohydrate boluses and correction boluses. The 500 Rule for carb boluses in Chapter 12 provides a close estimate of your insulin-to-carb ratio so that carbs in meals can be matched with precision. The number of carbs eaten is tracked by counting the grams of carbohydrate in meals and snacks. An individualized insulin-to-carb ratio or carb factor is used to determine how much rapid insulin to take to cover food.

When the blood sugar is high, an insulin-to-point drop ratio or correction factor is used to determine how much bolus insulin is needed to bring a high reading down to target. Correction boluses are determined with the 1800 Rule in Chapter 13. Precise dosing allows people to overcome the fear of taking too much insulin and crashing.

Summary

Adjusting insulin to need has distinct advantages. Better blood sugars lessen the risk of developing health problems and aid in the repair of mild to moderate organ damage. High blood sugars can be corrected rapidly and safely.

Insulin doses that are matched to need allow a more normal daily life. Skip meals, exercise when you wish, work varied schedules, eat late, and vary the carb content of your meals. Quick insulin adjustments can be made when blood sugars are out of range, exercise is disrupted, or illness occurs.

By closely mimicking the function of the pancreas, extra injections allow freedom. This may seem frivolous to someone without diabetes, but anyone who has to eat meals on a rigid schedule, gets irritable when high, has a carb snack every night before bed to avoid waking up in a soaking sweat, faces high blood sugars every morning, suffers from lows when they exercise, cannot eat spontaneously, or has returned to consciousness in an emergency room with an IV catheter in the arm, will find that insulin injections matched to need are a pleasure and provide a dramatic improvement in lifestyle.

The time you spend testing, injecting and analyzing will be more than offset by a greater sense of well-being and more flexibility in your life. Most people find this approach offers clear advantages in the quest for a healthy lifestyle with normal blood sugars.

2.3 The Insulin Dose Checklist

Find out where your control falters and where to fix it by answering these question. If you answer "No" to a question, correct your control at that step before proceeding. For example, if your basal doses have not been correctly set, correct this before attempting to set your carb boluses.

Check here when done:

Review

Overnight Basal Dose
☐ Can you go to bed with a blood sugar of 90 to 120 mg/dl (5.0 to 6.7 mmol), eat little or no snack and wake up in the morning with a normal reading? No → Chapters 10 & 11

Yes ↓

Daytime Basal Dose
☐ With a normal blood sugar before a meal, can you skip that meal, take no carb bolus and have your blood sugar rise no more than 15 mg/dl (0.85 mmol) and fall no more than 30 mg/dl (1.7 mmol)? No → Chapters 10 & 11

Yes ↓

Carb Counting
☐ Can you determine the grams of carbohydrate in foods you eat by carb counting, food exchanges or another dietary system? No → Chapter 8

Yes ↓

Carb Boluses
☐ With a normal blood sugar before a meal, can you cover carbs with a carb bolus so that your blood sugar is normal 3 $\frac{1}{2}$ to 4 hours later? No → Chapters 10 & 12

Yes ↓

Correction Boluses
☐ When you have a high blood sugar, can you take a correction bolus so that your blood sugar retruns to normal 3 $\frac{1}{2}$ to 4 hours later? No → Chapters 10 & 13

Yes ↓

Unused Boluses
☐ When you give 2 or more boluses within 3 hours of each other, can you give them without causing a low blood sugar? No → Chapter 14

Yes ↓

Insulin Reactions
☐ When you have a low blood sugar, can you recognize and handle it yourself, and keep your blood sugar from going above 150 afterwards? No → Chapter 20

Yes ↓

Terrific! No problems! Check again later!

What You Need To Start

In this chapter you will learn:

- How to have the right attitude
- Stages of change in diabetes
- That flexibility is key to control
- Who will make needed adjustments
- That it takes more than just testing your blood sugar
- How to set your blood sugar targets
- The tools you need for success

The Right Attitude

A healthy attitude is a great asset for controlling blood sugars. A healthy attitude leads to problem solving rather than self-blame when blood sugars are out of control. People often blame themselves for their poor eating habits as a cause for their control problems, but the impact and importance of the diet are often overemphasized relative to the impact of well-adjusted insulin doses. If your diet is harmful, definitely start here, but if your diet is generally healthy and your portions reasonable, do not assume that your diet is at fault when your blood sugars are out of control.

Stay positive – realize you can control your blood sugar given some time and effort. Seek information or help when you need it. Listen to your family and friends, and discuss your diabetes openly. Being positive and persistent brings results.

Daily life involves many things that directly and indirectly impact your control. Changes in

3.1 Methods For Managing Diabetes	
Old	**New**
Confusion	An organized system
Fixed insulin doses	Vary doses to fit carbs & activity
Doing what you are told	Learning to be in charge
Stiff rules not followed	Flexible rules that work
Eat meals on time	Eat when you wish
Retrospective analysis	Prospective analysis
React	Anticipate

eating, physical activity, work or school schedule, and stress all cause fluctuations in your blood sugar. To some extent, you can minimize life's changes, but many of the ordinary changes in life cannot be avoided. These changes, whether happenstance or planned, need to be balanced with adjustments in your insulin doses.

This book shows you how to make these adjustments, but it all starts with the right attitude. Are you willing to train yourself to make the adjustments you need to achieve better blood sugars?

Using correct insulin doses is the best but most overlooked tool in the quest for control. The body normally keeps blood sugars perfectly controlled by changing the insulin level in the blood. Someone on insulin has to learn how to make this happen by injecting the right amount of insulin at the right time. It takes a long time to learn this on your own, so use the advice of your doctor, other health professionals, and this book to make it happen faster.

Tools other than insulin, like improved diet, exercise, and diabetes medications, can do most of the work for some people with Type 2 diabetes and are certainly important in Type 1. However, for the millions of people with Type 1 or Type 2 diabetes who use insulin, adjusting insulin doses so they match the normal routines and the changes in your daily life remains the most important tool for achieving success.

How Do People Change

Research into how people change has produced the Stages of Change model. This shows that a change in behavior for most people occurs gradually, with a person moving from being unaware or uninterested, to considering a change, to

3.2 Stages of Change[12]		
Stage	**Explanation**	**Example**
Precontemplation	Getting ready to act	"I may have a problem with my blood sugars."
Contemplation	Thinking about what to do	"I know I need to work on my blood sugars but I don't have time."
Preparation	Having a concrete plan	"I'll start to count carbs at home and begin to record."
Action	Putting the plan into action	"I'm recording blood sugars, carbs, insulin doses, and looking for patterns in my readings."
Maintenance and Relapse Prevention	Staying on track.	"I didn't record this week because I was busy, but I'm back to it this morning. "

deciding and preparing to make a change. The person then takes action and adopts new behaviors, which must be maintained in the face of relapses. The person may go backwards and repeat previous stages at times.

Change is a process with several stages. Knowing which stage you are in regarding controlling your diabetes helps you not blame yourself. Regardless of where you are currently at, you can get to your goal by passing through all these normal stages.

> ## 3.3 Tips For Better Control
>
> - Lows and highs become less frequent when you test often and use your readings to make ongoing adjustments in insulin, food, and exercise.
> - Time and size all insulin doses to your needs.
> - If you live a varied lifestyle, vary your insulin doses accordingly.
> - Adjust your insulin doses as your life changes.
> - Know when to contact your physician or CDE and do not hesitate doing so.
> - Get involved in your blood sugar control. It is your life after all.

People change for a variety of reasons in diabetes. Reasons range from ones that are typical for many people to very individualized ones. With diabetes, people may change to solve control problems or to better manage health problems. Sometimes change occurs out of a desire for a better life, or a desire for more lifestyle flexibility. For other people, change may be motivated by people or situations outside of themselves, such as inspiration from a significant other or a reason to live after the birth of a child or grandchild.

Do More Than Test

Most people realize that simply checking blood sugars is not enough to improve control. Testing, recording, and waiting until your next doctor's appointment to make adjustments is not going to keep you healthy unless you happen to be already blessed with excellent readings. Most people require ongoing adjustments in their insulin doses and lifestyle based on the patterns revealed in their test results.

One interesting result from the DCCT study mentioned earlier was what happened to those who received "conventional treatment". Conventional treatment improved over the course of the study, so that by the end of the study 83 percent of the conventional control group were testing their blood sugar several times a day, and 91 percent were on at least two injections a day.[13] Despite the increased frequency of testing and injections, their blood sugar control measured by A1c results did not improve. Their physicians could not use the blood sugar data to tighten control because they had to uphold the agreed-upon design of the study.

Frequent testing is critical for improving control, but the control group in the DCCT shows that testing blood sugars alone may not be enough to improve the blood sugar or health outcomes. Other studies have shown modest reductions in A1c results when the frequency of monitoring is increased. It is very important to record blood sugar readings, carb choices, carb amounts, insulin doses, and activity. But once you have done this, you and your physician must take an active role in identifying and responding to the blood sugar patterns that arise. Adjustments in insulin and lifestyle have to be based on the patterns identified by analyzing this data. Otherwise, your A1c and your health will not improve.

> ### 3.4 Get Started
>
> Decide on a testing frequency and reasonable targets for your blood sugar that you and your physician are comfortable with. If you are not monitoring your blood sugar, starting to test once or twice a day might be the perfect first step.

Are you currently changing your insulin doses based on your readings? Are you testing your blood sugars and reviewing your test results? If you can answer "Yes" to questions like these, you have the right attitude to bring about optimal control. You may only need better tools to enable you to have great blood sugar readings.

Flexibility Is Key To Control

For optimal readings, insulin doses and their timing must be adjusted to bring the blood sugar level into a range that is comfortable, consistent and satisfactory to you and your physician. The best insulin doses are ones that are matched with precision and flexibility to your changing needs.

Even when blood sugars are well-controlled, it is important to reevaluate regularly whether changes in your insulin doses are needed. Driven either by a desire to stop recent ups and downs in your readings or to increase flexibility, periodic adjustments in your insulin doses help you stay in control from day to day and whenever a new life situation affects your control.

Any change in insulin doses may be larger and more frequent as you first begin this adjustment process. Your total daily insulin dose, how often injections are given, and the type of insulin you use may all need to be changed. Once these global issues are addressed, much of the really erratic control should be eliminated. People with a consistent lifestyle or with residual insulin production may do well on the same insulin doses each day, but even here stress, weight changes, or illness can alter a pattern of terrific readings and require that doses be changed.

To fine tune control, smaller changes will then be required. Carb and correction boluses can be tailored to match changes that occur in carb intake and activity from day to day. The good news is that matching insulin to need is easier today because we have new rapid and long-acting insulin analogs that offer more consistent action and timing than older insulins. Properly used, these newer insulins can provide better blood sugar control. Correctly matching insulin doses to varied situations takes some thought, planning, and experimentation. Success also requires good record-keeping.

Decide Who Will Make Adjustments

Since insulin adjustments are needed frequently, consider carefully who will make them. Has your doctor or nurse educator suggested that you think about adjusting your own insulin? Have you brought it up yourself with your doctor?

Have you received any instruction in how to change your insulin doses? Have you considered assuming this responsibility on your own?

3.5 Steps To Control Your Blood Sugar	
Know what to do	**And why**
Know your target	A clear goal makes it easier to get there
Test and record often	Good records let you see patterns
Identify patterns	Enables you to make corrections
Decide if major or minor adjustments are needed	Scope of change lets you focus on change in TDD versus a change in one dose
Decide what to adjust	A change in insulin dose or carbs is usually a good choice
Make the adjustment	To improve blood glucose
Repeat these steps	Adjust every 3 to 7 days until target is reached
Know when to get help	For frequent or severe lows or highs, get your doctor's help right away

© 2003 Diabetes Services, Inc.

Not everyone is able to make the decisions required to adjust insulin doses, especially at first. Many people are uncertain whether they can do this simply because they have never attempted to do it and have never received instruction on how to do it. Knowledge needs to precede action for the best chance of success. Are you up to the task of changing your own doses, or would you prefer to identify when change is needed and contact your physician or nurse educator to discuss what he or she would recommend?

If you feel overwhelmed by the thought of making your first insulin adjustments, ask your health care team if you are ready to take this step. Once you have their support, make small adjustments at first, usually one unit of insulin at a time, unless there is a clear need to make larger changes. Small adjustments carry far less risk than going too far at first and losing confidence. As you learn to make small adjustments, it becomes easier to make the larger changes needed when your life suddenly shifts.

How often insulin doses need to be changed varies greatly from person to person. Someone with Type 2 diabetes who retains some insulin production and lives a steady lifestyle may need only occasional adjustments, perhaps only for seasonal changes or an illness. People with Type 1 diabetes who travel frequently for work, and exercise when their schedule allows may need adjustments every day to match their insulin doses to the carbs and blood sugars at each meal, and then correct highs or lows as they occur.

If your readings are frequently out of your target range, it may be wise to get some focused attention from your doctor, rather than making numerous small adjustments on your own. If your readings vary between extremes of highs and lows and you are a beginner, speed things up by getting your doctor's help for adjusting more than one insulin dose at a time. Pay attention to their advice because you can use it as you begin to change doses yourself.

Using the tips, tools, and suggestions in this book will make your job easier, whether you want to know when to contact your health care team or whether you prefer to make most of these changes yourself. Be patient. Adjusting insulin is not something you learn overnight.

You will want to read **Using Insulin** thoroughly now and then reread it after two to six months when this information will make a lot more sense and be easier to apply effectively. After a few weeks of tracking your numbers, you will realize that the information you previously read can now help you get where you want to go. Most people using insulin will want to keep this book handy on a nearby shelf and refer to it when problems arise. It is a valuable reference tool, not a text that has to be committed to memory.

Set Clear Blood Sugar Targets

If you don't know where you're going, it's harder to get there. Before you begin matching your insulin to your needs, start by setting reasonable target ranges for your day-to-day blood sugars. Constantly aim for reasonable targets to make steady progress toward these goals.

Your target range covers the numbers you would like your blood sugars to stay within at least 75% of the time. With your health care provider's help, select a target range for before meals, 2 hours after meals, and at bedtime.

The first target ranges you select will likely not be "ideal" ones. Instead, they should be chosen to improve upon your current readings, whatever they may be. A range to start with would be one in which your current readings fall about 50% to 75% of the time. This starting range can be tightened and improved gradually until you are ready for a more ideal range.

If your blood sugars swing wildly between 30 and 400 mg/dl (1.7 and 22.2 mmol) before meals, your physician may suggest you first try to stay between 50 and 300 mg/dl (2.8 and 16.7 mmol). Once your readings improve into this range, your physician may want you to aim for 60 to 250 mg/dl (3.3 to 13.9 mmol). You or your physician can narrow your target range as you make progress.

Keep in mind that stopping lows is always the first goal for improving blood sugar control. This may mean running higher blood sugars for awhile, but will move you toward better control faster and more safely.

For adults and adolescents, an ultimate target range might be 80 to 120 mg/dl (4.4 to 6.7 mmol) before meals and 110 to 150 mg/dl (6.1 to 8.3 mmol) after meals and at bedtime. For children, an ideal range may be 100 to 180 mg/dl (5.5 to 10 mmol) before meals and bedtime, especially for those in whom small insulin doses make precise control difficult.

The targets you select, however, will depend on your current control, age, living conditions, employment responsibilities and ability to recognize low blood sugars. If you are a woman who wants to become pregnant, your blood sugar targets will be significantly lower than at other times in your life to ensure a successful pregnancy. If you have been having severe lows in the middle of the night, your target at

3.6 Ideal Blood Sugar Targets

Have a clear goal for your blood sugar. Below are three goals for different people to achieve over time. The first was used in the DCCT clinical trial, the second is recommended during pregnancy, and the last is for someone who has hypoglycemia unawareness.

Time/Test	DCCT Goal	Pregnancy	Hypo Unawareness
Before Meals	70 to 120 mg/dl (3.9 to 6.7 mmol)	60 to 90 mg/dl (3.3 to 5.0 mmol)	100 to 150 mg/dl (5.6 to 8.3 mmol)
2 hrs after meals	< 180 mg/dl (< 10 mmol)	< 120 mg/dl* (<6.7 mmol*)	< 200 mg/dl (<11.1 mmol)
2 a.m.	> 65 mg/dl (> 3.6 mmol)	60 to 90 mg/dl (3.3 to 5.0 mmol)	> 90 mg/dl (> 5.0 mmol)
HbA1c	< 7.0%	4.8% or 20% less than your lab's upper limit for normal	< 8.0%

* During pregnancy, the desired goal is less than 120 mg/dl (6.7 mmol) at one hour after eating

© 2003 Diabetes Services, Inc.

bedtime may first be set at a higher level and later lowered after your insulin doses have been readjusted to prevent the night lows.

Not everyone's ideal target range is the same. Table 3.6 shows three ultimate target ranges that cover specific situations. In the first column are target blood sugars used by the intensive control group (the group that developed fewer complications) in the DCCT. The second column shows the lower targets that are to be met before and during pregnancy. The third column shows higher targets that might be used by people who have hypoglycemia unawareness, as discussed in Chapter 21.

You are not expected to reach your target range immediately nor all of the time. Remember that targets like those in the DCCT column are tight, and it takes time for most people to achieve this degree of control, even with support and help.

To get the best A1c results, be sure to select a postmeal target and monitor at least occasionally two hours after eating. If your blood sugar frequently spikes above 180 mg/dl (10 mmol) after meals but you are not testing at this time, your A1c may remain elevated even though your premeal readings are in your target range. With Type 2 diabetes, the blood sugar at one or two hours after eating is often the most important one for achieving a normal A1c.

On your charts or logbook, remember to mark all blood sugars that are above or below your current target range with a colored pen or highlighter so they can be picked up quickly by you and your doctor.

Set Red Flag Limits

With your doctor, also decide what blood sugar readings or patterns of readings are so low or so high that you should call for help. When "red flag" readings occur, you need to call your doctor to discuss what needs to change so they do not continue.

3.7: Contract For Better Health With Diabetes

With your physician's help, set a starting target range for your blood sugar that improves upon your current control. Select targets for before meals, after meals, and at bedtime. Also select personal targets for testing frequency, A1c, weight and exercise.

Time	Target Blood Sugars		
	Starting Range	Better Range 1	Better Range 2
Before meals	____ to ____	____ to ____	____ to ____
2 hrs after meals	____ to ____	____ to ____	____ to ____
At bedtime	____ to ____	____ to ____	____ to ____

My blood sugar goals

☐ I will test my blood sugar _____ times/day before meals and _____ times/day after meals

☐ I will have no more than _____ readings below _____ mg/dl in a week

and no more than _____ readings above _____ mg/dl in a week

☐ I will have an A1c of _____ % by ___/___/___

My red flag readings

☐ I will call my health professional if my blood sugar levels are:

below _____ mg/dl for any reason

below _____ mg/dl _____ or more times a day/week/month

above _____ mg/dl _____ or more times a day/week/month

or my blood/ketone levels are above _____

My weight goals

☐ I will lose/gain _____ lbs. by ___/___/___

☐ I will eat 3-5 servings of fruit and vegetables a day

☐ I will choose low-fat meats and dairy products.

☐ To lose weight I will reduce calories to: _____ lbs X 10 = _____ − 500 = _____ cal/day
current weight

My exercise goals

☐ I will exercise ____ days each week. (3-5 days for 30 minutes recommended)

☐ I will exercise on: **S   M   T   W   T   F   Sat**

at _____ am/pm for _____ minutes.

_____   ___/___/___   _____   ___/___/___
My signature   Date   My physician's signature   Date

For instance, your doctor may request that you call immediately if your blood sugar goes below 40 mg/dl (2.2 mmol) unless there is a clear reason for the low, such as taking a meal bolus but becoming distracted so that you do not eat. A call may be warranted if two consecutive tests are over 350 mg/dl (19.4 mmol), accompanied by moderate or large amounts of ketones in your urine.

With your doctor, decide on current targets for your blood sugars and what red flag readings require a phone call for help. By setting targets and working toward them, you gradually learn when and how to change your own insulin. Fill in the blanks in Contract 3.7 with your target range, red flag readings, and weight and exercise goals.

Use The Right Tools

Besides a healthy attitude and clear goals, it helps to have the right tools. This book will magnify and sharpen your skills using these essential diabetes tools:

Carb counting: This tool should be close to the top of your list. Matching carb intake to insulin accounts for half of the day's blood sugar control. Making the match requires only that you know how much carb you are eating and how much bolus insulin you need to cover that amount. Some people may have difficulty with actual carb counts, but any method that stabilizes carb intake for each meal of the day will work.

Frequent testing: Finger poking or forearm testing will be essential and the more the better. Four tests a day, before meals and at bedtime, are needed for basic dose adjustments. More readings are needed for better control. After meal readings are required to set meal boluses to maintain and refine control. Occasional 2 a.m. readings are needed to verify overnight control.

Recording: Use a record system, meter, or PDA (Personal Digital Assistant) which allows you to put everything that affects your control — carbs, blood sugar readings, insulin doses, exercise and stress — on the same page. Complete records make analysis easier and are essential for making better control decisions. Using records well also means applying past experience so you make better decisions each time you inject insulin. See pages 67, 68, and 75 for examples of complete records.

3.8 Tools For Success
• Blood sugar targets
• Frequent injections using a basal/bolus approach
• Carb counting
• Frequent testing 4 or more times a day
• Lots of records
• Know your patterns
• Know your rules
• Know your insulins
• Insulin adjustments based on patterns and rules
• Ask questions
• Try new things
• Don't blame yourself or others
• Expect to succeed

You may also download the memory from your glucose meter onto your computer using software available from most meter manufacturers or onto an internet site designed for this purpose. Remember, though, that blood sugar readings by themselves do not explain why high or low readings occur. Only when the major factors that affect your blood sugar are recorded and analyzed will control fall in place. Activity, food choices, carb counts, insulin doses, stress levels, and the monthly period for women are common factors that need to be evaluated before the blood sugar can be controlled with confidence.

Recognizing patterns: Besides recording blood sugars, you want to know what they are telling you. If you continue to use correction boluses every time you encounter a high blood sugar, such as adding a certain number of units to your breakfast bolus to correct readings above 120 mg/dl (6.7 mmol), you may overlook the bigger picture that shows your blood sugars are too high every morning. If your readings are over 120 mg/dl every morning, you want to evaluate whether you are getting enough basal insulin during the night, whether you have a Dawn Phenomenon, or whether you are going to bed with high readings.

> ### 3.9 Common Patterns
>
> - Often low
> - Mostly high
> - High morning
> - Low → high
> - High → low

Many patterns occur several times a week. However, some important patterns, such as Low —> High, only appear after a low blood sugar. To find irregular patterns, a careful review of your records will be needed.

Using the rules: Certain basic rules make insulin a lot easier to use. An accurately determined average total daily dose of insulin or TDD is your most helpful tool. From an accurate TDD, your basal/bolus balance can be used to set up basal insulin doses, and the 500 and 1800 rules can be used to determine your carb factor for carb coverage and your correction factor for lowering high readings. The unused bolus rule helps prevent overdosing. These five fundamental rules can be applied with assurance after a few weeks of practice.

> ### 3.10 Rules To Use
>
> - TDD First
> - 50/50 Rule or
>   Basal/Bolus Balance
> - 500 Rule for carbs
> - 1800 Rule for highs
> - Unused Bolus Rule

Your basal doses are set up to keep your blood sugar flat when you are not eating. Carb boluses are matched to the carbs in each meal using a carb factor determined from the 500 Rule. The 1800 Rule determines how far your blood sugar will drop per unit of insulin for use in safely correcting highs. The unused bolus rule keeps you from overdosing when carb or correction boluses overlap. How to use these rules to determine your doses is explained in the chapters that follow.

The right insulins: Most people require two different insulins. A rapid insulin (Humalog or Novolog) is used to cover carbs and lower high blood sugars. An intermediate (Lente and NPH), long-acting (UL), or flat (Lantus or Detemir) insulin provides around-the-clock basal coverage to keep your blood sugar from rising when you are not eating. It is especially helpful to know how quickly each of the insulins you use begins to work, when it peaks, and how long it lowers your blood sugar. This information helps you determine which insulin is causing a control problem and what changes may help to correct unwanted patterns.

Insulin adjustments based on patterns and rules: When unwanted patterns are identified, an insulin adjustment is likely to be needed. An unwanted pattern requires that you change something. A change in your insulin doses or a change to a different timing or type of insulin should always be at the top of your list.

Unwanted patterns are not that hard to identify once you understand what you are looking for. Graphic record systems like the *Smart Charts* covered in Chapter 6 make patterns easier to see, but even enhanced logbooks can be used to reveal patterns, as described in Chapter 7.

The steps above provide the basic ingredients for success in using insulin. They are designed to restore both confidence and control. We will cover each of these and more in the chapters that follow.

3.11 Good Diabetes Care

- Keep your blood sugars as close to normal as possible.
- Regularly monitor your blood sugar.
- Inject three or more times per day or use an insulin pump if your blood sugar control is not excellent with fewer injections.
- Record your blood sugar readings. Use these results to adjust your insulin doses, diet, and exercise to maximize control.
- Have an A1c test every 3 to 6 months to monitor your level of control.
- Have a yearly urine microalbumin test to detect early kidney disease. If microalbumin is over 30 mg/gram creatinine, repeat the test to monitor treatments that will reduce the need for dialysis or transplant.
- Have a yearly total lipid panel to measure cholesterol, triglycerides and HDL ("protective cholesterol"). If abnormal, repeat every two months until treatment corrects this. Minimize all risk factors for heart disease.
- Get a yearly eye exam to detect eye damage and prevent vision loss. If abnormalities are detected, repeat eye exams as recommended by your eye doctor.

© 2003 Diabetes Services, Inc.

Summary

It takes most people a few weeks to a few months to learn to use these tools. Be patient but persistent. You will learn more and your skills will sharpen as time passes. As confidence grows from your experience, you will eventually become a pro at managing your blood sugar and health. You probably didn't know you could do so well! Luckily, an intense level of involvement in controlling your blood sugar is not needed all the time. Think of this control effort as a short, intense period of tracking and learning that will pay off every day from now on.

> ## 3.12 Frustration
> Everyone who tries to improve control encounters frustration at times.
>
> Remember:
>
> - You are able to change your insulin doses, carb intake, and activity to improve your control.
> - Success will not come with every decision, but every decision improves your chances for learning and success.
> - Diabetes control is not the only important matter in your life.
> - Take a break when you need one and come back to the challenge refreshed.

To paraphrase Thomas Edison, *"Great control is missed by most people because it is dressed in coveralls and looks like work."* This book is your coveralls with its pockets filled with tools. Use it to take care of your health and productivity. Read this book so you can tell others you are *Using Insulin.*

Caterpallor(n.): The color you turn after finding half a grub in the fruit you're eating.
Washington Post's Style Invitational

3.13 I'm High! Is It Me Or Is It My Meter?

Many meters have built-in protection against user failure, but even advanced meters can fail. You and your doctor depend on accurate readings to make critical decisions, so it makes sense to test your meter if you get any suspicious readings.

For example, one of our patients recently purchased a new meter and was very surprised to find that his old meter was giving him much higher readings than his new one. When he did side by side tests, his old meter showed 306 mg/dl (17.0 mmol) while his new one showed 188 mg/dl (10.4 mmol). On another occasion, it was 290 mg/dl versus 160 mg/dl. He realized this might be why he had started to have very erratic readings with severe lows when he treated his "highs" with Novolog.

When he brought his meters to the clinic, the first question the nurse asked was how long it had been since he had cleaned his old meter. The light and embarrassment appeared on his face at the same moment as he answered "I didn't know I was supposed to." Many new meters require little maintenance compared to older meters. Check with your diabetes educator to stay current with new meters.

Test your meter for accuracy

1. Do five blood tests, one right after the other, from a prick done on the side of the finger. An ideal range to test a meter is between 180 and 300 mg/dl (10 and 16.7 mmol). No two readings will be identical, but none of the five readings should be more than 10% below your highest reading. If your highest reading is 200 (11.1 mmol), your lowest readings should be no more than 20 mg/dl below this, or between 180 and 200 mg/dl (10 and 11.1 mmol).

2. Compare your meter to another meter by doing two or three tests right after each other on each meter (4 to 6 tests total). Although the readings between meters will not be identical, there should be consistency between them. You may get larger differences between meters if one meter reads whole blood glucose and the other reads plasma glucose. (See Table 1.7)

If there is a major difference in the readings, reread the user's manual carefully. Accuracy depends on how much blood is applied, how it is applied, whether the meter needs cleaning, and whether alcohol was used on the finger, as this can interfere with the reading. If your readings fall outside the 10% range, ask your physician or nurse educator to recommend another meter or call the meter manufacturer (number on back of meter) for clarification.

*"If the rich could hire people to die for them,
the poor could make a wonderful living."*

Anon.

Go Figure 3.14: Gauge Your Blood Sugar Program

Circle the numbers that best describe your attitude, attention to detail, and dedication to self-care. Total your score and check below to see where you are on the road to optimal control.

1. How motivated are you to control your blood sugars?

   not very　　0　1　2　3　4　5　very　　　　_____

2. Number of blood sugar tests you do each day:

   　　　　　0　1　2　3　4　5　(or more)　　_____

3. Number of injections per day:

   　　　　　0　1　2　3　4　5　(or more)　　_____

4. Do you record your test results?

   　　　　　yes (5pts)　no　(0 pts)　　　　_____

5. Do you use your test results to adjust your insulin?

   　　　　　yes (5 pts)　no　(0 pts)　　　_____

6. Do you match your carb boluses to each meal by carb counting or other means?

   　　　　　yes (5 pts)　no　(0 pts)　　　_____

7. Do you use correction boluses to lower highs?

   　　　　　yes (5 pts)　no　(0 pts)　　　_____

8. Do you adjust basal or background insulin doses?

   　　　　　yes (5 pts)　no　(0 pts)　　　_____

9. Do you get an A1c test to evaluate your control at least every 6 months?

   　　　　　yes (5 pts)　no　(0 pts)　　　_____

10. Do you call your doctor when control problems occur?

    　　　　yes (5 pts)　no　(0 pts)　　　_____

Total = _____

© 2003 Diabetes Services, Inc.

Assessment

Points	0-9	10-19	20-29	30-39	40-49
Meaning	A bit casual	Honesty pays	You've got the idea	Minor changes will help.	Your program is well tuned.

32

What Type Of Diabetes Do You Have?

CHAPTER

4

With diabetes, the body no longer moves glucose into cells for fuel because insulin production is very limited or nonexistent in Type 1 diabetes or because the cells have become resistant to insulin and insulin production is inadequate in Type 2 diabetes. A third type, called Type 1.5 diabetes, is becoming recognized as a form of Type 1 in adults.

Without insulin, those with Type 1 would die, so they must rely on injected insulin as their primary form of treatment. In contrast, someone with Type 2 who is insulin resistant but retains enough insulin production may require only a healthy diet and a daily walk to keep their sugar normal. But as insulin production falls over time, two or three medications as well as insulin may be required to keep the blood sugar normal.

This chapter will present:

- What diabetes is
- The different types of diabetes
- Some tests that aid accurate diagnosis
- Why misdiagnosis occurs

Type 1 Diabetes

With easily recognized symptoms, Type 1 diabetes has been known since ancient times. People with Type 1 usually died within a year of diagnosis until Leonard Thompson got the first injection of an impure insulin extract in 1922. Since then millions of children and adults with Type 1 diabetes have been placed on insulin. In the past, those with Type 2 developed diabetes in their later adult years and were harder to diagnose. Since their diabetes was not caused by a lack of insulin, they were rarely placed on it until late in the disease.

A marker was eventually found that clearly differentiated Type 1 from Type 2 diabetes. Large amounts of ketones in the urine or blood from an excessive metabolism of fat, became the first clear marker for Type 1 diabetes. Because of the need for injected insulin, Type 1 diabetes became known as insulin-dependent diabetes or IDDM. Then in the early 1980's, another breakthrough occurred. Antibodies were discovered which targeted insulin and the beta cells that make insulin in the blood of people who had Type 1 diabetes. The immune system is designed to defend the body against attack from foreign substances, but in Type 1 diabetes, a massive error occurs. The body's immune system begins to attack its own beta cells that appear to be foreign. Destructive antibodies appear in the blood long before enough damage has occurred to create symptoms. Testing for these antibodies allows an early diagnosis, but no definitive way has been developed as yet to stop the attack.

As an autoimmune disease, Type 1 diabetes has similarities to Hashimoto's thyroid disease, lupus, pernicious anemia, and rheumatoid arthritis. People with these diseases may have genetic markers similar to each other. Type 1 can start at any age, but most cases begin between early childhood and the early adult years. It occurs in those over fifty years of age, but this is less common.

> ### 4.1 Suspected Causes of Type 1
>
> - Vitamin D deficiency
> - Viruses
>   - coxsackie B
>   - cytomegalovirus
>   - Epstein-Barr
>   - mumps
>   - congenital rubella
>   - rotavirus
>   - Ljungan
>   - encephalomyocarditis
>   - echo
> - Nitrates
>   - lunch meat
>   - farm well water
>   - fertilizer
> - Cow's milk in infants

Medical experts believe that two defects are necessary to get Type 1: an imbalance in the immune system plus exposure to a toxin, such as a virus or an environmental toxin (see Table 4.1), that causes insulin or the beta cells to become a target for an immune system that is out of balance. One part of the puzzle appears to be heat shock proteins that, despite their unusual name, are involved in the proper folding of the insulin molecule into its natural, active form. When heat shock proteins get damaged or sidetracked during a viral or toxic event, insulin may be released into the blood with abnormal shapes that then attract the immune system.

An out of balance immune system does not realize it is making a critical error in targeting insulin molecules with a funny shape. A gradual destruction of the beta cells begins. After many months to a few years, when only 10% of the beta cells are left to make insulin, the blood sugar abruptly rises.

Insulin enables glucose transporters to be moved to the cell wall so that glucose can enter and be turned into energy. As insulin levels fall, glucose transporters are not moved and cells cannot use glucose for fuel. The blood sugar rises, while more and more fat gets released to compensate for the apparent lack of glucose. As fat levels rise, ketones also rise as a by-product of fat metabolism.

A child or adolescent feels fine until this point, but then rapidly develops extreme symptoms of Type 1 diabetes: excessive tiredness, excessive thirst, excessive hunger, rapid weight loss, and frequent urination. As ketones levels rise, the blood becomes acidic and the person begins to experience abdominal pain, dehydration, nausea, and vomiting. Severe symptoms may progress to a serious, life-threatening condition called ketoacidosis, which requires immediate hospitalization to save the person's life. Symptoms will worsen rapidly if an infection or other illness begins, if the person turns to sodas or other high sugar drinks to quench their thirst, or they begin eating sweets to compensate for their loss of weight and energy.

> **4.2 Type 1 Symptoms**
>
> • Excessive thirst
> • Frequent urination
> • Excessive tiredness
> • Irritability
> • Extreme hunger
> • Weight loss
> • Abdominal pain
> • Dehydration
> • Nausea
> • Vomiting

Genes play a role in placing a person at risk for developing Type 1 diabetes. The strongest genetic links are associated with the HLA-DR and HLA-DQ regions of DNA. These regions are 10 times more strongly linked to Type 1 diabetes than any other genetic region, but they account for only one third of the total risk. Most people who have these genes will never develop diabetes and many others who do not have them will develop it. When both parents have Type 1 diabetes, there is only a 20% chance that a child will get it. About 70% of those who develop Type 1 diabetes have a weak inheritance pattern or seemingly none at all. Most often, only one person in a family will have Type 1 diabetes.

In 25 to 30% of cases, however, a family has a strong inheritance pattern. Several members will have Type 1, such as half the brothers and sisters, or a parent, aunt, uncle, or several cousins. There seems to be little or no link between Type 1 and Type 2 diabetes as far as inheritance, even though a family may have both types.

Regardless of cause, once the autoimmune attack has destroyed the beta cells, life depends on replacing natural insulin with injected insulin. Good health results when this is done well. Though Type 1 diabetes cannot be cured at the present time, it can be well controlled with use of a flexible and accurate insulin delivery plan that mimics the pancreas' normal release of insulin.

Type 2 Diabetes

Many people discover they have Type 2 diabetes after a high blood sugar is found during a doctor's visit for another medical problem, such as a winter cold or a flu that drags on or leads to a secondary infection. Early diagnosis and treatment are facilitated by having an annual physical exam that includes a blood sugar test, but when this is not done, diagnosis can be delayed by 10 years or more.

Diagnosis of Type 2 diabetes occurs when the fasting plasma glucose is 126 mg/dl (7.0 mmol) or higher on two occasions, a random glucose is 200 mg/dl (11.1 mmol) or higher on two occasions, or a random glucose is 200 or higher with the presence of diabetes symptoms. Normal fasting glucose levels are 110 mg/dl or lower, with readings no higher than 140 mg/dl at any time. Readings between 110 and 126 mg/dl on a fasting test is considered prediabetes or impaired glucose tolerance.

A delay in diagnosis allows serious complications to get underway. High blood pressure or a cardiovascular problem affect nearly half the people with Type 2 when the diagnosis is made. Therefore, a complete checkup for complications and associated diseases should be done at diagnosis.

People who are sedentary and overweight, especially if the excess weight is around the abdomen, are those most likely to develop Type 2 diabetes, regardless of age. People who have a family history of Type 2 diabetes and those with a Hispanic, Black, Native American, or Asian background face an even greater risk of Type 2 diabetes when they gain extra weight.

Unlike Type 1, symptoms of Type 2 start gradually and can easily be confused with conditions common in normal aging. Symptoms include tiredness, irritability, blurred vision or changes in vision, numbness and tingling in the feet and legs, frequent infections, or sores that don't heal properly.

At the time of diagnosis, beta cells often are producing as much as or more insulin than is needed by someone of the same weight who does not have diabetes. This increased insulin production is caused by the body's attempt to overcome insulin resistance and normalize the blood sugar. Eventually the beta cells wear out and insulin production falls. Diagnosis may not occur until this stage of the disease. Type 2 diabetes typically involves problems in both insulin production and insulin sensitivity.

A whole spectrum of changes occur in the decade that precedes the diagnosis of Type 2 diabetes. Changes in liver, fat and muscle cells cause a gradual increase in insulin resistance, the primary cause of Type 2. As fat cells lose insulin sensitivity, more free fatty acids are released into the blood making insulin resistance worse.

The presence of insulin in the blood normally signals the liver to shut off production of glucose. After the liver becomes insulin resistant, it loses this signal and

4.3 Type 2 Symptoms

When Type 2 begins:
- None

10 years later at diagnosis:
- Weight gain
- Tiredness
- Irritability
- Blurred vision
- Numbness or tingling of the feet or legs
- Infections
- Slow healing

4.4 The Insulin Resistance Syndrome

A diagnosis of the Insulin Resistance Syndrome is established when 3 or more of these risk factors are present.

Risk Factor	Defining Level
Abdominal obesity* Waist circumference	
Men	> 102 cm (> 40 in)
Women	> 88 cm (> 35 in)
Triglycerides	≥ 150 mg/dl
HDL-C	
Men	< 40 mg/dl
Women	< 50 mg/dl
Blood Pressure	
systolic	≥ 130 mm Hg or
diastolic	≥ 85 mm Hg or current use of BP med
Fasting glucose	≥ 110 mg/dl or current use of diab. med.

* Abdominal obesity is more highly correlated with IRS than weight or BMI

Expert Panel on Detection, Evaluation, and Treatment of High Blood Cholesterol in Adults. JAMA: 285: 2486-2497, 2001 begins producing and releasing excess amounts of glucose, making the blood sugar rise. Muscle cells that normally pick up glucose from the blood have difficulty in moving this glucose into their interior for use as fuel. These changes can damage the body in a number of ways. The strain of overproducing insulin for several years in an attempt to control the blood sugar means that insulin production begins to falter at some point before or after diagnosis.

New oral agents have enabled many to delay the use of insulin, but nothing works as well as insulin for controlling blood sugars and keeping people healthy when blood sugars are staying high. About 36% of all Type 2 individuals require insulin to control their blood sugars. Of those diagnosed with Type 2, 15% to 20% actually have Type 1.5 or LADA, described on page 40, where the need for insulin occurs earlier than in Type 2.

Cleveland Clinic researchers studied 101 patients who had been diagnosed as having Type 2 for about 4 years. They were

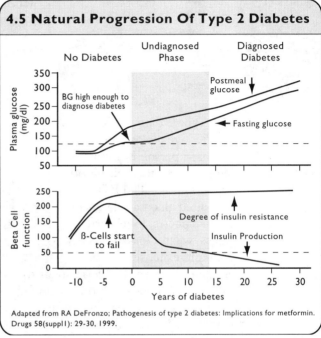

4.5 Natural Progression Of Type 2 Diabetes

Adapted from RA DeFronzo; Pathogenesis of type 2 diabetes: Implications for metformin. Drugs 58(suppl1): 29-30, 1999.

tested to find out how many might have antibodies that are typically found in Type 1 diabetes. The researchers found that 20 of the 101 people previously thought to have Type 2 diabetes had one or two of the many antibodies found in Type 1 diabetes.[14]

All 20 of the antibody positive people had GAD65 antibodies and 4 had a second antibody. This contrasts with Type 1 diabetes, where several antibodies are usually found. The presence of GAD65 antibodies in adult onset diabetes or in women with gestational diabetes identifies those who are likely to need insulin for treatment. Among those with antibodies, 80% required insulin compared to only 41% requiring insulin among those with no antibodies.

Although these individuals would have been identified as having Type 2 diabetes in the past, it is now clear that they possess distinctive features that are more common to Type 1 diabetes. Type 1.5 diabetes is one of several names that is used to describe people with this antibody-positive form of diabetes. In the past, 90% of all diabetes cases were considered to be Type 2 and the rest Type 1. Now that another type has been identified, Type 1.5, the percentage of true Type 2 turns out to be closer to 75% of all cases.

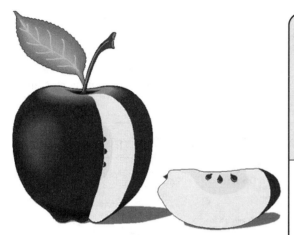

4.6 Do You Have An Apple Figure?

To find out if you have an apple figure, use a tape measure around your waist an inch above your navel. Then measure your hips at their widest point. Divide your waist measurement by your hip measurement. Ratios above 0.8 for women or above 1.0 for men suggest an unhealthy accumulation of fat in the middle.

What To Do:

• Eat fewer calories, especially less fat
• Eat less at each meal and leave food on your plate
• Eat smaller amounts of food more often
• Keep blood sugars normal before breakfast and two hours after meals
• Drink little or no alcohol
• Exercise regularly
• Do not smoke
• Reduce stress through lifestyle changes; learn to manage stress better

Type 2 diabetes is a progressive disease. Before it begins, a person have problems controlling their blood sugar. This is called IGT (impaired glucose tolerance) or prediabetes. In its early stages, weight loss, a healthy diet, and exercise may be enough to return the blood sugar to normal. In prediabetes, before Type 2 diabetes exists, more consideration is being given to early use of oral agents to delay the onset of diabetes. Acarbose, one of the glitazones, and metformin, which are discussed in Chapter 27, have all shown they can delay full-blown Type 2 diabetes.[15-17]

After a person has Type 2 for several years, insulin often becomes a necessary part of the treatment plan as production gradually declines. Some people may think that a Type 2 who is put on insulin becomes a Type 1, but this is not true. The differences between Type 1 and Type 2 are more complicated than this.

People with Type 2 diabetes are actually a subgroup within a larger group of those who have the Insulin Resistance Syndrome (IRS), which is also known as the Metabolic Syndrome or Syndrome X. This syndrome was first recognized in the 1960's and information about

4.7 Signs Of IRS

• Lack of physical activity
• Smoking
• High fat and calorie diet
• Obesity, especially an apple shape
• High blood pressure
• High cholesterol
• High triglycerides
• Low HDL(protective cholesterol)
• Prediabetes or Type 2 diabetes
• Polycystic Ovary Syndrome or PCOS
• Gout

4.8 Why Is An Apple Figure Dangerous?

Apples may be good for you, but an apple figure with excess weight in the middle is not. The apple figure is common in Type 2 diabetes and can also be seen in some adults with Type 1 diabetes. Risk of heart disease in men is two and a half times greater if they have excess weight in their midsection while for women the risk is eight times higher. Men and women with an apple shape share an equally higher risk for heart disease.

Before blaming your parents for this problem, realize that certain lifestyle factors cause fat to deposit in the middle. Drinking alcohol (especially beer), smoking, excess stress, lack of exercise, skipping meals, and diets high in fat or refined sugars contribute to the problem. People prone to Type 2 diabetes have higher levels of a stress hormone called cortisol in their blood, which increases fat deposits in the abdomen.

Fat within the abdomen is called "fast" fat because it is more quickly released into the bloodstream than fat located elsewhere. Fat starts to be released from the abdomen only three to four hours after the last meal, in contrast to a much later release from fat cells located in other areas of the body. This fast release provided rapid access to fuel for the exertion needed to fight, hunt, or flee from danger in early humans.

Today, people with an apple figure and abdominal fat who are mostly sedentary have higher triglyceride (TG) and free fatty acid levels in the blood. Excess fat in the abdominal cavity causes the insulin resistance that can lead to Type 2 diabetes and heart disease. Excess heart disease risks accompany an apple figure in the form of high triglyceride levels, low HDL (protective cholesterol), high blood pressure, and Type 2 diabetes. Often, these people also have a family history of high blood pressure, heart disease, diabetes or cholesterol problems.

it was first published in 1990. About 30% of all Americans have IRS,[18] of which about 30 or 40% of them will develop Type 2 diabetes at some time in their lives. Positive lifestyle changes can reduce the likelihood of IRS progressing to Type 2 diabetes when started early enough, and can often cause a marked reduction in health risk at any point.

Having an apple figure or upper body obesity, where excess weight is carried predominantly in the abdomen, turns out to be a critical indicator for IRS. Other critical indicators include high blood pressure, high triglycerides, high LDL and a low HDL. If any of these strong indictors are diagnosed early, this may lead to an earlier diagnosis of Type 2 diabetes. Ask your health care provider about these tests.

In the Insulin Resistance Syndrome, triglyceride levels are often above 150 and HDL levels below 45. High blood pressure is common and gout may be present. The cholesterol and blood pressure problems associated with IRS speed up cardio-vascular disease, which is responsible for 70% of the deaths in this group.

"She descended from a long line her mother listened to."

Gypsy Rose Lee

4.9 Polycystic Ovary Syndrome

Polycystic Ovary Syndrome or PCOS affects 6 to 10% of women in the United States and is part of the Insulin Resistance Syndrome. Women who have it typically experience two or more of these symptoms: obesity, acne, infertility, irregular menstrual cycles, ovarian cysts, and hair growth on the face, chest and back. They often have insulin resistance and other features of IRS, or even Type 2 diabetes. While all women produce some male hormones such as androgens and testosterone, women with PCOS typically produce higher levels than normal.

Because many of the symptoms of PCOS can be caused by other medical conditions, PCOS is diagnosed by comparing a person's history of symptoms and experiences with the results of a physical exam and lab tests. Ovarian cysts may be seen on a pelvic ultrasound and a blood test can be done to measure hormone levels to find out if PCOS is the cause.

PCOS is caused by a blend of genetics and lifestyle factors. Similar to insulin resistance and Type 2 diabetes, PCOS improves with weight loss, exercise and healthier eating habits. These lifestyle changes are often combined with hormones, insulin-sensitizing medications and sometimes androgen-blocking drugs. These, combined with low-estrogen birth control pills, help bring hormone levels under control, and can improve acne and unusual body and facial hair. Insulin sensitizing medications, such as Avandia or Actos, look promising for approval in the future to treat PCOS. Metformin is useful because it turns off production of glucose by the liver, and improves insulin sensitivity. Metformin may help weight loss and have the positive side effect of increasing fertility and enabling pregnancy.

Type 1.5 Diabetes Or LADA

When Type 1 diabetes starts, several different antibodies can usually be found in the blood which cause a gradual destruction of the beta cells. In contrast, when only one antibody called glutamic acid decarboxylase or GAD65 is present, destruction is slower and insulin may continue to be produced at a reduced rate for several years. This slower form of Type 1 diabetes is referred to as slow-onset Type 1 diabetes or Type 1.5. People who have Type 1.5 are often confused with those who have Type 2 diabetes because they are older at onset than those with Type 1 diabetes and they can usually do well on oral agents for a few years.

Type 1.5 is also called Latent Autoimmune Diabetes in Adults (LADA). Unlike people who have Type 2, people with Type 1.5 are often of normal weight, do not have an apple shape, have little or no resistance to insulin, and do not show the high triglyceride and low HDL pattern in their cholesterol test that is typical of Type 2. When a special blood test is done, GAD65 antibodies will be found to be present.

Compared to Type 1, Type 1.5 diabetes occurs at an older age where the immune system conducts a slower attack on the beta cells rather the more aggressive attack encountered in children or teens. Beta cells often function at a high level for a few years. Although insulin is required earlier than in Type 2, one benefit to having Type 1.5 is that when the blood sugar is controlled, people usually do not have the extra risk factors for heart disease seen in Type 2 diabetes. About 15% to 20% of people diagnosed with Type 2 actually have Type 1.5.

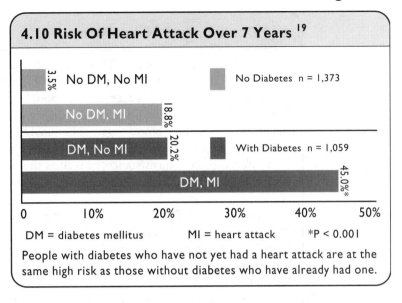

4.10 Risk Of Heart Attack Over 7 Years [19]

No DM, No MI — 3.5% — No Diabetes n = 1,373

No DM, MI — 18.8%

DM, No MI — 20.2% — With Diabetes n = 1,059

DM, MI — 45.0%*

DM = diabetes mellitus   MI = heart attack   *P < 0.001

People with diabetes who have not yet had a heart attack are at the same high risk as those without diabetes who have already had one.

Underdeveloped countries have higher rates of diabetes, especially Type 1.5, compared to the U.S. Although the U.S. currently has a lower prevalence of diabetes at 6% compared to 10% in the rest of the world, we are catching up quickly due to the rise in obesity. Because GAD65 antibodies are more common in the world at large, the number of Type 1s and 1.5s who require insulin to live is rising at faster rates in other countries than in the U.S.

Were You Correctly Diagnosed?

When you were diagnosed, you were probably told you had either Type 1 or Type 2 diabetes based on the understanding that diabetes usually falls into one of two categories. However, many people do not fit clearly into either type at the time they are diagnosed. Many others who do clearly have Type 1

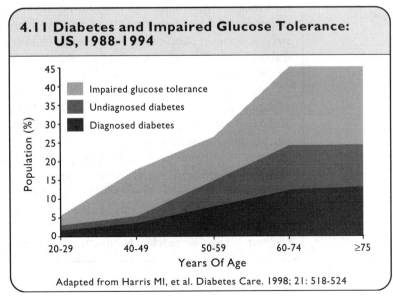

4.11 Diabetes and Impaired Glucose Tolerance: US, 1988-1994

Population (%)

Impaired glucose tolerance
Undiagnosed diabetes
Diagnosed diabetes

Years Of Age

Adapted from Harris MI, et al. Diabetes Care. 1998; 21: 518-524

4.12 Don't Have A Heart Attack

Cardiovascular disease (CVD) is the leading cause of death among people with Type 2 diabetes. The risk of death from CVD is twice as high for men and six times higher for women with diabetes than for people without diabetes. Most people with Type 2 diabetes suffer from the Insulin Resistance Syndrome (IRS), which can include insulin resistance, high blood sugar, abdominal obesity, high blood pressure and cholesterol problems. The cholesterol problems and excess blood pressure associated with insulin resistance, as well as the excess glycosylation and clotting caused by high blood sugars, magnify the high rates of CVD already found in the general population.

To prevent CVD and excess deaths from heart disease, all aspects of the IRS that are present must be treated aggressively. Although improved blood sugar control helps in small ways, prevention of CVD comes mostly through treatments directed at the underlying cholesterol, blood pressure, and clotting problems associated with this syndrome.

Guidelines for cholesterol levels in diabetes are to have the LDL ("bad" cholesterol) less than 100 mg/dl, triglycerides less than 150 mg/dl, and HDL ("good" cholesterol) above 40 mg/dl for men and 50 mg/dl for women.[20] Reaching the target for LDL is especially critical because when the LDL is high, it is likely to be made up of small, dense particles that increase the risk of stroke and heart attack. The LDL target for a person with diabetes is the same as for a person without diabetes who already has cardiovascular disease. As the LDL is brought down, the LDL particles become larger and fluffier, which reduces the risk of stroke and heart attack.

The statins and fibrates are two classes of drugs that are effective in reducing cholesterol problems in diabetes. Statins are so effective that some clinicians recommend them for all high risk individuals. This includes people with Type 2, regardless of their cholesterol level, because a large percentage of heart attacks and strokes occur in people who have normal cholesterol levels. In the high risk group of diabetes, statins lessen the risk of a heart attack by about 25% regardless of the cholesterol level.[21–24]

High blood pressure, another major risk factor for CVD, affects 20 to 60 percent of people with diabetes. Starting at 115/75, CVD risk doubles with each increment of 20/10 mm Hg. The goal in diabetes is a blood pressure less than or equal to 130/80 mm Hg. For those over the age of 50, the systolic or first number is more important than the diastolic number. High blood pressure is so common that one out of every four people currently has it. Someone who has a normal blood pressure at age 50 has a 90 percent probability they will develop HBP during their life.[25] Blood pressure control is important in diabetes because it helps to prevent CVD and kidney disease.

Taking an aspirin a day for those who do not have an intestinal or bleeding problem is another extremely effective way to prevent CVD.

Table 4.13 Differences In The Three Major Types Of Diabetes

	Type 1	Type 1.5 / LADA	Type 2
Avg. age at start	12	35	60
Typical age at start	3-40*	20-70*	35-80*
% of all diabetes	10% (25%**)	15%	75%
Insulin problem	absence	deficiency	resistance
Antibodies	ICA, IA2, GAD65, IAA	mostly GAD65	none
Early treatment	insulin is vital, diet & exercise changes helpful	pills or insulin vital, diet & exercise changes helpful	pills helpful, diet & increased activity essential
Late treatment	insulin, diet, exercise (occasionally pills)	insulin, pills, diet, exercise	insulin, pills, diet, exercise

* may occur at any age
** if all antibody positive cases are included, ie Type1 and Type 1.5

© 2003 Diabetes Services, Inc.

or 2 at diagnosis find the previously clear lines begin to smudge over time. Because of advances in understanding different types of diabetes, it may be wise to reevaluate your situation. Your treatment can be influenced by a clear diagnosis which is matched to how much insulin production you have, whether your insulin production can be increased, and whether you possess insulin resistance that can be reversed.

Misdiagnosis of diabetes and changes in the disease as you age may lead to mistreatment. A clear understanding of the type of diabetes you have is essential if the best treatment is to be followed. For instance, treatment of people with Type 1.5 diabetes with the sulfonylurea glyburide is associated with more GAD65 antibodies and perhaps a faster progression to beta cell failure,[26, 27] while early insulin use is found to protect the beta cells.[28]

When someone does not have the body type or age typical of Type 1 or Type 2 at the time of diagnosis, confusion is easy. Today, better lab tests and understanding help with diagnosis. For example, consider a person who is 51, slender, and has mildly elevated blood sugars. He is older at onset than most Type 1s and his blood sugars are not extremely high, but he appears to be too thin to have Type 2.

He may have developed true Type 1 at a later age, or have Type 1.5 with diminished insulin production but no insulin resistance. He may not appear overweight, but still have excess fat deposits in his abdomen that create insulin resistance causing true Type 2 diabetes. His physician can check a lipid panel for the low HDL and high triglyceride level that are characteristic of Type 2, and for antibodies that identify and differentiate Type 1 from Type 1.5. A C-peptide test can also be done to measure insulin production.

Or consider a child of 14 who is 40 pounds overweight and has high blood sugar. Due to overeating, poor nutrition habits, and a sedentary lifestyle, more and more children are developing Type 2. Some medical experts say that half of the people under age 20 with recently diagnosed diabetes have Type 2 diabetes, creating a new phenomenon in this country. The lab tests above, along with more traditional ones, can help to determine whether this child requires insulin right away.

Knowing your type gives a better understanding of the changes that may occur as you age and your disease progresses. For example, if someone has Type 1.5 diabetes for a couple of years and control is poor on a sulfonylurea medication because insulin production is now low, the use of insulin may be required. If, however, a person is insulin-resistent with poor control but insulin production measured by a C-peptide test is adequate, the addition of another medication or two plus paying closer attention to food and exercise choices may be all that's needed.

A selective use of the C-peptide test and other tests listed in Table 4.14 can assist in the treatment choice of medications or insulin. When someone does not match a typical profile or their insulin production is unknown, the C-peptide test can aid the creation of a successful treatment plan. The presence or absence of GAD65 antibodies can enable the early and appropriate use of insulin.

Can You Have More Than One Type Of Diabetes?

Blurring the lines further, people with one type of diabetes may acquire features of another as they age. For example, a person with Type 1 loses beta cell function while young, but as they age may gain weight around the middle and acquire insulin resistance. Their apple shape carries with it the extra cardiac risks associated with Type 2 diabetes and the Insulin Resistance Syndrome,[29] necessitating higher insulin doses. Although not normally used in Type 1 diabetes, medications like Glucophage, Actos, or Avandia in these cases may increase insulin sensitivity to improve blood sugar control and lower insulin requirements.

In Type 2 diabetes, insulin production may fail completely over time. Medications like the sulfonylureas which have helped to control blood sugar for years, may no longer work because the person cannot stimulate insulin production from depleted beta cells. As this happens, injected insulin becomes an essential part of treatment. Like Type 1s, Type 2s need injected insulin once this stage is reached. Stopping insulin during a surgical procedure, which is commonly done for most Type 2s, may have disastrous results in a select few. Hospital personnel need to be aware that high blood sugars or ketoacidosis can occur when insulin is stopped in older Type 2s who are now insulin-dependent, especially under the duress of surgery, a heart problem, or an infection.

Health In Diabetes Involves More Than The A1c

Although the focus of this book is how to keep high blood sugars from creating problems for you, this approach largely prevents microangiopathy or damage to small blood vessels. Preventing this can certainly make life more enjoyable in later years,

4.14 Lab Tests To Determine The Type Of Diabetes You Have

Because of the extra cost of some tests, ask that they be done only when a clearer diagnosis of diabetes type will lead to better health care treatment. These tests help, but they are not conclusive and may not provide everything needed for a clear diagnosis.

Ketones (indicates Type 1)

Ketones are a by-product from the use of fat as fuel. Fat breakdown increases as less glucose becomes available due to a lack of insulin. When someone's urine or blood shows large amounts of ketones, the diagnosis of Type 1 or insulin dependent diabetes is highly likely. One exception occurs in young black and Hispanic males who have ketones at diagnosis but when placed on insulin seem to regain insulin production.

Antibodies (indicates Type 1 or 1.5)

Both Type 1 and Type 1.5 diabetes appear to be largely auto immune diseases. At diagnosis, 80 to 90% of those with Type 1 will be producing characteristic antibodies against the beta cells. These include ICA-125 (an islet cell antibody), highly sensitive insulin antibodies, and GAD65. These antibodies can be detected in blood tests. When all these are present, the person has or is likely to develop Type 1 diabetes. Relatives of those with Type 1 diabetes can have antibody tests done to detect this type of diabetes as much as two or three years before the symptoms begin. In Type 1.5 diabetes, usually only GAD65 antibodies are found.

High Triglycerides Or Low HDL Levels (indicates Type 2)

Cholesterol problems characterized by high triglycerides and low HDL are typical of insulin resistance. These markers for Syndrome X are commonly found before the onset and during Type 2 diabetes. A detailed cholesterol or lipid profile test shows these levels.

C-peptide (normal or high: Type 2; low normal or low: Type 1)

If other tests fail to indicate the type of diabetes, a C-peptide test shows how much insulin someone is producing. C-peptide is the other half of the precursor molecule that splits to form insulin. If the C-peptide level is normal or high, Type 2 diabetes is indicated. If the level is very low, Type 1 diabetes is likely. If the C-peptides are in the low normal range, the person may have Type 1.5 or Type 2.

If insulin is being injected to control the blood sugar, the C-peptide may read low due to the suppression of insulin production in the beta cells by the injected insulin. This test is ideally done on blood drawn when the blood sugar is above 180 mg/dl (10 mmol) to drive insulin production as high as possible.

Uric Acid (indicates Type 2)

High uric acid levels are found in people with gout but also indicate Type 2.

but most people with diabetes do not die from microangiopathy. Most people with diabetes die of a heart attack or stroke caused by damage to large vessels or macroangiopathy, rather than microangiopathy.

Fortunately, there are excellent ways to prevent and treat a heart attack or stroke caused by macroangiopathy. Taking an aspirin a day reduces the risk by 25%, while use of an ACE inhibitor (a blood pressure medication) is nearly as effective, and use of a statin medication to lower cholesterol is slightly more effective. Stopping smoking is more effective than any of these. The way in which each method prevents cardiovascular disease is unique, so the benefits add up quickly when they are combined. One UCLA study combined these methods and found that the rate of death or a repeat heart attack fell from 14.8% to 6.4% in just one year.[30]

The Steno-2 Study in Denmark followed people with Type 2 diabetes over eight years with half receiving intensive management of blood sugar, blood pressure, cholesterol, and kidney disease. The combined treatment approach reduced heart disease by 53%, kidney disease by 61%, eye disease by 58%, and autonomic neuropathy by 63%.[31]

It is very important in diabetes, where over 50% of deaths occur as a result of CVD, that close attention be paid not only to blood sugar control but to control of blood pressure and lipids. Fortunately, today we have excellent tools to do this.

> ### 4.15 Besides Good Control, Remember To:
>
> - Control cholesterol, triglycerides, and HDL blood levels
> - Keep your blood pressure normal
> - Keep your weight down
> - Get regular exercise
> - Eat a variety of healthy foods
> - Limit intake of animal fat and protein
> - Eat more seeds and fish
> - Eat five servings of fruit and vegetables each day
> - Not smoke
> - Stay optimistic - attitude is everything
> - And most importantly, have fun!

Summary

A variety of lab tests and clinical signs can provide information that is helpful in determining which type of diabetes the person has and what type of treatment is currently needed. A list of helpful lab tests is shown in Table 4.14.

A clear understanding of the different types of diabetes continues to evolve. Stay aware of your situation as your body and pertinent information change and ask the right questions about your diagnosis and treatment, not only initially but again as time passes. An informed, questioning approach will increase your likelihood of receiving the best care during the many years you may be coping with diabetes.

"Time is nature's way of keeping everything from happening at once."

Anon.

Insulin Use

Most people with diabetes can achieve a level of control sufficient to prevent most or all damaging complications by using insulin well. However, many problems associated with diabetes arise from not understanding how to use insulin as an effective tool, and from not using it early enough in the treatment of Type 2 diabetes.

This chapter discusses:

- When to start insulin
- How to use insulin in Type 1, 1.5, and 2 diabetes
- Practical tips on insulin use
- How to combine insulins
- Which insulins can be combined and prefilled in a syringe
- How to inject
- How to use small insulin doses

When Is It Time To Start Insulin?

With Type 1 diabetes, knowing when to start insulin is easy – as soon as you are diagnosed. But with Type 1.5 or Type 2 diabetes, the answer becomes more complicated because the time to start insulin depends on lifestyle, retained beta cell function, and willingness to begin injections.

Some people will benefit from insulin use as soon as diet and exercise are no longer able to provide control as determined by an A1c that stays above 7%. Using insulin may protect remaining beta cells and prolong their activity by reducing glucose toxicity. Blood sugar control is easier when residual beta cells still function and are able to assist control by turning their insulin production on or off as needed.

Insulin is typically started after diet, exercise and oral medications are no longer able to control blood sugars. This may occur one to three years after diagnosis in Type 1.5 diabetes, while in Type 2 insulin may be started later because other treatments work considerably longer. The move to insulin often occurs when the person is on maximum doses of two medications but they no longer control the A1c. The higher an A1c test is above 7.5%, the less likely it becomes that a third medication will bring the blood sugar to target. Adding a third medication generally lowers the A1c by 1% or less, making insulin a better choice. When insulin is started, con-

5.1 Short Term Insulin Use To Overcome Glucose Toxicity

If you have Type 2 diabetes, short-term insulin treatment might be one way to improve your control. Research studies suggest that even a few days' treatment with an insulin pump can aid those with Type 2 diabetes. In one French study, 82 people with Type 2 diabetes who could not control their blood sugars with a low calorie diet and maximum doses of Glucophage (metformin) were temporarily placed on insulin pumps for periods of 8 to 32 days. Their blood sugars rapidly improved on a pump, but what was of interest was that their control continued to be excellent long after the pump treatment was stopped. Brief use of insulin appears to allow an overworked pancreas to rest and then resume production of the amount of insulin required, sometimes for weeks or months afterward.[32]

A similar Turkish study tried two weeks of pump treatment for people with newly-diagnosed Type 2 diabetes who did not respond well to diet control alone. After a brief period of insulin pump use, six of the 13 people were able to stay well controlled on diet alone for between 16 and 59 months. Four later required a second two-week treatment, and one required a third.[33]

A larger Korean study followed 91 people with Type 2 diabetes who were placed on insulin pumps after they were unable to maintain control while on a variety of therapies. Of these, 31 were able to remain in good control for over 13 months following a few weeks of pump use. Those who succeeded had diabetes a shorter period of time (3.3 versus 9.1 years), had lower post meal blood sugars, and were able to gradually reduce their pump doses after 2 weeks without losing control.[34]

Whether a short, intense period of treatment with multiple daily injections of insulin would achieve the same benefit is not known. If you have Type 2 diabetes, you may want to discuss using an insulin pump or basal/bolus injections with your physician. If one of these brings your blood sugars back into the normal range, and your pancreas has a chance to recuperate, it may again produce adequate amounts of insulin. The chances for success is greatly increased by losing some weight and becoming more active.

This approach assumes that a person can still produce enough insulin. Insulin production can be measured with a C-peptide test, discussed on page 45. Temporary insulin treatment would not work for someone with Type 1 diabetes and becomes less likely to work when someone has had Type 2 diabetes for a long time.

tinuing the current medications is important because it allows less insulin to be used for the same degree of control. Use of insulin can also entitle people on Medicare to receive more coverage for testing supplies. Rather than coverage for one test strip a day, a single daily injection of insulin allows coverage for four tests a day.

Insulin Use In Type 1

Two injections a day is the bare minimum in Type 1 diabetes, but this rarely provides optimum control. It may work for some children or adults shortly after diagnosis if they still produce insulin during a "honeymoon phase." The key to control is to base the number of injections and types of insulin used on how well the blood sugar is controlled. If your A1c stays below 6.5% with no significant hypoglycemia on twice a day injections of Regular and

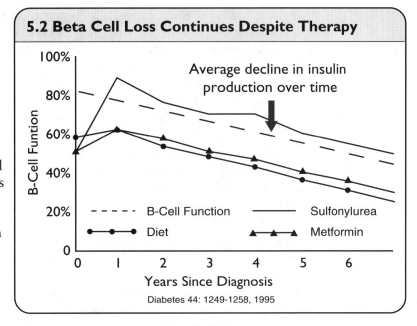

5.2 Beta Cell Loss Continues Despite Therapy

Average decline in insulin production over time

B-Cell Funtion

- - - - - B-Cell Function   ——— Sulfonylurea
●——●——● Diet   ▲——▲——▲ Metformin

Years Since Diagnosis

Diabetes 44: 1249-1258, 1995

NPH, there is no need to change, but control with this approach is quite rare. Most Type 1s feel better and have better control when they use a basal/bolus approach with three or four injections as soon as diabetes is diagnosed.

Two injections a day are unable to mimic the action of a normal pancreas which puts out a steady supply of background or basal insulin and then gives short bursts or boluses of insulin precisely timed and matched to a meal's carbohydrate content. Giving insulin in doses that are matched to food and activity and mimic the normal action of the pancreas usually requires three or more injections a day.

Insulin Use In Type 2

Determining when insulin is needed in Type 2 complicated. The pace at which people lose their insulin production varies greatly. There are also several lifestyle changes and medications that can help to maintain control. Diet changes, weight loss, increased activity, and medication combinations can all delay or reduce the need for injected insulin as long as sufficient internal insulin production remains. Medications that stimulate the pancreas to produce insulin, slow the digestion of carbs, or reduce excess glucose production by the liver are often effective in controlling the blood sugar until insulin injections are needed to support the failing beta cells.

In the first phase of Type 2 diabetes soon after diagnosis, control can often be achieved by changes in diet and exercise. Oral medications can be added and a combination of medications can favorably impact the dual problems of insulin resistance and insulin deficiency.

When the blood sugar rises as a result of physiologic insulin resistance, and oral agents are no longer adequate for control, an insidious psychological form of insulin resistance often appears. Insulin is rarely used early enough in Type 2 diabetes and, once started, it is not used aggressively enough to bring blood sugars to goal. Many diabetes specialists believe that over half of those who have Type 2 diabetes would be better controlled if they were on insulin rather than the 36% or so currently using it.

Among those who are not yet on insulin, 57% say that they fear injections. This drops to only 6% among those who currently inject insulin, [35] a 10-fold difference. Some 58% of U.S. physicians say that the fear expressed by patients is the most common reason that they delay insulin therapy. This compares to only 20% among British physicians. [36]

The sharp drop in fear once a person tries injecting insulin, as well as the marked differences in attitude toward this among physicians in different parts of the world, show how much the fear of injections is mental and cultural rather than real. Especially in the U.S., insulin seems to be feared rather than accepted for what it is, an extremely useful health tool.

One way some physicians bridge this mental gap is to give an injection of insulin, usually a 70/30 mixed insulin, to anyone whose blood sugar is higher than 200 mg/dl (11.1 mmol) when they are diagnosed. This single injection is usually all that is needed to overcome the fear most people have of injections. In addition, the rapid drop in blood sugar from the injection gives rise to well-being and relief.

Diabetes medications are far more limited in their ability to lower the blood sugar than insulin. Medications are able to lower A1c levels between one half percent and two percent. Insulin, on the other hand, has an unlimited ability to lower blood sugar and A1c levels. When insulin is used early in Type 2 diabetes, one injection of insulin a day is often all that is needed to enable a return to optimal control.

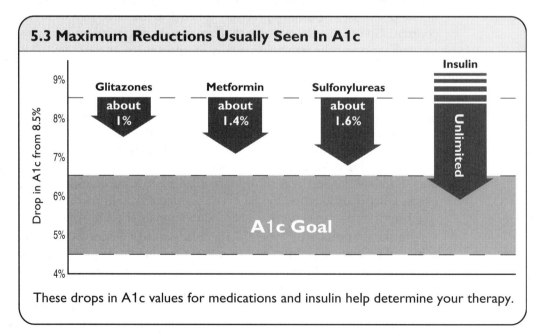

5.3 Maximum Reductions Usually Seen In A1c

Glitazones — about 1%
Metformin — about 1.4%
Sulfonylureas — about 1.6%
Insulin — Unlimited

Drop in A1c from 8.5%

A1c Goal

These drops in A1c values for medications and insulin help determine your therapy.

The choice of therapy is also influenced by cost. One study found that metformin (a generic form of Glucophage) plus insulin provided equivalent control to taking three oral medications for diabetes. However, the daily cost was only $2.70 with metformin plus insulin, compared to $10.30 using three medications.[37]

A common way to start insulin in Type 2 diabetes is to give one injection of a long-acting insulin before bed. Peaking insulins (NPH, Lente, or UL) or newer non-peaking ones (Lantus or Detemir) may be used at bedtime to control the breakfast reading. Doses can be gradually increased until the breakfast reading is in the normal range.

Another common situation early in Type 2 diabetes is to have high readings at bedtime from the dinner meal, followed by high readings at breakfast. In this situation, one injection can be taken before dinner with a combination of a rapid insulin to cover the meal and lower the bedtime reading, plus a long-acting insulin to work during the night and lower the breakfast reading. Doses of each insulin can be adjusted to cover their respective tasks.

Another injection is added before breakfast when pre-lunch and pre-dinner readings are high. To remedy this, an injection with both fast and long-acting insulins can be started before breakfast. The long-acting insulin from breakfast peaks early in the afternoon and can be used to cover carbs at lunch. Again, each insulin is adjusted to cover its respective task.

For many people with Type 2 diabetes, the best treatment option is three injections a day. When a rapid insulin is added at lunch to the breakfast and dinner or bedtime injections, a person is able to vary the amount of carbs they have at lunch or have a late lunch. Here, the breakfast long-acting insulin can be changed to Lantus or Detemir which do not peak during the afternoon.

Can You Get Off Insulin If You Have Type 2 Diabetes?

If you have Type 2 diabetes, you may have been placed on insulin when you were diagnosed. If your blood sugar was quite high or if you had major symptoms, insulin may have been started to quickly bring your blood sugar down and reestablish control. It is important to realize that being put on insulin at the time of diagnosis does not mean that it will always be needed.

For people with Type 2 diabetes, the best way to get off insulin, when this is possible, is to lose weight and become more active. Once the toxic effects of past high blood sugars lessen and internal insulin production improves, weight loss, diet changes, and oral medications may be able to keep the blood sugar normal without the need for external insulin.

In the late 1990's, Dr. David Bell, a clinician and researcher in Birmingham, Alabama, wanted to see if he could eliminate insulin use in a group of people with Type 2 diabetes by using a combination of oral medications. Most of these people had been placed on insulin a few years earlier when the older sulfonylurea drugs lost their effectiveness before the newer medications were available to try.

Dr. Bell first tested C-peptide levels and chose only those people who had normal levels for his study. Of the 130 people with adequate C-peptide levels in his study, 100 were able to discontinue insulin use altogether and control their diabetes on various doses of glyburide and metformin.[38] He found that their overall control, as measured by their A1c levels, was actually better on two oral medications than it had been previously on two daily doses of insulin. Others in the study were able to improve their A1c levels by using glyburide and metformin together with a single dose of insulin at dinner or bedtime.

Researchers have determined that the Type 2 patients who are most likely to control their blood sugars on a combination of oral agents are those least over-weight (BMI of 30 or less), with the shortest duration of diabetes, and C-peptide levels normal or only slightly low.

To determine whether insulin is required, doses may be gradually reduced over a few weeks' time. If the blood sugar rises as this is done, the insulin doses can again be raised. But if the blood sugar remains controlled as insulin is gradually stopped, oral medications are adequate for control.

Insulin Use In Type 1.5

Most people with Type 1.5 diabetes start with medications when they are diagnosed. Since insulin resistance is minimal or nonexistent, medications designed to reduce insulin resistance, such as Avandia and Actos, will have little or no effect. The sulfonylureas, which stimulate insulin release from the beta cells, will help as long as there are enough beta cells left to respond. Other medications like Precose, Glyset, or Glucophage can also be helpful for control.

Destruction of the beta cells in Type 1.5 by the immune system occurs much faster than the loss of beta cell activity seen in Type 2 diabetes. Insulin is required in half of those with Type 1.5 diabetes within four years of diagnosis, compared to over ten years in those who have true Type 2.[14]

The number of injections required in Type 1.5 diabetes depends on how much residual insulin production remains and how much assistance oral agents are able to provide. One injection of mixed insulins before dinner or a bedtime injection of long-acting insulin will occasionally work in early stages. More typically, an injection of rapid plus long-acting insulin before breakfast and another before dinner is needed. Eventually three or more injections are necessary to maintain control and allow a flexible lifestyle.

How To Mix Insulins

Be sure to mix any cloudy insulin before each use by vigorously rolling and turning the bottle at least 20 times. The potency of a cloudy insulin in a bottle or pens can vary greatly from injection to injection if it has not been mixed well. A cloudy insulin should look like milk when used. If it cannot be mixed so it has a uniform color, or if particles appear on the inside of the bottle, discard the bottle.

Insulins which can be mixed together are shown by the Xs in Table 5.4. Rapid and long-acting insulins can be mixed to give a single injection with one exception. Lantus insulin should never be mixed with any other insulin or even exposed to a syringe that has been used with another insulin. This contamination with another insulin can cause Lantus to come out of solution and vary in activity or become inactive. Because it cannot be mixed, an additional injection is required. Many users find the extra injection worthwhile because of Lantus' consistency of action. Detemir also provides consistent action and can be mixed with rapid insulins.

How To Mix Two Insulins In One Syringe

1. See Table 5.4 for allowed insulin combinations. Collect both insulin bottles and the smallest syringe you can use, i.e., a 30-unit syringe if your dose is less than 30 units. Check the insulin's expiration date and use opened bottles within 30 days.

2. Wash your hands in warm, soapy water. Do not touch or breath on the rubber stopper of the insulin vial or the syringe needle. Clean the rubber stopper with an alcohol swab if the stopper comes in contact with something or you require extra protection against infection.

3. Mix any cloudy insulin vigorously by rolling the vial between the palms of your hands and turning it end to end at least twenty times.

4. Remove the plastic cover from the needle. Pull the plunger out and draw air into the syringe equal to the units of insulin to be withdrawn from the long-acting insulin bottle. Inject the air into the upright insulin vial. Remove the syringe without drawing out any insulin.

5. Pull the plunger out again to draw air into the syringe equal to the units of rapid insulin to be withdrawn. Inject the air into the rapid insulin vial with the bottle upright. Then with the syringe still in the vial, invert the bottle so the stopper is down. Pull back on the plunger, withdraw about 5 units of insulin

5.4 An X Means Insulins Can Be Mixed In The Same Syringe								
	Detemir	Humalog	Lantus	Lente	Novolog	NPH	Reg	UL
Detemir		X			X		X	
Humalog	X			X		X	X	X
Lantus								
Lente		X			X		X	X
NPH		X			X		X	
Novolog	X			X		X	X	X
Reg	X	X		X	X	X		X
UL		X		X	X		X	

into the syringe, and push the insulin back into the bottle to get rid of small air bubbles. Do this once or twice until no visible air bubbles remain in the syringe. (Air bubbles are not dangerous, but they reduce the dose slightly.)

6. Now pull back on the plunger to draw the rapid insulin into the syringe until the top of the plunger reaches the mark on the syringe equal to the number of units of rapid insulin you need for this injection. Remove the syringe and set the rapid insulin bottle down.

7. Next, insert the syringe into the upside-down long-acting insulin bottle and pull the plunger down until the top of the plunger reaches the mark equal to the total units of insulin (rapid plus long-acting) that you need for this injection. Do this carefully. If you go past this line, do not return any insulin to the bottle, but push the insulin out of the syringe into a sink and start over.

8. Remove the syringe from the vial. If you set the syringe down before injecting, be sure the needle does not touch anything. Inject as described below.

How To Inject

1. Wash your hands with soap and water.

2. Choose an injection site. The skin may be cleaned with an alcohol swab if your immune system is suppressed or the site is dirty.

3. Recheck the dose in your syringe to be sure it is correct for the time of day, the number of carbs you plan to eat, and the current blood sugar.

4. Hold the syringe like a dart. Pinch the skin between the thumb and index finger, then quickly push the needle through the skin at a 90° angle. Pinching helps prevent injecting into muscle where insulin may be picked up by the blood more quickly. Inject 1/2 inch beyond the tips of your thumb and finger to lessen pain.

5. Push the plunger in as far as it will go. Release the pinched skin, but leave the needle in place for five seconds before pulling it out of the site.

6. You may press the injection site lightly with a finger or alcohol swab if you want, but do not rub it.

7. Place the used syringe in a plastic container with a screw top for disposal.

Injection Tips

1. Be sure to pinch up the skin. The layer of fat or soft tissue you inject into should be thicker than the length of your needle when the needle is pushed straight in. A 1/4 inch (5 mm) needle can be used by small children and very thin adults. A 5/16 inch (8 mm) needle is recommended for average weight adults, and the 1/2 inch (12.7 mm) needle is better for adults with extra padding. A 1/2 inch needle provides better blood sugar control than a 5/16 inch needle in those who are overweight with a BMI over 27. Normal weight adults can use either 5/16 inch or 1/2 inch needles. If you fear needles, use an automatic injector, like the Inject-Ease, to keep the needle out of sight.

2. Inject into the upper abdomen to speed absorption and action time, or into the thigh or buttocks to slow the action time or lessen the risk of a night low. However, do not use muscle areas if you plan to exercise, since blood flow may increase absorption.

3. Try to inject into the same area of the body at the same time of day. If you rotate areas, use the abdomen before breakfast, the buttocks before bed, etc. to get more consistent action from your insulin each day.

4. You may inject within an area, such as the abdomen, all the time, but rotate sites so that scarring does not interfere with insulin absorption. To rotate, move injections two "fingerwidths" to the left or right of the last spot. When you reach the side of an area, do a U turn and move back across either above or below line used before.

5. When using an insulin pen, be sure no airlock or blockage forms in the needle if the pen has not been used recently. Give a 3 to 5 unit dummy injection into the air to ensure that insulin is flowing freely through the needle. After pushing the pen plunger into the skin, wait 5 to 10 seconds before withdrawing the needle on the pen to make sure the insulin stays below the skin.

5.5 What About Premixed Insulins?

Premixed combinations of Humalog and NPH, Regular and NPH, and Novolog 70/30 are available at pharmacies in bottles and insulin pens. Premixed solutions are an advantage for those who are visually impaired, people who have limited dexterity, and those who have difficulty mixing insulins. They can work well for people who produce much of their own insulin and have relatively stable blood sugars, such as those with Type 2 diabetes. They offer convenience and can be effective for people who have a regular lifestyle.

The disadvantage of premixed insulins is that the ratio of each type of insulin is fixed and cannot be altered. Set ratios do not allow someone to match each insulin to a particular need. Premixed insulins in fixed ratios may not be effective if:

- your blood sugar varies
- you have a varied or irregular schedule
- you need to add extra Humalog, Novolog or Regular for extra carbs or high blood sugars

All cloudy insulins need to be carefully mixed before use. The pen or bottle needs to be rolled at least 10 times and tapped end to end at least 10 times before use.

Ways To Reduce Injection Pain

1. Use insulin that is at room temperature, but do not use insulin kept at room temperature longer than a month.

2. If you use alcohol on the skin, wait until it evaporates before injecting.

3. Allow muscles in the area to relax for an easier injection.

4. Use an ice cube or Emla Cream on the skin to numb it before injecting.

5. Penetrate the skin quickly. Practice on an orange or lemon until you feel confident with your technique.

6. Go straight in. Do not change the direction of the needle during insertion or removal.

Small Insulin Doses

Measuring insulin doses accurately can be a problem for those who require very small doses, such as 25 units a day or less. People on small doses are likely to have blood sugars that fluctuate because they are sensitive to insulin. Even slight dose variations can make a large difference in the blood sugar. For instance, people using 20 units of Humalog a day will find that their blood sugar may drop 100 mg/dl (5.6 mmol) or more on one unit. A half unit mistake in their dose will make their blood sugar rise or fall by 50 mg/dl (2.8 mmol). Some syringe manufacturers have 25 unit syringes with half-unit markings on the barrel. These syringes are very helpful in addressing the need for exact doses. An insulin pump will help people who use small doses because measurements are more accurate and insulin can be given in tenths of a unit or less. This offers greater assurance against overdosing.

> ### 5.6 Diabetes Supplies To Have On Hand
>
> - A rapid insulin (Humalog, Novolog, or Regular)
> - A basal insulin (Lente, NPH, Ultralente, Lantus, or Detemir)
> - Ultrafine lancets and a lancing device
> - A blood sugar meter, strips, and cotton balls
> - Fast-acting carbs like glucose tablets, Sweet Tarts®, other dextrose candy, or Monojel®
> - The *Smart Charts* in Chapter 6 are one example of an advanced record system you can carry with you.
> - Computer software and internet analysis and your meter readings can also provide an overview of your control
> - A glucagon injection kit should be available for anyone on insulin who may experience severe low blood sugars

Is Your Insulin OK?

Insulin is a protein which degrades when exposed to heat or freezing temperatures. Unopened bottles of insulin should be refrigerated above 36 degrees F. Opened bottles can be left out at room temperature below 86 degrees F for up to 30 days. Prefilled pens should not be used longer than 10 days to avoid a fall in potency.

Check your insulin anytime you have high readings for no apparent reason. Bottles of clear insulin like Humalog, Regular, and Lantus can be checked by grasping the bottle at the neck, turning it upside down, and rocking it gently back and forth or swirling it. If the insulin is potent, it will be as clear as water with no clumps or particles in it and no clumps on the sides of the bottle.

Cloudy insulin, like Lente, NPH and Ultralente, should be rolled vigorously in the palms of your hands and turned end to end 10 times each to put the insulin completely into solution. No clumps or particles should appear in the insulin or on the sides of the bottle. If there is any question of potency, use a new bottle with a different lot number. Give yourself a day or two to troubleshoot for other causes for your high readings. If you believe a bottle of insulin has gone bad, show it to your pharmacist or physician to confirm this.

I'm Fat, But Only Where I Inject!

A side effect of insulin is the growth of fat cells, especially near the injection site. When insulin is injected into the same area repeatedly, this tissue begins to plump up. Rotation of injection sites helps prevent this "localized lipohypertrophy" and also lessens the formation of scar tissue that might over many years make needle penetration and insulin absorption more difficult.

Which Insulins Can Be Used To Prefill Syringes

Only a few insulin combinations can be mixed together in a syringe and then placed into a refrigerator for later use.

- If prefilling of syringes is required, Regular and NPH insulins can be combined in the same syringe and stored up to 3 weeks in the refrigerator without changing their potency.
- Lente and Ultralente cannot be used with Regular in prefilled syringes because the zinc binder in the Lente insulins delays the onset of Regular's action.
- Humalog and Novolog should not be used with NPH or Lente insulins when prefilling syringes. Prefilling may delay their onset of action.

Insulin Pens

The basal/bolus approach of matching insulin to need requires a convenient, precise way to take doses of insulin anytime anywhere. The answer to this requirement for many is an insulin pen. Pens have been available and very popular in Europe for several years, but have been little used until recently in the United States. Insulin pens allow discrete injections on a just-in-time basis. With a pen, there is no need to carry a syringe and bottle of insulin and no need to draw up a dose of insulin before injecting. Insulin doses are usually given more accurately with a pen, so medication errors are less likely.

An insulin pen looks like a fountain pen and is similar in size. It has a disposable needle on one end, a cartridge that holds insulin in the middle and a dial that is used to select the insulin dose. Pen cartridges hold 150 or 300 units of insulin. Some

---

5.7 Expiration Dates

Keep an eye on the expiration date of your insulin and how long the bottle has been open. Although its strength falls gradually, insulin should retain full strength at room temperature for at least 30 days after opening. People who use small insulin doses will want to discard any insulin after it has been open for 30 days. If you notice that your blood sugar starts to run higher as you near the end of a bottle, discard the bottle and use a fresh one.

pens are entirely disposable and are thrown away once the insulin is gone, while others have disposable cartridges which can be replaced. Different pens can deliver insulin in half unit, one unit or two unit increments. The half-unit pens are particularly well suited for children and adults on low doses, and come in bright graphic designs. The needle on the pen is pushed into the skin and a button is

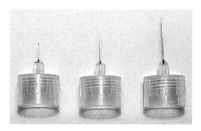

pressed to give the selected dose. Pen needles are available in different lengths and sizes, as shown here. The needle may be discarded after each use or at the end of the day.

One disadvantage of using a pen compared to a syringe is that the pen cannot be used to mix a rapid insulin with a basal insulin in the exact doses you may prefer. Pens and pen cartridges will have either one type of insulin in them or a premixed ratio of rapid to long-acting insulin. Prefilled cartridges are available for common insulins, such as NPH, Regular 70/30, Humalog , Humalog 75/25, Novolog, and Novolog 70/30 insulins. See Table 9.1 for a list of the premixed insulin ratios that are available.

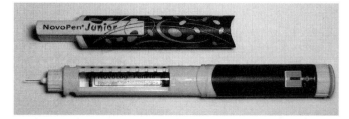

Those who love the convenience of a pen and prefer to mix their own doses will usually use a pen with a rapid insulin to cover carbs and correct high readings, and then take one or two doses of a flat basal insulin as separate injections.

Before using a pen that contains one of the cloudy insulins, hold the pen in the middle and flip it back and forth at least 20 times to fully resuspend the insulin. To prepare the pen for use, always prime it first. Before dialing a dose, purge three to five units of insulin into a sink or the air to ensure that the pen is functioning, not clogged, and has insulin in it. Put a needle on before each injection and take the needle off after using it for an injection to avoid insulin loss or evaporation of insulin inside the needle. When the pen is not in use, the cap should be kept on it to prevent contamination of the insulin.

Do not clean a pen with alcohol as this may damage it. After you inject, leave the needle under the skin as you count to eight. It takes longer for insulin to enter the skin from a pen than from an injection by a needle. If insulin is dripping out of the needle when you take it out, you probably have not received your full dose. Leave it in longer next time.

In storing a pen, avoid freezing and exposure to heat, just as you would with a bottle of insulin. A pen with insulin should be kept unrefrigerated only as long as the insulin in the pen can be kept unrefrigerated.

Better Records With Charts

Charts help you visualize a complete picture of the interactions between insulin doses, food intake, carb counts, and activity. They can also help pinpoint other things that affect your blood sugar, such as menses, stress, or an infection. Having a complete picture enables you to sort out what is causing unwanted changes in your blood sugar.

This chapter describes

- The value of charting
- How to chart
- How to spot your blood sugar patterns
- A sample chart with analysis

The information recorded on your charts will be used in the chapters that follow to assist you in gaining control and having more consistent readings.

Benefits Of Charting

Life changes constantly and so do blood sugars. Days lengthen and shorten, activity increases and decreases, weekends differ from weekdays, stress rises and falls, food intake shifts from more carbs in the summer to more fat in the winter, and meals may be delayed or skipped. In spite of these changes, your goal in diabetes is to have smooth blood sugar control without exposing yourself to lows and highs.

Changes in daily life affect how much insulin you need, while your control is determined by how well your insulin is matched to these changes. Though charting takes some time and effort, it lets you see clearly how insulin and carbs can be adjusted to control your blood sugars.

Charts have these advantages over traditional logbooks:

- they let you record in one place everything that affects your control,
- they provide a graph in real time of the rise and fall in your blood sugar,
- they reveal patterns in your readings,
- they reveal the time of day when problems typically occur, and
- they help pinpoint the causes of control problems.

Over time, charts tell you if you are getting where you want to go. They can be used as a guide to let you know whether the changes you make are really helping you gain better control. Writing things down as they occur improves your decisions.

This chapter shows you how to use *Smart Charts* to identify patterns and correct them. Whatever recording device you use, you want to identify patterns easily and be able to record in one place all the things that affect your control. If your current recording tool does not do this, try using *Smart Charts* or ask your doctor whether a more complete logbook is available. The sample *Smart Chart* on page 62 shows how much information you can record to help you spot patterns and take action.

What Do I Put On My Charts?

A tried and true rule is that the more information you place on your charts, the easier it is to control your blood sugars. Keep your charts or other recording tools handy so that recording and reviewing are easy to do. Use colored markers to quickly spot differences in activities, events, and readings. Highlighting highs and lows is particularly valuable. For each high and low, record what you think led to the particular problem.

> ### 6.1 What If I Prefer A Logbook?
>
> Standard logbooks, though usually not as helpful as a graphic system, are widely available. For tips on how to get the most out of and recognize patterns in a standard logbook, see the next chapter.

Activity

Record physical activity, exercise, or work that is greater than normal in the activity area at the top of the graph. With an ink pen or felt pen, block in the time and intensity of your activities and add a word or two to specify what you did in the comments section.

Rank your extra activity on a personal 1 to 5 scale. A "1" is used for a mild increase in activity, while a "5" is given to activities that are far more strenuous than usual. For instance, if sitting behind a desk is your usual work activity, but you spend the day moving your files and records to a new office, you would block in an area between "1" and "5" during the appropriate workday hours, based on how much extra activity this moving required.

If you begin a running program and become quite winded because of the running, you might mark a "5" on your chart at the time of the run. After you have run the same route for a few days, this activity may no longer be strenuous and would be listed progressively as a "4" and then a "3."

If some control problems are caused by changes in activity, you can see how to adjust your insulin doses or food to maintain control rather than stopping these activities. Make note also when your activity drops below normal. For instance, if you do aerobic exercises each day, but strain your knee and skip class for a week, put a short note like "resting knee, no aerobics" on your charts in the comments section.

See area A on Figure 6.2 for an example of how to chart physical activity.

Blood Sugars

Graphing your blood sugar readings in the top half of the *Smart Chart* allows patterns to be revealed clearly so that insulin doses can be adjusted correctly. Discuss with your physician how often to monitor your blood sugars. A minimum of four tests a day, before meals and at bedtime, are needed to make basic insulin dose adjustments. To gain critical information about how foods affect your readings, test also at 1 or 2 hours after meals.

A complete picture of your blood sugar is best provided with seven tests a day with an occasional 2 a.m. reading. In general, the more varied your readings, the more you will learn through frequent monitoring. If the cost of test strips prohibits frequent monitoring, vary the timing of your tests so you get a better overall picture of changes in your blood sugar, even though you may not do an ideal number of tests.

Although meter readings can be downloaded to a computer, writing these readings down as they appear in your life allows you to quickly spot trends and avoid highs or lows that are part of a current pattern. A written record that is evaluated frequently allows unwanted patterns to be identified before they become established.

Always test when you believe your blood sugar is low, unless symptoms are so severe that waiting to test would be dangerous. Check when you feel low because excitement, fatigue, stress, anxiety, and even a high blood sugar can all mimic the symptoms of a low blood sugar. If a severe low occurs, eat fast-acting carbs and then test or ask someone else to do the test while you are treating the low.

Record all suspected low blood sugars on your charts even if monitoring was not done. Highlight all lows on your charts with a circle, an arrow, or a specific color. Show the severity of a low blood sugar with the size of the mark. For instance, if symptoms are mild, use a small circle or arrow. If severe, use a large one.

Never be reluctant to show all your lows. You can't improve patterns if you don't acknowledge them, nor can you study them if you don't make note of them. The first step for improving control is to eliminate severe and frequent lows. Identifying patterns of lows allows insulin doses and carb intake to be adjusted correctly. If you are experiencing lows that you can't seem to eliminate, consider wearing a continuous monitor, which is able to warn you even before your blood sugar goes low.

Area B in Figure 6.2 shows the values and a graphic record of blood sugars.

Insulin Doses

On the top line for insulin doses near the middle of the *Smart Chart*, record how many carb bolus units you take for meals and snacks. On the third line for extra insulin, record all correction boluses used to lower high blood sugars. Note when each dose is given by putting the number of units at the correct vertical time line. You can also place a dash on the time line at the exact time the dose is taken. Basal insulin doses are recorded on the middle insulin line.

Area C in Figure 6.2 shows a record of all insulin doses for the day.

6.2 Sample Smart Chart

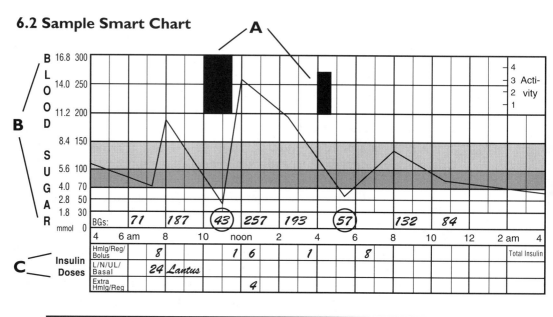

B - BLOOD SUGAR

Activity scale: 4, 3, 2, 1

	16.8 / 300
	14.0 / 250
	11.2 / 200
	8.4 / 150
	5.6 / 100
	4.0 / 70
	2.8 / 50
	1.8 / 30
mmol	0

| BGs: | 71 | 187 | (43) | 257 | 193 | (57) | | 132 | 84 | |

Time scale: 4, 6 am, 8, 10, noon, 2, 4, 6, 8, 10, 12, 2 am, 4

C - Insulin Doses

Hmlg/Reg/ Bolus		8			1 6		1		8			Total Insulin
L/N/UL/ Basal		24 Lantus										
Extra Hmlg/Reg					4							

D - Foods and carbs

	Breakfast			**Lunch**			**Dinner**	
Time	Food	Carb Grams	Time	Food	Carb Grams	Time	Food	Carb Grams
7:00	Cheerios	40	1:00	1 c nonfat milk	13	6:00	pasta and clams	64
	1 c nonfat milk	13		tuna sandwich	34		green salad	11
	strawberries	10		apple—154 gms	23		Chardonnay	6
	2 rye toast	30			70		vanilla ice cream	17
	applebutter	8						98
	poached egg	0						
	Morning Snacks	101		Afternoon Snacks			Evening Snacks	
11:00	2 blueberry muffins	70		crackers	12			
	banana	25		cheese	4			
	diet soda	0		glucose tabs	10			
		95			26			

Day: **Saturday**
Date: **05 / 24 / 03**
© 1994, 2003 Diabetes Services, Inc.

Comments: *Biked 21 miles in a.m., but ate too much! Noon, blew my fuse at nursery store clerk??? 4 pm - helped Fred load dirt into his trailer.*

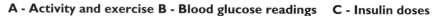

A - Activity and exercise B - Blood glucose readings C - Insulin doses
D - Foods and carbs E - Comments

Foods and Carb Counts

Carb counting provides an easy way to measure how a meal or snack will raise your blood sugar. Carbs can be counted directly from food labels, or by weighing a food on a gram scale and multiplying its weight by its carb percentage, or by looking up a food's carb content in a book that lists carbs. If you are not counting carbs yet, learn how in Chapter 8. It is easier than you think and is a very important step to control.

When control problems appear, it helps to record the foods you eat and the number of carbs in them. Be as specific as you can. A general word like "cereal" won't do, unless you eat the same cereal every day. All cereals are not equal. Cheerios®, Grape Nuts®, Cornflakes®, and oatmeal have very different effects on blood sugars. A sandwich can have a very different effect if it is "sandwich: whole wheat/tuna/tomato, 32 grams," "sandwich: white bun/hamburger, tomato, 45 grams," or "sandwich: ice cream with cookie covers, 68 grams."

Do not overlook what you eat to correct low blood sugars. If you don't record the four full-size graham crackers (44 grams) and 16 ounces of milk (24 grams) that you took for a nighttime low, you won't know why your blood sugar rose to 307 mg/dl (17 mmol) the following morning.

List all foods you eat and the time you eat them on the bottom half of the chart. You may discover that foods with only a little carb in them, like cheese or nuts, may cause your blood sugar to climb gradually for several hours after they are eaten. By listing what you eat in addition to its carb content, you begin to see the whole effect these foods have on your blood sugars. You may find some "good" foods have undesirable effects, while others thought to be "bad" may be perfectly fine. It helps to estimate the amount of the non-carb foods you eat. Record amounts on the chart, such as 2 ounces of cheese or 10 ounces of prime rib, since the protein and fat in foods like these may affect blood sugar levels.

A dietician can help you improve your blood sugar and health through your food choices. A dietician can provide you with precise recommendations for your daily carb need and how to distribute it to suit your lifestyle. You can do it yourself by looking at the section for figuring how many carbs you need in Chapter 8. How to match your carb boluses to the carb content in meals is covered in Chapter 12.

Area D in Figure 6.2 shows a list of foods eaten and their carbohydrate content.

Comments: Emotions, Stress, Medications. Other Factors

At the bottom of the chart, in the Comments section, you can record any other information you feel is relevant. Changes in weight, emotions, stress and illness can all impact your blood sugars and should be noted. This information might be "Asthma worse – used steroid inhaler," or "I woke up with a headache, may have gone low during the night."

An unusual high blood sugar before dinner might be explained by a comment like "stressed at work today." Comments like these may let you and your doctor see that there's a logical reason for a high reading which appeared to have no relationship to the food you ate. Understanding the reasons for highs and lows may involve factors other than food and insulin.

Emotions and blood sugars are a two-way street. Understanding their relationship can help in your blood sugar control. The brain controls the secretion of various stress hormones that can interfere with insulin's effectiveness. On the other hand when high or low levels of sugar reach the brain, the result may be impaired memory, anger, irritability, slowed thinking, or depression. As blood sugars rise, the levels of hormones that prevent depression may be lowered. This can worsen symptoms of depression and leave a person with less interest in doing the things needed to improve control, such as thoughtful selection of food, regular exercise, and rest. A vicious cycle of growing depression and worsening control can arise.

The Comments section is the place to begin connecting your emotions and illnesses to your blood sugars. Area E in Figure 6.2 shows an example.

6.3 Write Down Reasons And Excuses

Excuses may not always be desired, but they can be very helpful in diabetes. If your blood sugar falls outside a reasonable range, such as when it goes below 50 mg/dl (2.8 mmol) or above 200 mg/dl (11.1 mmol), always write down a reason or excuse in your chart or logbook.

It may be excess insulin, excess snacking, too few carbs, being impatient and overdosing, overtreating a low, stress, a change in activity, or anything else you think might have triggered it. Never let an unwanted reading go without a reason or excuse. Leave no stone unturned before shrugging your shoulders and saying, "I don't have a clue."

Writing your reasons down makes a remedy more likely. Review them regularly to reduce the frequency of problem readings. Show them to your doctor. Let your doctor know you are cogitating and trying to find solutions. This motivates your doctor to help you!

Spot Your Blood Sugar Patterns

Once a week, review your completed charts for patterns of high and low blood sugars. For instance, every Saturday morning review the last seven days' charts. Look carefully at your charts for the patterns that are discussed in Chapters 17 and 18.

Charts allow you to see patterns in your readings so that you become aware of any consistent rise or fall in your blood sugars. As you gather information on your charts, patterns will become apparent to you and your health care team. You may be amazed at how satisfying it is to finally see logical explanations for ups and downs you were not previously able to explain. You will no longer feel at the mercy of your readings.

Charting any change in blood sugar and correcting unhealthy patterns leads to freedom from the worry about internal damage, freedom from the annoyance and frustration of test results that show blood sugars out of control, and freedom from the mood swings caused by high and low blood sugars. Your moods can be affected by the body's response to highs and lows, but it can also be impacted by your emotional response to out of control readings. Charting gives you the freedom to eat, work and exercise the way you want and to deal with what really impacts your control.

Patterns to look for:

- Severe lows
- Frequent lows
- Frequent highs
- Highs that follow lows
- Lows that follow highs
- Repeated highs or lows at a particular time of day, such as high blood sugars when you wake up
- High or low blood sugars following particular foods
- High or low blood sugars after eating out
- Drops and rises in blood sugar with exercise
- Differences between weekend and workday blood sugars
- How stress affects your blood sugar

> **6.4 Look For Patterns**
>
> Blood sugar patterns can be seen in your charts related to:
>
> - time of day
> - insulin doses
> - food
> - activity
> - stress
> - particular events, such as low blood sugars, exercise, or eating out

How to identify the patterns in your charts is shown in Chapters 17 and 18.

Percent of Blood Sugars Within Your Target Ranges

A good way to monitor your overall control is to find the total percent of your readings that fall within your target ranges. Once a week, add up the total number of readings you have recorded. If you test 4 times a day, you will have 28 readings. Circle all the readings above your target range in one color and all the readings below in another color. Then add up the number of highs and lows outside your target ranges.

Divide the number outside of your range by the total number of readings. For example, if you had four readings in a week above and below your target range, divide the 4 outside readings by 28 total readings. Your answer is .14 or 14% which means you're within your target ranges 86% of the time. Aim for being inside your current target ranges at least 75% for the week. You can also add up the number of lows and highs at each period of the day, such as before breakfast. Aim for 75% success at each period of the day.

Sample Charts

Sara injects three times a day before the main meals and gives other injections as needed to bring down high blood sugars or cover extra carbs. She weighs 160 pounds, leads an active lifestyle, and eats about 2000 calories a day, with 1000 of these calories coming from carbohydrates.

Her total daily insulin dose (background and rapid insulins) averages 44 units a day. Sara takes 14 units of NPH before breakfast and 9 NPH before dinner as her basal insulin, and 17 to 24 units of Humalog each day to cover carbs, and another 3 to 5 units a day to lower occasional high blood sugars. Her target range is 70 to 130 mg/dl (3.9 to 7.2 mmol) before meals and 120 to 170 mg/dl (6.7 to 9.4 mmol) two hours after meals.

She counts carbs and uses one unit of Humalog for every 11 grams of carbohydrate. If she has a high blood sugar, she uses 1 unit of Humalog for every 40 points (2.2 mmol) above 100 mg/dl (5.5 mmol) to bring it down. On average, she eats 250 grams of carbohydrate a day with about 70 grams for breakfast, 60 for lunch and afternoon snack, 90 for dinner, and 20 for a bedtime snack. Her carb boluses for meals vary from day to day according to her carb choices and activity.

6.5 Why Blood Sugars Go:	
High	**Low**
too little insulin	too much insulin
too many carbs	too few carbs
snacking	missed meal
inactivity	delayed meal
stress	exercise

Take a look at four of Sara's *Smart Charts* on pages 67 and 68. These four days of charts provide a sample pattern followed by an analysis of Sara's charts and the options she can take. Take a close look to spot any patterns in her readings. Decide what you might change if you were Sara and these were your charts. When are her readings out of the normal range? Why do highs or lows occur and what would you do about them? Write your suggestions down, then look at the analysis that follows on page 69 for confirmation of your thinking. Don't peek!

Can you raed Esnilgh?

Aoccrdrnig to a rscheearch at an Elingsh uinervtisy, it deosn't mttaer in what order the ltters in a word are, the only iprmoetnt thing is that the frist and lsat ltteer is at the rghit pclae. The rset can be a total mses and you can still raed it wouthit a porbelm. This is bcusae we do not raed ervey lteter by it slef but the word as a wlohe.

Ins't that good to kown, now we dn'ot have to worry aobut seplilng aynomre!"

6.6 Sara's Charts

Monday Chart

Insulin scale: B 16.8 300 | L 14.0 250 | O 11.2 200 | D 8.4 150 | S 5.6 100 | U 5.6 100 | G 4.0 70 | A 2.8 50 | R 1.8 30 | mmol 0

	4	6 am	8	10	noon	2	4	6 pm	8	10	12	2 am	4	TDD	Wt
BGs:				137 / 172	113			103		118					
Carb Bolus H/Nov/R		7			4			7.5		2					
Basal Lan/L/N/U		14						9							
Correction Bolus		1													

Breakfast — Time 8:00

Food	Carb Grams
large muffin	36
6 oz yogurt	30
Soy latte	9
	75

Lunch — Time 1:00

Food	Carb Grams
4 crackers with peanut butter	36
apple	30
cheese	9
	75

Morning Snacks

Afternoon Snacks

Food	Carb Grams
1 1/2 graham crackers	16

Dinner — Time 6:00

Food	Carb Grams
roast beef	20
2 bread	32
potato	26
carrots	8
asparagus	5
1 cup milk	12
	83

Evening Snacks — Time 10:00

Food	Carb Grams
1/2 cup of ice cream	26
	102

Comments: Good Day

Day: Monday Wt: ____ Date: 05/19/03

Tuesday Chart

Insulin scale: B 16.8 300 | L 14.0 250 | O 11.2 200 | D 8.4 150 | S 5.6 100 | U 5.6 100 | G 4.0 70 | A 2.8 50 | R 1.8 30 | mmol 0

	4	6 am	8	10	noon	2	4	6 pm	8	10	12	2 am	4	TDD	Wt
BGs:			201		173			49		148					
Carb Bolus H/Nov/R		5.5			4			8		2					
Basal Lan/L/N/U		14						9							
Correction Bolus		2								1					

Breakfast — Time 8:00

Food	Carb Grams
2 waffles	30
blueberry	12
1 cup of milk	9
Soy latte	11
1/2 cup yogurt	62

Lunch — Time 12:30

Food	Carb Grams
lentil & veget. soup. 1 cup	24
1/2 cup of beets	24
	48

Morning Snacks

Afternoon Snacks

Time	Food	Carb Grams
4:00	apple	20
5:30	Sweet Tarts	16
		84

Dinner — Time 6:00

Food	Carb Grams
2 beef franks	4
2 buns	48
salad, greens	12
milk	26
potato	90

Evening Snacks — Time 10:15

Food	Carb Grams
1/2 cup of ice cream	26

Comments: Packed supplies in heavy boxes and moved to another office at work. Made me low at 5:30. Ate Sweet Tarts to bring me up and then ate dinner. High at bedtime, added 1 unit to bring me down.

Day: Tuesday Wt: ____ Date: 05/20/03

Wednesday — 05/21/03

Insulin / Blood Glucose chart

mmol / BGs	6 am	8	10	noon	2	4	6 pm	8	10	12	2 am	4
B 16.8 / 300												
L 14.0 / 250												
O 11.2 / 200												
O												
D 8.4 / 150												
S												
U 5.6 / 100												
G 4.0 / 70												
A 2.8 / 50												
R 1.8 / 30												
BGs			172/187	77	129		136	183		143		

TDD: , Wt:

Insulin	6 am	noon	6 pm
Carb Bolus H/Nov/R	7	4	8
Basal Lan/L/N/U	14		9
Correction Bolus	2	2	2

Breakfast

Time	Food	Carb Grams
8:00	2 eggs	
	Eng Muffin	26
	Orange Juice	30
	Soy latte	9
	1/2 cup of yogurt	11
		76

Morning Snacks

Lunch

Time	Food	Carb Grams
12:00	salad, greens	2
	2 bread	32
	cheese	1
	milk, 1 cup	12
		47
		76

Afternoon Snacks

	1 1/2 graham crackers	16
		63

Dinner

Time	Food	Carb Grams
6:15	1 cup rice stir fry	46
	veggies	11
	3/4 cup of carrots	2
	green beans, corn	32
	2 breads	89

Evening Snacks

Day: Wednesday Wt:
Date: 05/21/03

Comments: Tested at 2 am to check overnight blood sugar – about same as bedtime reading. Needed 2 units of Humalog before dinner to bring down a high (Mary's BD party at work)

© 1994, 2003 Diabetes Services, Inc.

Thursday — 05/22/03

Insulin / Blood Glucose chart

mmol / BGs	6 am	8	10	noon	2	4	6 pm	8	10	12	2 am	4
B 16.8 / 300												
L 14.0 / 250												
O 11.2 / 200												
O												
D 8.4 / 150												
S												
U 5.6 / 100												
G 4.0 / 70												
A 2.8 / 50												
R 1.8 / 30												
BGs	203		168	71	132		106		77	104		

TDD: , Wt:

Insulin	6 am	noon	6 pm
Carb Bolus H/Nov/R	6	4	9
Basal Lan/L/N/U	14		6
Correction Bolus	3	1	2

Breakfast

Time	Food	Carb Grams
7:30	Bagel	45
	1/2 cup yogurt	11
	Soy latte	9
		65

Morning Snacks

Lunch

Time	Food	Carb Grams
12:00	cottage cheese	5
	1 cup grapes,	
	blueberries, and	14
	raspberries	26
	Eng Muffin	45

Afternoon Snacks

	1 1/2 graham crackers	16
		61

Dinner

Time	Food	Carb Grams
6:00	pizza	62
	6 oz pepperoni	34
	1 cup of corn	96

Evening Snacks

10:00	1/2 cup cherry garcia ice cream	20
		20

Day: Thursday Wt:
Date: 05/22/03

Comments: High at 10:00 pm, took 2 units to bring it down overnight. Got up at 1 am to check.

© 1994, 2003 Diabetes Services, Inc.

Analysis

Overall, Sara's readings are adequate. Monday's readings are largely in the normal range. On Tuesday afternoon, she moved her office at work with extra activity packing and moving file boxes and desk utensils. Because her blood sugar had been high at lunch, she had not expected this activity to cause her to go low, but by 5:30 that afternoon she was 49 mg/dl (2.7 mmol). This activity combined with the carb coverage and correction bolus taken at lunch was enough to make her feel nervous and check her blood sugar earlier than usual that day before dinner. She ate 16 grams of glucose from Sweet Tarts right away to feel better fast.

After talking to her doctor, she realizes her major pattern is being high in the morning when she gets up. Three of her four charts show her breakfast readings above 170 mg/dl (9.4 mmol) and an overnight basal test on Wednesday night through Thursday morning shows that her blood sugar rises in the early morning hours.

On Wednesday, Sara's reading at dinner was higher than usual after she underestimated the carbs in a piece of birthday cake at work. Because her blood sugar had been rising overnight for several weeks, Sara decided to check her overnight basal insulin dose. She covered her dinner carbs so that she got to bedtime with a reading of 136 mg/dl (7.6 mmol). She skipped having a snack that evening so that no rapid insulin would be active after she went to bed. When she awoke at 2 a.m., her blood sugar had remained steady at 143 mg/dl (7.9 mmol), but by breakfast it had risen to 203 mg/dl (11.3 mmol).

Sara knows she needs to increase her basal insulin during the night, but when she raised her dinner NPH dose in the past she would start to have nighttime lows before reaching a dose that would bring her breakfast reading into a normal range. She decides to increase her evening basal dose from 9 units to 10, but not give it all before dinner. She changes to 6 NPH at dinner and another 4 units at bedtime on Thursday evening. The peaking action of the bedtime NPH will occur in the early morning when she needs it. If her breakfast reading continues to stay high, she can then increase her bedtime NPH dose with little risk of nighttime lows.

Sara has other minor problems but these don't add up to a pattern. She needs to consider the effect of unplanned activity. When unexpected activity occurs, such as moving boxes in her office on Tuesday, she decided in the future it would be a good idea to take a little time out and check her blood sugar an hour and a half or so into the activity even though she started high that day at lunch, and also to test as soon as the activity was finished.

"Some things have to be believed to be seen."
Ralph Hodgson

Summary

As you begin to fill out charts, you may have difficulty remembering to record everything. As you do more recording, it becomes easier to correct problems as you run into them. With practice, charting becomes a small distraction that pays off by helping prevent low blood sugars and lessening the time you spend at high blood sugar levels. Palm devices, enhanced meters, and software help make carb counting easier and simplify recording.

> ### 6.7 Continuous Monitors
>
> A continuous monitor can make blood sugar collection and analysis easier. The large number of readings collected by these devices allow patterns and trends to be spotted. They display trends in your blood sugar and let you know whether your reading is going up or down, so you can make better decisions about the actions you need to take. Continuous monitors allow basal and bolus doses to be tested quickly as outlined in the next few chapters.

Review your charts regularly for patterns, and bring them to every visit with your physician/health care team. Flipping *Smart Chart* pages back and forth can help you pick up patterns. Be sure to look at and evaluate the data you are collecting on a regular basis to eradicate unwanted patterns and increase your confidence that you can manage your diabetes well.

Show your charts to others and listen to their suggestions. Other people, especially those trained in diabetes care and experienced with glucose control, will see things that you may miss. Diabetes professionals, in particular, understand the complexities of dealing with diabetes in daily life. If you have any uncertainty about how to correct an unwanted pattern or need advice on adjustments, be sure to contact your physician or health care team. Use the knowledge and experience of others to simplify your path toward normal readings.

A fully detailed *Smart Chart* may be more extensive data than you need all the time. Although charting allows factors that influence your blood sugars to be understood and changed quickly, once you have stabilized your blood sugar with improved insulin doses, you may be able to maintain your control with a simple logbook. **Anytime that your control starts to slip, use a comprehensive recording system like *Smart Charts* to help you get back where you want to be.**

"Take notes on the spot, a note is worth a cart-load of recollections."

Ralph Waldo Emerson

6.8 Technology And Blood Sugar Control

With new technology, there are many additional tools to aid your charting. Enhanced meters, PDAs, meters that communicate current readings via a cellphone, software programs for your computer, and internet downloads are all available. Some tools aid pattern identification, allow you to record carb and correction factors to give suggestions for improvements, and identify what actions may remedy the problem.

Some provide real-time reports to your health care team over the internet so they can reply quickly with helpful advice about your diabetes care. Internet sites allow you to download your meter, record events using your keyboard, and send the data directly to your doctor.

PDAs Or Personal Digital Assistants

Many people find the convenience, organization, and portability of PDAs make their record keeping easier. Enhanced data analysis, dietary software to assist carb counting, and even dose calculations with individualized carb and correction factors can be found.

Use of a PDA with an add-on meter module can be a quick fix to the problem of testing, as well as record keeping and analysis. Inexpensive carb counting software is available for Palm and PocketPC devices. Some programs allow users to select their carb and correction factors for easier dosing using a basal/bolus approach.

Smart Charts

Despite their advances, electronic devices do not display as conveniently or as concisely all the data you need to improve your blood sugars as *Smart Charts*. *Smart Charts* let you see that a blood sugar rise was caused by eating a scone, or that your blood sugar plummeted because you walked the golf course. A chart merges all the relevant data on one page, displays the causes, and makes answers easy to find.

"The art of living is more like wrestling than dancing."
Marcus Aurelius

6.9 Better Monitoring Tools Could Help You Find Patterns

Home blood glucose monitoring created a major advance in diabetes care 25 years ago, but its full benefits have been slow to be realized. Testing has certainly become easier, but many people with both Type 1 and Type 2 diabetes continue to test infrequently or not at all. One reason for infrequent testing is that most people do not know how to use their readings and receive little help from physicians who have only a brief opportunity to glance at them every 3 to 6 months.

Testing allows users to treat high or low blood sugars immediately, but in the long term, testing does little good unless readings are analyzed for patterns to allow adjustments to be made for better control.

Blood sugar readings are displayed in most meters as a disjointed series of numbers without any connection to their causes. This simplistic approach makes corrections nearly impossible. By the time the meter's memory is reviewed and readings below 50 mg/dl (2.8 mmol) or above 300 mg/dl, (16.6 mmol) are seen, the user no longer remembers the circumstances which generated that reading.

Finding meaning in meter data is similar to the problem seen in the early days of EKGs. Barry Ginsberg, M.D., Ph.D., of Becton Dickinson Technologies describes this problem as looking at the points or trees in an EKG, rather than the vector or forest. Few physicians could correctly identify EKG patterns in early machines. They lacked critical information, such as how to distinguish between an inferior wall MI and a normal heart beat.

EKG companies quickly recognized the problem and organized the data so doctors could make decisions more easily. Rather than having to look for a deep Q-S segment and inverted T wave in leads 3 and AVF to identify a heart attack in the bottom wall of the heart, a doctor can simply look at the computer analysis printed on the EKG printout that says "inferior wall MI". The readout from a quick pattern analysis, which machines do better than humans, enables the physician to make quick and appropriate clinical decisions that can save someone's life.

Instead of showing you a jumble of unrelated numbers, your meter might tell you: "Your results show you are having too many low blood sugars. Discuss this with your doctor right away." or "Following your last 3 low blood sugars, your next reading averaged 425 mg/dl. You appear to be over treating your lows." or simply that your blood sugar is trending upward at this time rather than downward.

Patterns are obvious to those who have an eye for spotting them. You may be good at this and your physician may occasionally have the time to do it for you, but your meter should be able to do this type of analysis as well as display helpful solutions.

New devices and software are moving in the right direction. Meters can be downloaded over the internet for faster access by a physician or nurse. Even better, software could enable pattern analysis and advice based on rules similar to those found in this book. Integration of this analytic software into PDAs, meters, meter-PDA combos, and internet sites is beginning. Be on the lookout for devices that can help you spot problematic blood sugar patterns and assist you to improve your control.

Visit www.diabetesnet.com/diabetes_technology/ for the latest developments in this area.

Better Records With Logbooks

Testing your blood sugar at least four times a day and recording your readings on a chart or in a logbook is one of the most important tools you can use to improve your control. Testing blood sugars by itself will not lead to better control unless other data related to control is considered.

Many people use a logbook to record and track their blood sugar readings. One problem with standard logbooks is that they lack sufficient space to fill in everything that affects your blood sugar. An enhanced logbook, as shown on page 75, improves the traditional logbook by enabling the recording of other important data. If you use a logbook, always be on the lookout for patterns, but be mindful that logbooks may not be as useful as charts for finding causes and solutions.

People who are visual may prefer to use charts for their graphical approach to analyzing records. Others will prefer to use a logbook where they can add up the numbers that fall outside their target range. Either approach can be used to adjust your insulin to better match your lifestyle. Analyzing records for patterns takes only a bit of time, but must be done with care so that your decisions will be good ones. Luckily, the more analysis you do, the faster it becomes.

This chapter helps in showing:

- Benefits of using an enhanced logbook for better control
- How to find patterns in logbooks

Enhanced Logbooks

The logbooks that are handed out in doctor's offices usually provide only a simple format for recording blood sugars, insulin doses, and time of day. An enhanced logbook allows more information to be written down so that everything that affects control can be tracked. Enhanced logbooks include room to record food choices or at least the grams of carb eaten, the length and type of exercise, room for comments about things like stress or illness, and pattern analysis.

The enhanced logbook on page 75 provides space for important details and a system for recognizing patterns. Blood sugar results before each meal, one to two hours after each meal, and at bedtime can be recorded. Tests can be done anytime

7.1 Tips For Using Logbooks To Improve Control

- Although recording is done across a logbook, patterns are found by looking up and down the page. Check whether your readings remain in your target range at each time of day.

- Give your best excuse for every reading that is out of your target range. Write related information in the margins or wherever space is available.

- Look for lows first. Circle every low in your log book in red so they stand out. If frequent or severe lows are happening, these should always be stopped before attempting to stop other patterns.

- Do highs often follow lows? Try eating 20 grams of fast carbs (glucose tabs, Sweet Tarts, etc.) to treat your lows instead of unmeasured amounts of carb.

- After stopping lows, control the pre-breakfast reading next. A good pre-breakfast reading helps control the rest of the day.

- Look for the time of day when your readings are highest. Adjust your insulin to bring these high readings down.

- Do particular foods have specific effects on your blood sugar? Adjust insulin doses or carb amounts for foods that do.

- After one insulin dose has been increased or decreased, watch for a few days to see if other insulin doses are affected and how they need to be changed.

you think you may be low, more often when you are ill, and occasionally at 2 a.m. to see what happens during the night. Extra testing can be done when you start a new insulin, change an insulin dose, or increase your exercise. Any extra tests done can be written in the nearest box or in the margin.

Space is provided to write down the doses of bolus and basal insulin you use so you can see their effect on your blood sugars. Record the number of units and types of insulin, such as 6H/17N (representing 6 units of Humalog and 17 units of NPH). Once you know the action time for each insulin, you can determine its effect on your blood sugar during the time it is active.

Circle all low blood sugars in red to make them stand out better. If you have a low but do not test before eating fast carbs, mark it down as a low and circle the time that it happened in red ink. Mark all highs in a different color. Even though space is limited, it helps to record the types and quantities of foods, especially carbs and the time they are eaten. Make note of the times and duration of exercise. You may have to write in the margin.

Current target ranges for before and after meals can be written in at the bottom and then analyzed at the end of the week right above it. When a reading falls outside your target range, write an explanation for it in the margin of your logbook or on the back of the page using numbers to signify where each note belongs on the front side of the log. Write down anything that might have influenced your blood

Enhanced Logbook		Breakfast Before	Breakfast After	Lunch Before	Lunch After	Dinner Before	Dinner After	Night Bedtime	Night 2 a.m.
Sunday 5|18|03 (walk)/run/bike at 7 am/(pm)	BG	167				181		93	
	Time	9:30				7:00		10:30	
	Carbs	88				66			
	Insulin	8+2H,14N				6H, 9N			
Monday 5|19|03 walk/run/bike at ___ am/pm	BG	137	172	113		103		118	
	Time	8 am	10:30	1:00		6:00		10:00	
	Carbs	75		44		83		26	
	Insulin	7+1H,14N		4H		7.3H,9N		2H	
Tuesday 5|20|03 walk/run/bike at ___ am/pm	BG	201		173		(49)		148	
	Time	8:00		12:00		5:30		10:00	
	Carbs	62		48		90		26	
	Insulin	5.5H,14N		4+2H		8H,9N		2+1H	
Wednesday 5|21|03 walk/run/bike at ___ am/pm	BG	172	187	77		183		136	143
	Time	8:00	11:00	12:00		6:00		10:00	2:00 am
	Carbs	76		47	24	89		0	0
	Insulin	7+2H,14N		4H	2H	8+2H,9N		night basal test	
Thursday 5|22|03 walk/run/bike at ___ am/pm	BG	203	168	71	138	106		171	104
	Time	7:00	10:00	12:00	4:00	6:00		10:00	1:00 am
	Carbs	65		45	16	96		20	
	Insulin	6+3H,14N		4H	1	9H,6N		1+2H,4N	
Friday 5|23|03 (walk)/run/bike at 4 am/(pm)	BG	141	196	128		87	135	102	93
	Time	7:30	10:00	12:30		6:15	8:30	10:30	
	Carbs	55		60		83		20	
	Insulin	5+1H,14N	1H	5.5H		7H,6N		1H,4N	
Saturday 5|24|03 walk/run/(bike) at 7 (am)/pm	BG	134		77		111		(86)	
	Time	8:00		12:30		6:00		10:30	
	Carbs	89		52		80		30	
	Insulin	8+1H,14N		4H		7H,6N		2H,4N	
# below target						1		1	
# above target		7	3	1		2		2	

PATTERNS

My target ranges:		
Before meals 70 to 130	At bedtime 90 to 140
After meals 120 to 170	At 2 a.m 90 to 140

sugar that day. Extra stress, unusual exercise or activity, large meals, or high carbo-hydrate meals are things worth recording. Write the note in your logbook close to the time it happens, or draw a line from the time for your comment to the margin where you have more room to write. You can also place comments on the back of the log sheet, but this time use letters to indicate where on the logbook it belongs and that it is a comment. Be consistent and thorough in your records.

Look For The Patterns In Your Readings

After testing and recording for a week, review the last seven days' records and look for any patterns in your readings. Logbook patterns can be spotted by looking up and down the page for errant readings at a particular time of day. The pattern section at the bottom of the *Enhanced Logbook* helps you pick up patterns by having you record how many readings that week were above or below your target range. Add up all the highs that fall outside your target range for each time of day and do the same for all the lows. Write these numbers at the bottom of each column on the *Enhanced Logbook*. High readings at the same time of day on three or more days in one week, or low readings on two or more days can be considered a pattern.

When unwanted patterns occur, ask yourself if there is any reason other than the doses of insulin you are taking. Are you eating too many or too few carbohy-drates, engaging in more or less activity than usual, feeling more or less stress than usual, or in the midst of an illness?

If you identify something other than your insulin doses that is causing un-wanted readings, it will be easier to deal with this directly first. If your insulin doses are not correct or need to be adjusted to match other things in your life, read this book carefully and work with your doctor to learn how to adjust your doses to match your lifestyle needs. After you make a change, record blood sugars, carb intake, and insulin doses to guide your changes and verify improvements.

Look at Sara's logbook. As noted on page 65, she is on 3 shots a day with Humalog and NPH at breakfast, Humalog at lunch and Humalog and NPH at dinner. Her target range is 70 to 130 mg/dl (3.9 to 7.2 mmol) before meals and 120 to 170 mg/dl (6.7 to 9.4 mmol) two hours after meals. She marks all lows with a circle and highs with an upright triangle.

At the bottom of Sara's logbook, there is a "below target" and "above target" analysis area that help her spot patterns. Here, she adds the numbers of highs and lows at the same time each day and writes the number at the bottom of the column at the end of the week. From this analysis, it is easy to see that her readings tend to be high, especially before breakfast, with relatively few lows. This lets us know the overnight basal dose probably needs to be increased. See the previous analysis on page 69 for more information.

"The only normal people are ones you don't know very well."

Joe Ancio

Carb Counting Made Easy

"I never met a carbohydrate I didn't like." is the way many people feel about pasta, potatoes, pastries, fruit, and all the other wonderful foods in this food group. One of the great things about flexible therapy is the opportunity to match any carbohydrate you chance to eat with an appropriate injection of Humalog or Novolog.

To take advantage of the flexibility that insulin adjustments afford, you need an approach to food that is as exact and as flexible as your injections. Carb counting offers the most precise and flexible approach available today. It is more precise than the exchange system, can be applied directly to the foods in your meal, and is relatively easy to learn and use. It takes some practice, but if you are persistent, you will see the results you want over time.

This chapter describes the following:

- Why you want to count carbohydrates
- What are carbs and grams
- How to calculate your daily need for carbs
- How to count carbs
- Three ways to count carbohydrates
- Is carb counting the only way
- The "bigger picture" in healthy eating
- The glycemic index and carbs

The exchange system that many people have learned is based on estimates of the average nutrient values for each of six classes of foods: breads, fruits, vegetables, milk, fats, and meat (or protein). This diet approach is an excellent way to provide balance in nutrient intake, but it does not provide an exact way to measure carbohydrates. Bagels get bigger every day, but exchanges don't. A half a bagel is still called a bread exchange whether it has 15 grams or 32 grams.. If someone using the exchange system has well-controlled blood sugars, this imprecision does not matter, but it may cause others to experience unexpected high blood sugars.

Carb counting is recommended for people who want to improve their blood sugar control. It is especially important for those trying to adjust their insulin to match the food they eat.

Why Count Carbs?

Carbs from food provide a large part of the energy that our cells use. Counting carbohydrates lets us quantify how much a meal will raise the blood sugar. Counting carbs and covering them with insulin account for about half the day's blood sugar control. Get started right away with this great tool if you are not already using it.

Food is made up of three main fuels: carbohydrate, fat, and protein, but the carbohydrate is the primary part that affects blood sugars. Over 90 percent of the calories from digestible carbohydrates (starches and sugars) end up as glucose. Thus, glucose raises the blood sugar rapidly following a meal. Knowing the grams of carbohydrate eaten provides a useful guide to how high that meal will drive the blood sugar.

To keep your blood sugar in control after you eat, the carbs in your food must be balanced with insulin or exercise. After you have counted how many grams of carbohydrate are in the foods you plan to eat, you want to know how large a carb bolus or how much exercise is needed to balance these carbs. To determine the size of your carb insulin bolus, you want to first determine how many grams of carb you need to match each unit of fast insulin. How to do this is covered in Chapter 12.

Carb boluses generally make up 40 to 55% of your TDD, the total insulin taken in 24 hours. Carbs do not need to be covered with an insulin bolus if they are used to balance exercise or to raise a low blood sugar. If your blood sugar is 50 mg/dl (2.8 mmol) before a meal and you need 15 grams of carbohydrate to raise your blood sugar to 100 mg/dl (5.6 mmol), this would not be counted in your premeal bolus. Similarly, carbs eaten to replace those burned during a bike ride would not be covered with a bolus.

When the blood sugar is normal before a meal, a carb bolus of rapid insulin can be taken 10 to 20 minutes before eating begins, but if the reading is high, the meal can be delayed longer to allow the combined carb and correction bolus to lower the blood sugar. Care must always be taken so that the meal is not delayed any longer than planned after the injection since this is the most common cause of low blood sugars.

Counting carbohydrates lets you measure the impact a meal will have on your blood sugar. Though you might not eat them often, counting carbs can enable you to eat "splurge" foods like ice cream, cake, pie, and candy. These can be counted and covered by a carb bolus or by exercise so that they don't destroy your hard-won diabetes control.

Carb counting is especially helpful to those who have a small total daily insulin dose, smaller body size and weight, greater insulin sensitivity, or a higher level of activity because these people have less margin for error.

Carb counting presents some challenges. In starting, you will need to check labels, books, or a database in a PDA; weigh and/or measure unpackaged foods;

8.2 What About Fat And Protein?

Food contains three fuels – carbohydrate, fat, and protein. All affect glucose in the blood, but their effects are not equal. For instance, the fat in certain foods may delay absorption of carbohydrate from the intestine and reduce the expected rise in blood sugar.[13] The fat in old-fashioned ice cream that has a low glycemic index (raises the blood sugar slowly) is a good example of this. On the other hand, certain high fat meals create a rapid, temporary state of insulin resistance for up to 8 to 16 hours, making the blood sugar rise more than expected.[38, 39] The fat content of many chips and pizzas cause a greater than expected rise.

High fat and calorie diets lead to weight gain and can create permanent insulin resistance such as that found in Type 2 diabetes, particularly in those prone to an apple figure or male pattern obesity.[40–42] Insulin resistance makes it harder for sugar to enter cells and be used as fuel. Although fat's effect on blood sugar after most meals or snacks is small,[43] dietary fat, especially saturated and hydrogenated or trans fat, should be reduced in the diet for better heart health.

Normal portions of dietary protein have little impact on blood sugar.[44] Making up only 10 to 20 percent of calories in most diets, protein affects less than a tenth of the total blood sugar control.

Large portions of protein, however, can cause blood sugars to rise. Half of the calories in protein are slowly converted to glucose over a period of several hours. For instance, a high-protein dinner such as an eight-ounce steak or a bean burrito may cause blood sugars to rise 4 to 12 hours later and create an unexpected high reading the next morning.

The delayed rise caused by high protein meals may be covered by a small increase in the dinner or bedtime basal dose. This should be considered only if the meal consistently raises the next morning's blood sugar. A better plan for blood sugar control and better protection for the kidneys is to limit how often this much protein is eaten. Talk to your doctor or dietician if you think your intake of fat or protein may be affecting your blood sugar.

keep food records; do some basic arithmetic; and test the blood sugar more often. It is important to determine what effect the carbs you eat have on the blood sugar, especially when you are having problems with your control.

If you are like most people, you eat the same food frequently. Keep a list of the foods that you eat often, your portion sizes and how much carbohydrate they contain. In about two weeks, you will have a list of most of the foods you eat and know most of these numbers by heart. If you have any difficulty, ask your dietician to help you over this learning curve.

Carb counting is worth the effort when you consider how many years you will want to have optimal control. You won't have to repeat this learning process, but you may want to refine it somewhat later.

Where's The Carbohydrate?

Healthy diets often contain 50 to 60% of the day's total calories as carbohydrate. An important exception comes during pregnancy when a 40 percent carbohydrate diet is recommended as a way to improve blood sugar control which is so critical to the health of the child. The American Diabetes Association does not recommend any specific carbohydrate intake but states that the diet for any person with diabetes needs to be individualized. For you to know how much carbohydrate you eat, you need to be clear about which foods are primarily carbohydrate and which contain enough carbs that they need to be considered.

Carbohydrate is found in:

- Grains (breads, pasta, cereals)
- Fruits and vegetables
- Root crops (potatoes, sweet potatoes, and yams)
- Beer and wine
- Desserts and candies
- Most milk products, except cheese
- -ose foods, like sucrose, fructose, maltose

Healthy Carbohydrates

In a healthy diet, most carbohydrate comes from nutrient-dense foods like whole grains, fruits, legumes, vegetables, nonfat or low fat milk, and yogurt. Nutrient-dense foods and complex carbs contain a high volume of vitamins, minerals, fiber, and protein in proportion to their calorie content. They also tend to be lower on the glycemic index.

Low-nutrient foods like candy and regular sodas contain carbohydrate, but lack the other nutrients your cells require for health. Because they contain simple sugar or refined grains, they are more likely to cause the blood sugar to spike. Nutrient-dense foods like brown rice and broccoli are better for both your health and your blood sugars.

Remember that it is the total amount of carbohydrate, either nutrient-dense or otherwise, in a meal that determines what impact a meal will have on your blood sugar. Low-nutrient carbs may be eaten in small amounts and have only a minor impact on blood sugars. For blood sugar control, it is best to always include high-nutrient carbs in meals that contain low-nutrient ones. This helps keep the blood sugar within your target range after a meal.

What Are Grams?

Carbs are counted in grams. A gram is a unit of weight like pounds or ounces, but because of its small size (28 grams make a single ounce), grams can be used to measure components of food precisely. Simply weighing foods does not tell how much carbohydrate they contain because most foods are not purely carbohydrate.

For example, even though 224 grams (one cup) of milk, a 160 gram slice of watermelon, one 14 gram rectangular graham cracker (two squares), and 12 grams (one tablespoon) of sugar have different weights, they all contain exactly 12 grams of carbohydrate. The milk and watermelon contain water, graham crackers have other ingredients, while the sugar is all carbohydrate.

Despite their different weights, they all require the same carb bolus to cover them because they each have 12 grams of carbohydrate. Knowing a food's weight and what percentage of its weight is carb allows precise carb measurement. Knowing your carb factor, which is how many carbs are covered by one unit of insulin, allows precise insulin dosing.

> ### 8.3 Long-Acting Carbs
>
> Just like long-acting insulins, there are long-acting carbs. Such carbs are useful at bedtime and during lengthy exercise to keep the blood sugar from dropping over a long period of time.
>
> Examples of long-acting carbs include beans (lima, pinto, etc.), green apples, PowerBars, raw cornstarch, pasta al dente, barley, cracked wheat, parboiled long grain and whole grain rice, and whole-grain rye bread.

How Many Carbs Do You Need A Day?

Although a healthy diet gets 50 to 60% of its calories from complex carbohydrates, most people actually eat only 40% of their calories as carbohydrate, another 40% from fat and 20% from protein. If your current diet has less than 50 to 60% as carbs, you may have difficulty consuming this much carbohydrate at first. On the other hand, you may find a higher complex carb meal plan allows you to feel full at every meal, which can be a welcome change. You will, however, need to reduce the other components of your diet if you don't want to be adding calories.

Try eating your usual meals for a few days and keep a record of how much carbohydrate you actually take in. Some computer software programs will help in analyzing your daily diet for you. If you are eating significantly less carbohydrate than that recommended in Go Figure 8.6, try increasing your carb intake by 10% while reducing fat and protein calories by the same amount.

Because carbohydrate plays such a major role in setting your insulin doses, it is best to make gradual changes in how much carbohydrate you eat so that you can adjust your insulin more easily. You may find that abruptly increasing the amount of carbohydrate you eat makes blood sugar control more difficult. Don't let this stop you from working toward a healthy diet but realize that your progress will be somewhat slow. That actually is an advantage since fast changes of food patterns seldom become permanent ones.

8.4 Ideal weight

For this height	Optimum weight
4'10"	91-119 lbs.
4'11"	94-124 lbs.
5'00"	97-128 lbs.
5'01"	101-132 lbs.
5'02"	104-137 lbs.
5'03"	107-141 lbs.
5'04"	111-146 lbs.
5'05"	114-150 lbs.
5'06"	118-155 lbs.
5'07"	121-160 lbs.
5'08"	125-164 lbs.
5'09"	129-169 lbs.
5'10"	132-174 lbs.
5'11"	136-179 lbs.
6'00"	140-184 lbs.

A higher complex carb diet helps reduce fat and protein calories because it fills you up and makes you feel satisfied. Less fat and protein in your diet reduces your risks for heart disease and kidney disease respectively, risks which are quite high in people with diabetes. Over 70% of people with Type 2 diabetes, for instance, die as a result of cardiovascular disease, while some 30% of those with Type 1 diabetes die directly or indirectly from kidney disease. If you find you have a problem balancing your carbs with injections of rapid insulin, be sure to discuss how to do this with your physician or dietician because it is well worth making the switch to a healthier diet.

8.5 Weight Goal If overweight	
Current weight	Wt goal ↓ by 10%
150 lbs.	135 lbs.
160 lbs.	144 lbs.
170 lbs.	153 lbs.
180 lbs.	162 lbs.
190 lbs.	171 lbs.
200 lbs.	180 lbs.
210 lbs.	189 lbs.
220 lbs.	198 lbs.
230 lbs.	207 lbs.
240 lbs.	216 lbs.
250 lbs.	225 lbs.
260 lbs.	234 lbs.

Your daily carbohydrate goal is based on how many total calories you need. A person who needs 2000 calories a day ideally would get 1000 to 1200 of those calories from the carbohydrate in breads, grains, vegetables, fruits, low-fat milk, and so on. There are four calories in each gram of carbohydrate, so a person eating 2000 calories a day would need 250 to 300 grams (1000 to 1200 calories divided by four) of carbohydrate.

The number of grams of carbohydrate needed daily becomes the basis of a carb counting meal plan. This amount is divided among the meals and snacks the person normally eats. Table 8.7 shows three examples of how 225 grams of total daily carbohydrate can be divided among meals and snacks. Your own pattern can be based on your personal preferences and needs.

One nice thing about flexible insulin therapy is that snacks are optional. Once the basal insulin has been correctly set, you have the freedom to enjoy snacks and cover them with an injection when you want, not when your insulin says you must.

How To Count Carbohydrates

A few foods like table sugar and lollipops are entirely carbohydrate, so their weight on a gram scale will be exactly the same as the number of grams of carbohydrate they contain. Most foods, however, have only part of their total weight as carbohydrate. The carb content of these other foods can be determined by food labels, reference books or software, or a scale and a list of carb factors.

Like any new skill, counting grams of carbohydrate will take a couple of weeks to master. You will need to consult books or software in a Personal Digital Assistant (PDA) and weigh and measure foods consistently for a while. As time passes, you will train your eye to estimate accurately both serving sizes and weights, whether eating out or at home. As you look up the foods you commonly eat, make a list of them for easy reference. Keep that list next to your Smart Charts or food log, and use it to figure the carbs in a meal before you decide how much insulin to take.

Eventually, you'll be able to look at a piece of fruit, a bowl of pasta, or a plate of stir-fried veggies and rice at home or in your favorite restaurant and estimate its

Go Figure 8.6: Determine Your Carb Requirement Per Day

Steps:

1. Enter your current weight or desired weight in pounds below. If overweight, a 10% reduction in weight is an ideal goal.

2. Choose a <u>calorie factor</u> that best describes your activity level from the table below.

3. Multiply your weight times your calorie factor to determine your <u>daily calorie need</u>.

4. Divide your daily calorie need by 10 if you want 40% of your calories to come from carbs. Divide by 8 to have 50% of your calories as carbs or by 6.67 if you prefer a 60% carb diet.

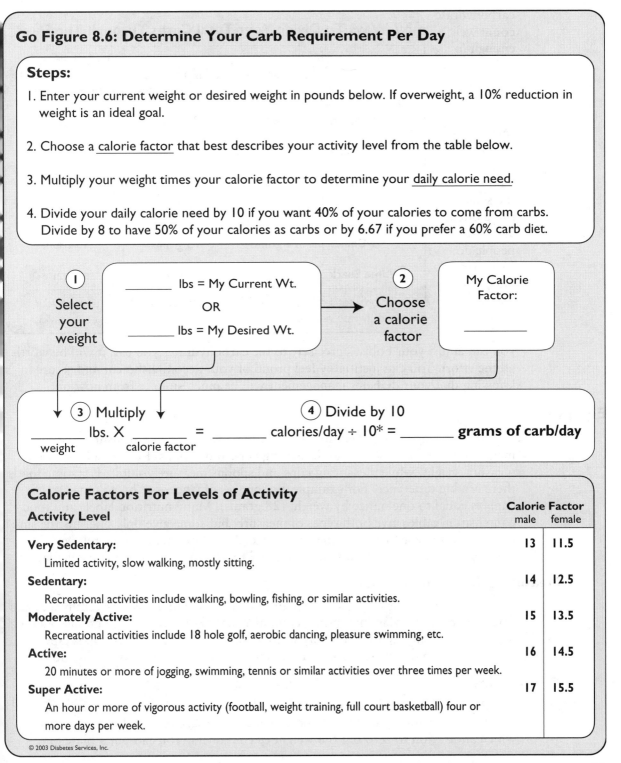

| ① Select your weight | _____ lbs = My Current Wt.
 OR
 _____ lbs = My Desired Wt. | ② Choose a calorie factor | My Calorie Factor:
 _____ |

③ Multiply   ④ Divide by 10

_____ lbs. X _____ = _____ calories/day ÷ 10* = _____ **grams of carb/day**
weight   calorie factor

Calorie Factors For Levels of Activity

Activity Level	Calorie Factor male	Calorie Factor female
Very Sedentary: Limited activity, slow walking, mostly sitting.	13	11.5
Sedentary: Recreational activities include walking, bowling, fishing, or similar activities.	14	12.5
Moderately Active: Recreational activities include 18 hole golf, aerobic dancing, pleasure swimming, etc.	15	13.5
Active: 20 minutes or more of jogging, swimming, tennis or similar activities over three times per week.	16	14.5
Super Active: An hour or more of vigorous activity (football, weight training, full court basketball) four or more days per week.	17	15.5

carbohydrate count well enough to take the right amount of insulin for the food you eat. This, of course, is easier if you tend to eat the same thing often, as many people do. Be patient but persistent as you develop this skill. When

Meal	Carbs divided among 3 meals	Light breakfast, frequent snacks	Big breakfast & lunch, light dinner & bedtime snack
8.7 Ways To Divide Your Total Carbs Through The Day*			
Breakfast	75 grams	30 grams	75 grams
Morning Snack		15 grams	
Lunch	75 grams	45 grams	70 grams
Afternoon Snack		30 grams	
Dinner	75 grams	75 grams	40 grams
Bedtime Snack		30 grams	40 grams

* Based on a total daily carb need of 225 grams. See pg 93 to determine your own daily carb requirement.   © 2003 Diabetes Services, Inc.

you can adjust your boluses precisely to the carbohydrates you eat, it will be worth all the effort. You can justifiably feel proud of your accomplishment and secure in knowing that your diabetes management will be much simpler from now on.

Equipment

Truly accurate carb counting requires some weighing and measuring equipment, such as a gram scale and measuring cups and spoons. Remember that scales measure weight, while measuring cups and spoons measure volume. For some foods there is a big difference. For example, ten ounces of Cheerios® by volume (1 1/4 cups) is equal to one ounce by weight (28 grams). Many nutrition labels and food composition tables give both types of measure, but some give only one. Just be sure to match your type of measurement, i.e., weight or volume, with the reference material you are using. To do otherwise will require considerable extra calculation.

Measuring Cups and Spoons

Accurate measuring cups and spoons are available in many different places and price ranges. Use a glass measuring container that allows you to "sight" across the top for measuring liquids. You may want a second one that will let you scrape a knife across the top to get the exact measure for dry items such as cereal and rice.

Gram scales

A gram scale measures the actual weight of a food in grams. An ideal scale will weigh food accurately within one or two grams. Be sure to look for a tare feature which allows you to zero out the weight of containers. You can put a plate or serving bowl on the scale, press the tare button, and the scale goes back to zero. Then place the food you want to eat into the serving bowl. The weight that is then registered on the scale is the weight of the food alone. This eliminates the hassle of weighing foods on the scale and then moving them into your bowl.

If you can afford a few extra dollars, a computerized gram scale can save a lot of effort. These scales are pre-programmed with the percentage of nutrients contained in each food. You simply enter a code into the scale for a food from a list of codes, and then place that food on the scale. The scale can then give you the total weight of the food, and the grams of carbohydrate, fat, protein, cholesterol and calories it contains. You can also program your own food choices into the scale.

Several brands of scales are available, ranging in price from $35 to $100 for simple digital scales to $130 for the computer scales which are pre-programmed. Scales can be found in gourmet and kitchen shops, or online at sites such as www.diabetesnet.com/ishop/.

Just remember that carbs in foods can be determined in three ways: food labels, reference books and software, or with a gram scales with a list of carb factors.

Food Labels

Almost all packaged foods today have a "Nutrition Facts" label. Besides providing nutritional information, including the number of calories and the grams of protein and fat, they also give the exact number of grams of carbohydrate contained in a serving and the size of this serving.

If you're eating a food that has all the information you need on the label, you can calculate the amount you should eat and the carb bolus required to cover it. For example, an 8-ounce carton of Elsie's Lowfat Yogurt has a label to the right that tells you that a one cup or 8 ounce serving contains 17 grams of carbohydrate. Once you know this and also know how many grams of carbohydrate you cover with one unit of insulin (from Chapter 12), you can figure the bolus dose needed to cover the yogurt. If the serving you eat differs from the serving size listed on the package, you will have to weigh or measure your actual serving and do some calculations.

Serving Size

Total grams of carb

Nutrition Facts	
Serving Size 1 cup (225 g)	
Servings Per Container 4	
Amount Per Serving	
Calories 120	Calories from Fat 0
	% Daily Value *
Total Fat 0 g	0%
Saturated Fat 0 g	0%
Cholesterol 5 mg	2%
Sodium 180 mg	8%
Total Carbohydrates 17 g	6%
Dietary Fiber 0 g	0%
Sugars 17 g	
Protein 12 g	

Advantage: Very easy, little or no calculation required.

What you need: Food label, measuring cup, and a calculator to calculate the carbs in an amount you plan to eat when it differs from the portion size on the label.

8.8 Use Labels To Count Carbs

Let's say you want to eat a cup of Uncle Bob's Wild Rice.

1. Look at its Nutrition Facts label to the right. The label says one serving size is a half cup, so you will be eating 2 servings.

2. The label shows one half cup serving contains 27 grams of carbohydrate.

3. Multiply 27 grams by two servings to determine the total grams of carbohydrate you will be eating:

Carbs in a 1/2 cup portion	=	27 grams
Times 2 for one cup serving		X 2
Total Carbs	=	54 grams

Nutrition Facts

Serving Size 1/2 cup cooked (38 g)
Servings Per Container 8

Amount Per Serving

Calories 130   Calories from Fat 0

% Daily Value *

Total Fat 0 g	0%
Saturated Fat 0 g	0%
Cholesterol 0 mg	0%
Sodium 0 mg	0%
Total Carbohydrates 27 g	6%
Dietary Fiber 0 g	0%
Sugars 3 g	
Protein 4 g	

Focus on the Total Carbohydrates, usually in bold, but also pay attention to the Dietary Fiber. Although fiber is carbohydrate, it has no effect on your blood sugar since it is not digested. Subtract the grams of fiber from the total carb grams before calculating your bolus.

What To Do: Food labels contain all the information needed to do carb counting. Just be sure your serving is the same size as the serving on the label, or be sure to do some calculating on the basis of the amount you'll be eating.

Nutrition Books, PDAs with Software, and Cookbooks

Nutrition books, software in a PDA or Palm device, and newer cookbooks, similar to nutrition labels, list the amount of carbohydrate in a typical serving size of each food. If what you eat varies from this serving size, you may need to weigh or measure your actual serving, and you'll need to do the necessary calculations to convert your serving into the grams of carbohydrate eaten.

Cookbooks usually list the number of grams of carbohydrate in a serving. You only need to calculate the number of carbs in your serving if it differs from the portion size referred to.

Advantage: Nutrition books and software may provide information useful for food eaten at home and in restaurants. They also provide an easy way to look up brand name foods. Many cookbooks provide carb information for easy counting when preparing meals at home.

8.9 Books For Healthy Eating

At Home:

1. **The Diabetes Carbohydrate and Fat Gram Guide** by Lea Ann Holzmeister (American Diabetes Association, $14.95)—includes carb and fat grams, exchanges, and many fast food restaurants

2. **Doctor's Pocket Calorie Fat and Carbohydrate Counter** (Family Health Publications, $6.99)—lists over 11,000 foods

3. **Convenience Food Facts** by Arlene Monk (IDC, $12.95)—gives the grams of carbohydrate in 1,500 popular brand name products

4. **ADA Complete Guide To Carb Counting** by Hope Warshaw and Karmeen Kilkarney (ADA, $16.95)—master the food part of control with carb counting

Eating Out:

1. **Guide to Healthy Restaurant Eating** by Hope Warshaw (American Diabetes Association, $17.95)—gives calories, carbohydrates and exchanges of the healthy choices in 100 chain restaurants across America, such as Denny's, Round Table Pizza, etc.

2. **Eat Out, Eat Right!** by Hope Warshaw (Surrey Books, $11.95)—gives strategies and specific food choices for controlling calories, carbohydrates, fat, cholesterol and sodium in the 14 most popular kinds of restaurants

3. **Fast Food Facts** by Marion Franz (IDC, $6.95)—gives grams of carbohydrates in 1,000 menu items from 20 restaurants

Look for these books at discount at www.diabetesnet.com/ishop/   © 2003 Diabetes Services, Inc.

What you need: Books or software programs with a food database, or a PDA. You may also need measuring cups, spoons, and scales to determine serving size.

What To Do: Look for books and cookbooks in the "Nutrition and Diet" section of your local bookstore and library, or in online sources like the Diabetes Mall (www.diabetesnet.com). Online sources and diabetes product guides from diabetes magazines, such as Diabetes Interview and Forecast, also list software and written sources. Look for recipes that have the carb content in the "Food" section of your local newspaper and in magazines related to health.

A Gram Scale and a List of Carb Percentages or a Computer Scale

Most carbohydrate foods have only part of their total weight as carbohydrate. When you eat a food like fruit that has no label, you can calculate how many grams of carb are in your serving by weighing the food on a gram scale and then multiplying its total weight by a carb percentage, which is the percentage of that food's total weight that is carbohydrate. A list of carb percentages is in Appendix A at the end of this book.

If you weigh food on a computer scale, just put in the code for the food, push the button for "carbohydrate," and the computer scale does the calculation for you. You can even program computerized scales to give you the percentage of carbohydrate of your favorite combination foods, such as stir-fried vegetables with rice.

Advantage: Convenient for measuring carbs in odd-sized foods like fruits, unsliced bread, soups, or casseroles.

What you need: A gram scale, a calculator, and a list of carb percentages like those in Appendix A at the back of this book, or a computer scale.

What To Do: Find the amount of carbohydrate in a serving of food:

1. Weigh the food to find its total weight in grams. Note that the total weight of the food is not how many grams of carb in the food.

2. Find the food's carb percentage in one of the food groups listed in Appendix A.

3. Multiply the food's total weight in grams by its carb percentage.

4. The result of this multiplication gives the number of grams of carbohydrate that the food contains.

8.10 Use a gram scale to count the carbs in cooked spaghetti.

You want to count how many carb grams are in a plate of spaghetti.

With a standard gram scale and list of carb factors:

(1) Zero out your plate on the scale, then place the amount of cooked spaghetti you want to eat on it.

(2) Let's say your scale shows that the portion you want weighs 200 grams on the scale. From Appendix A, you find that cooked plain spaghetti has 26 percent of its weight as carbohydrates.

(3) Multiply the spaghetti's total weight by its percentage of carbs.

$$\underset{\substack{\text{weight of}\\\text{spaghetti}}}{\underline{200 \text{ gm}}} \times \underset{\substack{\text{carb}\\\text{percent}}}{\underline{.26}} = \underset{\substack{\text{total carbs}\\\text{in this portion}}}{\underline{52 \text{ gm}}}$$

(4) So when you eat 200 grams of cooked spaghetti by weight, you'll actually be eating 52 grams of carbohydrate.

With a computer gram scale:
Computerized gram scales already contain information about the nutrition content of spaghetti and other foods.

(1) Zero out your plate on the scale.

(2) Enter the food code for spaghetti into the scale.

(3) Put the portion of spaghetti you want onto your plate.

(4) Press the carb key on the scale to find out how many grams of carbohydrate are in the spaghetti.

Gram scales are available at www.diabetesnet.com and kitchen supply stores.

If you find this detailed calculation is more than you are willing to tackle, you may benefit by requesting a list of foods that contain approximately 15 grams of carbohydrate from a dietician. You can also get an ADA exchange list and use the section for carb serving sizes. For example, this list may contain 1 cup of milk, 1 ounce slice of bread, 1 medium fruit, etc. This is not as exact as counting carbs, but it may help you estimate how much insulin to use if you don't need or want to count carbs precisely.

Is Carb Counting The Only Way?

No. There are other ways to improve your matching of food and insulin for good control. These include the exchange system, counting calories, and the TAG (total available glucose) system.

Food exchange lists prepared by the American Diabetes Association give the approximate carbohydrate content of foods. This system was the basis for food planning taught to people with diabetes in the past. It can still be used by people whose control does not require exact carb calculations. In some cases, the exchange system will describe a particular food accurately and in some cases it will not. Consider, for example, that the exchange value of one slice of bread is 15 grams of carb.

Example 1: A slice of Wonder bread (1 bread exchange) = 15 grams of carb
Actual carb value = 15 grams of carb

The value above equals one exchange, so there's no problem.

Example 2: A slice of Lieken bread (1 bread exchange) = 29 grams of carb

In the second example the carb value for Lieken bread, which is similar in size to Wonder bread, has twice as many carbs. With many food items, the differences between the exchange system value and the actual grams of carbohydrate won't be this large. However, when estimating an insulin bolus for a meal, if the carbohydrate content of several items in a meal is different from those found with the exchange system, the differences may cause control problems. The exchange system may be less accurate than counting carbs because it divides foods into broad categories like breads, meats, and fruits, and then gives portion sizes having about the same nutritional value.

If the exchange system works well for you, don't change a thing. On the other hand, if your control is not what you desire, or you're interested in a more logical and exact approach to food management, learn carb counting.

Weight Gain

Horror stories about people gaining weight when they begin to control their blood sugars certainly exist. However, weight gain does not have to happen with improved control. The road to real blood sugar control lies in eating only what you need and adjusting your insulin to handle that amount of food. This will not cause

8.11 The Carb Container Problem

Your body holds 5 liters or quarts of blood. This blood is distributed through 60,000 miles of large and tiny blood vessels with a surface area equal to three tennis courts. When your blood sugar is normal, the blood scattered over this large area has only 5 grams of glucose in it!

One 12 ounce can of soda contains eight times as much sugar as your entire bloodstream! Luckily, the interstitial fluid surrounding the cells helps soak up some of this excess glucose before insulin shifts it into the cells' interiors.

Typical meals contain many times the amount of glucose that would be found at one time in the blood. Eating a healthy, carb-rich breakfast of pancakes or cereal can present a challenge to control. Whether you plan to consume 15 or 150 grams of carbohydrate, proper insulin dosing becomes critical to maintaining control by moving glucose into cells quickly.

weight gain. You can lose excess weight and still maintain good control if you follow a healthy, sensible diet at every meal, keep portion sizes small, and stay active. It is vital to match the calories you take in with those you use as energy if you want to avoid gaining weight.

Once your blood sugar is in good control, your body will use food just like it did before you had diabetes. If you eat too much, you gain weight. If you eat less, you lose weight.

If your recent control was poor, your body will have flushed away many of the calories you were eating. You may have been used to overeating and not gaining weight. Once you attain good control, you will have to reduce the amount of food you eat if you wish to avoid gaining weight. This change can be a challenge, but it will contribute to the overall good health you want.

Keep track of your weight and your appetite. These tell you whether you're actually eating the right amount of food, provided you are eating healthy foods. Keep fat and protein calories at moderate levels. Research has shown that meals that are higher in fat actually are less satisfying and will trigger hunger sooner than high carb meals, especially if the carbs are complex ones. Maybe you do not need all the food you have been consuming. Focus on an appropriate food plan, consider your carbohydrate and calorie intake, and recognize that you can make changes that will cause weight loss without losing good control.

The Bigger Nutrition Picture

When you have mastered the art of carbohydrate counting and can figure your insulin-to-carb ratio or carb factor, you will be an expert in balancing your insulin and food intake to achieve blood sugar control. As important as this is, however, blood sugar control is not the only health goal you have. Your overall health depends on eating a wide variety of nutrient-rich foods.

The amount and type of fat in your diet appears to be very important to health. High intake of saturated, trans, or hydrogenated fats has been found in more and more studies to create greater risks for heart disease, cancer, and obesity. Heart disease is especially common in people with diabetes, especially in those who have insulin resistance, where a two- to sixfold increase is seen over those without diabetes. A fat intake of no more than 20% to 30% of total calories is recommended by the American Heart Association and the American Dietetic Association, and the fats preferred are unsaturated or monounsaturated.

8.12 Skipping Meals

When a person has a habit of eating only once or twice a day, the body learns to store extra fat in an easy-to-access area known as the abdomen. The fat stored here is a variety that can be quickly released to enable survival when food is unattainable.

However, when meals are skipped and while fasting overnight, larger abdominal fat stores increase circulating fat and triglycerides in the blood. This, in turn, increases insulin resistance and may accelerate damage to blood vessels. Eating reasonable amounts of complex, low glycemic index carbohydrates through the day helps to reduce circulating fat and may assist weight maintenance.

This focus on reducing fat intake, especially of saturated and hydrogenated fats, may be one reason for the gradual reduction in the number of heart attacks over the last few years.

To reduce cardiovascular risk, most people cut back by using less fat on their foods (butter, margarine, sour cream, salad dressings, oils, and shortening used for frying, etc.). When they eat fat, they try to choose polyunsaturated ones (like safflower oil), monounsaturated oil (olive oil), or nuts. They also focus on eating protein foods that are lower in fat or that contain better types of fat (fish, skinless chicken, nonfat milk, and nonfat cheese products, for example).

Diets that are lower in animal protein have been shown to slow the development and progression of diabetic kidney disease, an important consideration when deciding what to eat. Because about one third of people with Type 1 diabetes develop kidney disease, keeping red meat portions small is highly recommended. This automatically lowers fat intake, a secondary benefit of major importance.

Good news in the diabetes diet is that we do not have to avoid sugar. The old taboo on sugar was relaxed in recent years after research showed that it is possible

8.13 Online Resource For Carb And Nutrition Information

A great resource for nutrition information is the USDA National Nutrient Database at http://www.nal.usda.gov/fnic/foodcomp/Data/ The database can be searched, or you can go to Nutrient List, then Carbohydrates to select an alphabetical 30 page pdf list of almost every food you can think with its carb content to download.

to retain glycemic control when eating some splurge foods if we know how to manage their carbohydrate content. This has become even easier with today's rapid insulins which quickly counteract the extra carbs in desserts, ice cream, and candy.

Sugar is no longer banned from coffee, nor jelly from toast, nor an occasional small piece of pie from the dinner table. It appears that it may, in fact, be healthier to have applebutter (which contains some sugar but no fat) on your waffle rather than butter or margarine.

No one with or without diabetes really benefits nutritionally from an excess of high-calorie, low-nutrient foods. However, small amounts of sweets can add flavor to a diet and, if chosen wisely, make avoiding fatty foods easier. Be careful though: sugar almost always travels with fat. For instance, a chocolate candy bar gets about 60 percent of its calories from fat!

If you find that sweets are addictive for you and a little is never enough, you may find it easier to eliminate splurge foods entirely. A very good cure for sweet craving is to eat only whole grain foods for six to eight weeks, then gradually allow small amounts of refined foods back into your diet.

Whether you include some sweets in your meals or not, the key to blood sugar control is to determine the amount of carbohydrate in your food and cover it with an appropriate amount of insulin. This and a nutrient-rich, low-fat, low-protein diet is a vital part of any healthy lifestyle.

8.14 Three Approaches To Control With Diet

Tom uses carb counting:		Matt uses exchanges:		Mike eyeballs his diet:
1/2 banana	15 grams	1/2 banana	1 fruit	1/2 banana
1 cup milk	12 grams	1 cup milk	1 milk	milk in an 8 oz. glass,
8 oz tomato juice	12 grams	8 oz. tomato juice	1 fruit	tomato juice in 8 oz glass,
1 oz. cheese	0 grams	1 oz. cheese	1 protein	1 slice of packaged cheese
Brand X Cereal	45 grams	Brand X Cereal	3 breads	Brand X Cereal in a bowl that holds 3 cups

"There are some things only intellectuals are crazy enough to believe."
George Orwell

THE GLYCEMIC INDEX

The glycemic index is a well-researched ranking of carbohydrate foods based on how quickly they are digested and how quickly and how high they raise the blood sugar. [47-50] Knowing this can be very helpful for preventing unwanted spikes after meals or raising low blood sugars quickly.

For example, when your blood sugar is already low or rapidly dropping due to exercise, you want carbs that will raise it quickly. You want a high glycemic index food. On the other hand, to prevent a gradual blood sugar drop during a few hours of mild activity, you might prefer to eat carbs with a low glycemic index and long action time. If your blood sugar tends to spike after breakfast, you may want to change your cereal to one with a lower glycemic index. Lower glycemic index foods also help to prevent overnight drops in the blood sugar because their digestion and effect on the blood sugar lasts for a longer period of time.

A food's glycemic index is a number that indicates the food's effect on the blood sugar. The number shows how quickly that food will raise the blood sugar relative to the action of glucose, which is the fastest carbohydrate. Glucose is given a value of 100, and then other carbs are given a number relative to glucose. Fast carbs have higher numbers and are great for raising low blood sugars or for covering periods of moderate or strenuous aerobic exercise. They also are good for restoring glycogen stores after exercise. Slower carbs have lower numbers and are the best choices to maintain good control in your day-to-day diet.

A food's ranking is compiled from more than one research study if possible. More than one glycemic index list exists. Each list will be close to, but may not be identical to other lists. The glycemic index of a food can be lowered by adding vinegar to it or by adding a healthy fat such as olive oil to pasta. The actual impact a food has on your blood sugar also will depend on factors other than the glycemic index, like ripeness, cooking time, fiber and fat content, time of day eaten, blood insulin level, and recent activity. Use the glycemic index as just one of the many tools you have available to improve your control.

Research studies have drawn mixed conclusions on how well the glycemic index measures a food's effect on blood sugar control. However, many people who adjust their insulin to match need have found they can improve their blood sugar control through wise use of the glycemic index. If you are using a continuous blood glucose monitor, you can quickly create your own personalized glycemic index based on how different foods affect your blood sugar.

An excellent book that provides more information on this topic is **The New Glucose Revolution**. The authors of this highly readable and scientifically sound book are respected nutrition experts who have taken their findings from nearly 20 years of research regarding hundreds of people's blood sugar responses to foods.

See www.diabetesnet.com/ishop/ for this book and the **Glucose Revolution Pocket Guides** to heart disease, diabetes, weight loss, and more.

8.15 Glycemic Index

Foods are compared to glucose, which ranks 100. Higher numbers indicate faster absorption and a faster rise in the blood sugar, while lower numbers indicate a slower rise.

Cereals		Snacks		Fruit	
All Bran™	51	chocolate bar	49	apple	38
Bran Buds +psyll	45	corn chips	72	apricots	57
Bran Flakes™	74	croissant	67	banana	56
Cheerios™	74	doughnut	76	cantalope	65
Corn Chex™	83	graham crackers	74	cherries	22
Cornflakes™	83	jelly beans	80	dates	103
Cream of Wheat	66	Life Savers™	70	grapefruit	25
Frosted Flakes™	55	oatmeal cookie	57	grapes	46
Grapenuts™	67	pzza, cheese & tom.	60	kiwi	52
Life™	66	Pizza Hut™, supreme	33	mango	55
muesli, natural	54	popcorn, light micro	55	orange	43
Nutri-grain™	66	potato chips	56	papaya	58
oatmeal, old fash	48	pound cake	54	peach	42
Puffed Wheat™	67	Power Bars™	58	pear	58
Raisin Bran™	73	pretzels	83	pineapple	66
Rice Chex™	89	rice cakes	82	plums	39
Rice Krispies™	82	saltine crackers	74	prunes	15
Shredded Wht™	67	shortbread cookies	64	raisins	64
Special K™	54	Snickers™ bar	41	watermelon	72
Total™	76	strawberry jam	51	**Pasta**	
Root Crops		vanilla wafers	77	cheese tortellini	50
French Fries	75	Wheat Thins™	67	fettucini	32
pot, new, boiled	59	**Crackers**		linguini	50
pot, red, baked	93	graham	74	macaroni	46
pot, sweet	52	rice cakes	80	spagh, 5m boil	33
pot, wht, boiled	63	rye	68	spagh, 15m boil	44
pot, wht, mash	70	soda	72	spagh, prot enr	28
yam	54	Wheat Thins™	67	vermicelli	35

8.15 cont. Glycemic Index

Breads		Beans		Soups/Vegetables	
bagel, plain	72	baked	44	beets, canned	64
banana bread	47	black beans, boil	30	black bean soup	64
baquette, Frnch	95	butter, boiled	33	carrots, frsh, boil	49
croissant	67	cannellini beans	31	corn, sweet	56
dark rye/blk br	76	garbanzo, boiled	34	green pea soup	66
hamburger bun	61	kidney, boiled	29	green pea, frzn	47
muffins		kidney, canned	52	lentil soup	44
apple, cinn	44	lentils, gr or br	30	lima beans, frz	32
blueberry	59	lima, boiled	32	Parsnips, boil	97
oat & raisin	54	navy beans	38	Peas, fresh, boil	48
pita	57	pinto, boiled	39	splt pea sp w/ham	66
pizza, cheese	60	red lentils, boil	27	tomato soup	38
pumpernickel	49	soy, boiled	16	**Cereal Grains**	
sourdough	54	**Milk Products**		Barley	25
rye	64	chocolate milk	35	Basmati whi rice	58
white	70	custard	43	Bulgar	48
wheat	68	ice cream, van	60	Couscous	65
Drinks		ice milk, van	50	Cornmeal	68
apple juice	40	skim milk	32	Millet	71
colas	65	soy milk	31	**Sugars**	
Gatorade™	78	tofu frozen dess	115	fructose	22
grapefruit juice	48	whole milk	30	honey	62
orange juice	46	yogurt, fruit	36	maltose	105
pineapple juice	46	yogurt, plain	14	table sugar	64

8.16 Who Discovered Insulin?

In 1788, Dr. Thomas Crawley was the first person to identify the pancreas as the cause of diabetes. He did an autopsy on a patient who had died of the disease and found multiple calculi in the pancreas. Over a hundred years later in 1889, another researcher isolated the area of the pancreas responsible for diabetes, which now carries his name as the islets of Langerhans. That same year, a third researcher named Minkowski was able to create diabetes in dogs by surgically removing the pancreas.

Minkowski theorized that a dog's pancreas could be minced and an extract obtained that would cure diabetes. Unfortunately, his lab techniques were unable to isolate insulin and his discovery was ignored for over 30 years until a young surgeon in Canada revitalized his work.

In 1921, the surgeon, Frederick Banting, who had recently returned from World War I in France, and his assistant, a medical student named Charles Best, worked at the University of Toronto to isolate a crude extract from dog pancreases. Once this extract was purified and tested in animals, insulin became the first hormone discovered and isolated successfully. It was given to humans and found to cause a mild lowering of the blood sugar. Banting and Best were fortunate. The insulin molecule is remarkably similar from one species to the next, and extracts obtained from different animals worked in humans without triggering an allergic reaction.

Once early experiments showed some progress, biochemist James Bertram Collip was asked to help purify a crude mixture from oxen into a solution that would no longer cause abcesses when it was injected as the dog extract did. While Collip worked, Leonard Thompson, who was close to a diabetic coma, received the first injection of insulin derived from dogs at Banting and Best's lab. Although dog extracts had little impact, Collip's cleansed oxen extract had the desired effect.

The Eli Lilly Company offered to help with insulin modifications and production in early 1922, and by November of that year a method for purifying insulin from cows had been developed. By January of 1923, insulin became available in sufficient quantity to distribute to universities and hospitals, where experimentation with the new drug was started in humans.

A Nobel prize was awarded in 1923 to Banting and to Professor John J. McLeod, head of the physiology department at the University of Toronto, who supplied lab space and support for the experiments. Banting gave half of his prize money to his collaborator, Charles Best.

For additional information, see **The Discovery of Insulin** by Michael Bliss, Univ. of Chicago Press, 1982, and Dr. F. G. Banting's article "Medical Research and the Discovery of Insulin" on page 288 of the May, 1924 issue of *Hygeia* or visit www.discoveryofinsulin.com.

"I will always cherish the initial misconceptions I had about you."

Anon.

Which Insulin To Use And How To Start

CHAPTER

9

In the quest for better control, today's new insulins offer distinct advantages. Doctors and consumers have welcomed these insulins that have a more consistent action along with their faster or longer action times. New insulins allow the normal pancreas to be mimicked more closely, with better control as the outcome.

This chapter covers

- New choices for bolus and basal insulins
- Benefits of rapid bolus insulins
- Why rapid bolus insulin is not that rapid
- Basal insulin choices and which may be best for you
- What to do if you forget a dose
- Variable insulin absorption and what to do about it
- Cautions about temperature and storage
- How to start insulin in Types 1, 1.5, and 2 diabetes

Rapid Bolus Insulins

Humalog, produced by Eli Lilly and Company, was released in the U.S. in 1996. Novolog is made by Novo Nordisk and was released in 2001. Both insulins offer quicker action time than short-acting Regular insulin, which was first produced as a crude extract in 1921.

Humalog and Novolog provide better coverage for meals and snacks, and are able to lower a high blood sugar quicker than Regular. Most meals cause the blood sugar to rise over a period of two to three hours. In contrast, Regular insulin starts working in 30 minutes, peaks at three to four hours, and continues to lower the blood sugar for six to eight hours after the injection. Novolog and Humalog, on the other hand, begin to work in 10 to 20 minutes, peak at one to two hours and are mostly gone in four hours.

The activity of Humalog and Novolog matches the "action time" for most meals, creating a tremendous advantage almost everyone using insulin, but especially for mothers of small children and people on the go. Those feeling ill can wait to cover food until they are sure of keeping it down. Kids who are picky eaters can be given their dose after they finish the meal and still maintain reasonable control.

Humalog and Novolog taken before a meal are lowering the blood sugar at the same time food is raising it. Blood sugar levels measured one to two hours after eating do not spike as high as with Regular. After four hours the blood sugar can be close to its starting point. The fast action of a rapid insulin means that insulin from the previous meal bolus is gone before the next meal begins, so doses can be accurately calculated. Compared to Regular, rapid insulins given at dinner have less residual insulin activity at bedtime and cause fewer lows in the middle of the night.

One advantage of faster insulins is convenience. Although a 10 to 20 minute lead time is ideal, carb boluses can be taken with the first bite of food and still result in reasonable postmeal control. Of course, their quick action means that eating must not be delayed! If the premeal blood sugar is high and eating is delayed to allow the blood sugar to drop, the food must be eaten at the planned time to avoid a low blood sugar.

Foods that have a high glycemic index and raise the blood sugar quickly, like cold cereals or a scone for breakfast, are easier to cover with a rapid insulin. On the other hand, when low glycemic carbohydrates like pasta al dente or a bean burrito are eaten, the blood sugar may go low after a bolus of rapid insulin before these foods can completely digest and enter the bloodstream.

For occasional foods that have a low GI, carb boluses can be split with half taken before the meal and the second half an hour or two after eating. Another option is to use an injection of Regular to match slow carbohydrates. High fat content in a meal may slow down the digestion and require a slower insulin for coverage like Regular. If your blood sugar is low at mealtime, the meal can be eaten and then covered with a slightly reduced dose of rapid insulin afterward.

As you first start using Humalog or Novolog, it is wise to test before eating, two hours after eating, and anytime you experience unusual symptoms. Use extra caution when lowering a high blood sugar. Be alert for a low blood sugar one to two hours after a meal in which a low glycemic index food was eaten or a meal that had too few carbs for the carb bolus that was given.

Humalog and Novolog are excellent for lowering high blood sugars and avoiding lows. Their faster action means less time is spent at high levels and little residual insulin remains after four hours to cause a delayed low blood sugar. The consistent action time of these rapid insulins makes them easier to troubleshoot when control problems occur.

One benefit of rapid insulins is that fewer lows are experienced during the night. In the past when people used Regular to cover dinner, they often needed a bedtime snack to avoid a low during the night. In contrast, Humalog and Novolog can be used at dinner with little need for a bedtime snack if four hours have passed since bolusing and the nighttime basal insulin is correctly set.

Although Humalog and Novolog are relatively similar in action, they do have minor differences. The two insulins are interchangeable for most users, but an occa-

9.1 Insulins Available In The U.S.

Type	Made by	Introduced	Starts in*	Peaks in*	Gone by*
Rapid					
Humalog®	Lilly	1996	10-20 min	1.5-2.5 hrs	4-5 hrs
Novolog®	Novo Nordisk	2001	10-20 min	1.5-2.5 hrs	4-5 hrs
Short					
Regular	Lilly, Novo Nordisk	1922	30-45 min	2-4 hrs	5-7 hrs
Intermediate					
NPH	Lilly, Novo Nordisk	1946	1-3 hrs	4-9 hrs	14-20 hrs
Lente®	Lilly, Novo Nordisk	1951	2-4 hrs	6-12 hrs	16-24 hrs
Long with peak					
Ultralente®	Lilly, Novo Nordisk	1951	2-4 hrs	8-14 hrs	18-24 hrs
Long with little peak					
Detemir	Novo Nordisk	2003	1 hr	8-10 hrs	18-24 hrs
Lantus®	Aventis	2001	2 hrs	6 hrs(slight)	18-26 hrs
Mixtures of Rapid and Intermediate					
75/25 Hum/H-Pro	Lilly	2000	10-20 min	1.5-3 hrs	14-18 hrs
70/30 Nov/N-Pro	Novo Nordisk	2002	10-20 min	1.5-3 hrs	14-18 hrs
70/30 Reg/NPH	Lilly, Novo Nordisk	1999	30-45 min	3-5 hrs	14-20 hrs
50/50 Reg/NPH	Lilly	1999	30-45 min	2-4	14-20 hrs

* Dynamic action times at which insulin affects BG   © 2003 Diabetes Services, Inc.

sional user may find that Novolog has a slightly stronger action than Humalog. If this occurs, slight bolus dose reductions of 10% or less may be required.

One disadvantage to rapid insulins is their price. The price of a bottle of Humalog or Novolog is typically three times the price of a bottle of Regular.

Rapid Insulin Is Not That Rapid

One problem associated with the use of rapid insulins is that situations occur that cause people to perceive them as faster than they really are. For example, a person may feel perfectly normal at 70 mg/dl (3.9 mmol), take a bolus of rapid insulin for a meal, and a few minutes later begin to shake, sweat and have trouble thinking. Though the timing of the symptoms gives the impression that the rapid insulin is responsible and acts very quickly, the symptoms are unlikely to be caused by the rapid insulin just given. More likely, another insulin given earlier is causing the blood sugar to drop. A drop of only a few mg/dl causes the person to go from feeling normal to feeling low. Because the meal bolus was just given, it often receives the blame for a low caused by an insulin that was given earlier.

Once injected, a rapid insulin will not begin to work for 15 or 20 minutes. It does not reach any significant level of activity until 30 to 60 minutes have passed. See Figure 9.3 which shows the actual glucose lowering action of Humalog and Novolog. The kinetics of an insulin are when that insulin can be measured in the bloodstream, whereas an insulin's dynamics are when it actually affects the blood sugar.

Another situation often seems to confirm for many the false impression that a rapid insulin is really rapid. This occurs when a carb or correction bolus is given and a low blood sugar begins only an hour or two later. Here, the rapid insulin is likely at fault, but again the low blood sugar is not caused by any rapid action. Rather, the quick drop in blood sugar seen in the blood sugar is more likely to have been caused by a carb or correction bolus that was too large.

For instance, if enough Novolog is taken to cover 100 grams of carbohydrate, but only 50

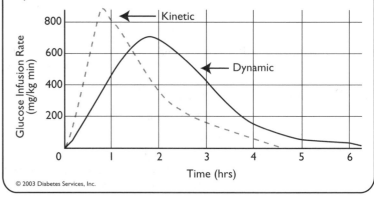

9.3 When Do Humalog And Novalog Insulins Really Work?

After an injection, peak levels of Humalog and Novolog insulins are seen in the bloodstream about 45 minutes later, as shown by the dashed kinetic line below. However, the effect on your blood sugar is not nearly this quick. The solid dynamic line to the right shows when these insulins are actually lowering the blood sugar. The maximum effect on lowering the glucose level is not seen until 2 hours after an injection and continues for over 4 hours.

© 2003 Diabetes Services, Inc.

9.4 Action Times For Insulins				
Insulin	**Starts in**	**Peaks at**	**Ends after**	**Lows likely at**
Hum/Nov	10-20 mins	1.5-2.5 hrs	4-5 hrs	2-5 hrs
Regular	30-45 mins	3-4 hrs	5-7 hrs	3-7 hrs
NPH	1-3 hrs	4-10 hrs	14-20 hrs	4-16 hrs
Lente	2-4 hrs	6-12 hrs	16-24 hrs	6-16 hrs
Ultralente	2-4 hrs	10-18 hrs	18-24 hrs	8-18 hrs
Detemir	1 hrs	5 hrs	18-24 hrs	8-16 hrs
Lantus	1-2 hrs	6 hrs	18-26 hrs	5-10 hrs

grams are eaten, the excess insulin makes the blood sugar drop quickly, giving the false impression that the insulin acts quickly. A rapid fall in blood sugar may also be caused when a bolus overlaps with another recent bolus or basal dose.

When a low blood sugar occurs less than three hours after a bolus dose has been given, consider the cause carefully. There may be an error in carb counting, an overlap of two or more boluses, an excessive basal insulin dose, excess physical activity, a low glycemic index carbohydrate, or another factor such as delayed gastric emptying from gastroparesis that is responsible. Remember to note a reason for all unexpected lows and highs in your record book.

Basal Insulin Choices

Intermediate, long, and flat are the basal insulin choices now available. The action times of these different basal insulins can be used to your advantage when you understand them.

NPH and Lente are intermediate insulins that last for 14 to 24 hours and usually peak in action at 4 to 12 hours after they are given. NPH tends to peak earlier and taper off faster than Lente, which has a flatter peak and a longer period of action. When injected before breakfast, the peak in NPH or Lente can be used to cover lunch instead of using a carb bolus at that time. However, because the timing of these peaks can be inconsistent, this approach can often create control problems. The long-acting insulin, Ultralente or UL, lasts up to 24 hours and has less peak action than NPH or Lente. A flat profile insulin, Lantus, begins working earlier at one to two hours and has an almost peakless profile that lasts 18 to 26 hours in most users. Another insulin soon to be released, called Detemir, achieves an almost flat profile when it is taken twice a day.

Correct basal doses let you:

- skip meals without encountering lows or highs
- eat meals later than usual without worrying about a low blood sugar
- precisely cover carbs and lower high blood sugars with boluses

Which Basal Insulin Is Best For You?

Research and clinical experience show that about 70% of people with Type 1 and Type 2 diabetes will experience some rise in the blood sugar during the early morning hours. On average, a 20% increase in basal insulin in the early morning hours is needed to offset a Dawn Phenomenon using the precise delivery of an intravenous infusion pump.[51] Insulin cannot be delivered this precisely with injections, but the timing, doses and types of basal insulin can nonetheless achieve good results when carefully planned. How to cover the rise while avoiding a low earlier in the night is important for many.

9.5 Number of Injections Required For Smooth Basal Coverage			
Basal insulin	# of injections needed	24 hour action profile	Typical % of TDD for basal coverage
NPH	2-3		50% - 60%
Lente	2-3		50% - 60%
Ultralente	2		50% - 60%
Detemir	2		45% - 60%
Lantus	1-2		45% - 55%

© 2003 Diabetes Services, Inc.

To counteract a rising morning blood sugar, the blood insulin level needs to rise before the liver starts its production of glucose at around 3 a.m. If a peaking insulin is used, the evening dose of this insulin should be given at the appropriate time and set high enough to stop the liver, while avoiding a rise in the blood insulin at 1 a.m or 2 a.m. when it would cause a low.

Because NPH peaks faster than Lente or UL, it works well when given at bedtime to match a strong Dawn Phenomenon. If nighttime lows are occurring with NPH because its peak is too sharp, switching to Lente with its flatter and more rounded peak may help prevent these lows. Lente, which has less peak than NPH, may work well when given before dinner, in those with Type 2 diabetes to prevent a rise in the morning blood sugar. To create an even flatter insulin profile during the night, a split dose of Lente can be given, with part at dinner and the rest at bedtime. UL has a flatter peak than NPH or Lente and works well for those who have little or no Dawn Phenomenon. However, UL's action can be inconsistent, and Lantus or Detemir may be preferred.

Although Lantus has almost no peak, one injection a day given at dinner or bedtime appears to be able to shut off glucose production by the liver during the night and stop the rise in the morning blood sugar that is seen with a Dawn Phenomenon. Its lack of a peak and more consistent action means it is less likely to cause lows in the middle of the night.

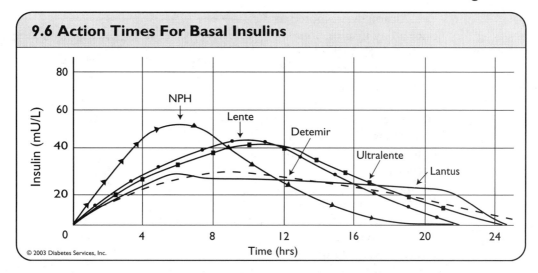

9.6 Action Times For Basal Insulins

© 2003 Diabetes Services, Inc.

If hypoglycemia does occur in the middle of the night but the morning blood sugar is still rising on an evening dose of Lantus, the dose of Lantus should be split into a morning and an evening injection. For those who have a strong Dawn Phenomenon and for those with Type 2 who experience a sizeable blood sugar rise during the night, the higher peaking action of NPH or Lente can be used to supplement the flat profile of Lantus.

The bedtime dose of NPH or Lente can be increased by one unit every four to seven days until the pre-breakfast reading is no longer high. Combining different basal insulins is unnecessary for most, but it can be a perfect choice for people who experience lows in the middle of the night but still have breakfast highs.

Once overnight basal doses are set well enough to allow a person to wake up with a normal blood sugar, the daytime basal doses will be easier to set.

Lantus And Detemir Insulins – Extra Benefits And Cautions

Lantus (glargine) is the newest basal insulin to come on the market, with Detemir awaiting final FDA approval in the U.S. No tradename is available for Detemir yet.

Lantus is approved for use by anyone over the age of six with Type 1 or Type 2 diabetes. It is not approved for use in younger children or in women who plan to become or are pregnant. Detemir will likely not be approved for use in pregnancy when it reaches the market, but it is not known whether there will be other restrictions. Either insulin is a good choice when first starting on insulin or as a fresh starting point for those who have tried various insulin combinations in the past but continue to have control problems.

Lantus can be taken at any time of day, but it is important to take Lantus at the same time each day. Taking the dose at the same time each day when only one dose is given a day helps to prevent a gap in activity or a doubling of activity that may occur when a dose is taken an hour earlier or later than usual.

Although promoted as a once a day insulin, some users may find that Lantus' action ends after about 18 hours, a full 6 hours before the next dose. When Lantus is given at bedtime and its activity lasts less than 24 hours, a gap in insulin action occurs around bedtime. As shown in Figure 9.8, the Lantus taken the night

9.7 Why New Basal Insulins Are Better

The new analog basal insulins, Lantus and Detemir, offer distinct advantages over NPH, Lente, and Ultralente insulins.

- More consistent action from day to day
- Nearly peakless profile
- Less variability in fasting blood sugars
- Fewer nighttime lows
- Improved quality of life

before begins losing its power around dinner time. The dinner carb bolus provides insulin activity for three to four more hours following dinner, but the bedtime Lantus takes two hours to reach full activity, creating an insulin gap near bedtime.

When Lantus works less than 24 hours, if someone takes a carb bolus for dinner at 6 p.m. and a bedtime dose of Lantus at 11 p.m, a gap appears in the insulin coverage between 10 p.m. and 1 a.m. The person may experience erratic breakfast blood sugar readings and not understand what is causing the loss of

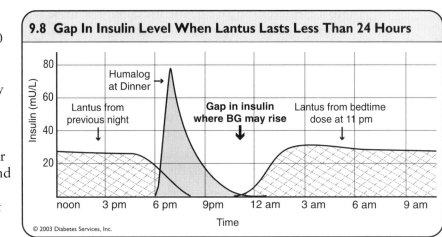

9.8 Gap In Insulin Level When Lantus Lasts Less Than 24 Hours

Humalog at Dinner

Lantus from previous night

Gap in insulin where BG may rise

Lantus from bedtime dose at 11 pm

Insulin (mU/L)

noon   3 pm   6 pm   9pm   12 am   3 am   6 am   9 am

Time

© 2003 Diabetes Services, Inc.

control. Those who find they have a short action time can improve their control by taking Lantus twice a day to eliminate the gap in action.

Taking Lantus in the morning may work better for those who suffer from nighttime lows. Lantus has a slight peak in action about six hours after it is taken and has slightly more activity during the first 12 hours after an injection. Having this extra activity occur during the daytime is safer for anyone who prefers to use more than 50 percent of the TDD as basal insulin. When Lantus is taken as a morning injection, the carb bolus for lunch can be reduced if Lantus does have some peaking of activity during the afternoon hours.

An occasional user may find that for them Lantus has a distinct peak in action about six hours after it is given. This more pronounced peak is often seen in people who experience a shorter action time with Lantus. If low blood sugars occur during

9.9 Basal Choices For Night Lows And Morning Highs		
Night lows?	**AM highs?**	**Best basal insulin choice**
no	no	NPH, UL, L, or Lantus before dinner or at bedtime
yes	no	Lente at bedtime or Lantus before breakfast
no	yes	NPH or Lantus at bedtime or Lente before dinner
yes	yes	NPH, Lente, or Lantus at bedtime

the night when Lantus is given at bedtime or dinner, either the dose needs to be reduced or the Lantus dose needs to be split into two equal injections.

About two of every three Lantus users take this insulin once a day at breakfast, dinner or bedtime. The rest split the dose into two injections. Taking Lantus twice a day also helps smooth out its activity when someone is unable to take one injection at the same time each day.

Lantus cannot be mixed with other insulins. It typically loses activity if it comes in contact with any amount of another insulin. Do not give a dose of Lantus with a syringe that was previously used to inject another insulin. When inactivated, Lantus becomes hazy, so use only Lantus that is crystal clear. About 3% of Lantus users experience mild discomfort at the injection site, but this is almost never serious enough to discontinue its use.

Because of its shorter action time, Detemir requires two injections a day, but it can be mixed in the same syringe with any of the rapid insulins. Given twice a day, Detemir will not have any gap in activity during the day as may be seen when NPH is given twice a day. Detemir, however, is a less active insulin with only about 30% of the activity of other insulins. This may create some confusion when selecting doses to give.

Unlike older basal insulins, Lantus and Detemir are clear, so care has to be taken not to confuse them with a clear, rapid insulin. The Lantus bottle has a tall distinctive shape, but even so, some users have mistakenly injected a bedtime dose of Humalog or Novolog rather than Lantus! Be careful also to not use Lantus or Detemir to cover a meal or a high blood sugar by mistake. A large rubber band can be wrapped around the Lantus or Detemir bottle to make it easy to distinguish from Humalog or Novolog. To help avoid this mix-up, Dr. Paul Davidson of Atlanta recommends use of a Humalog or Novolog insulin pen for boluses, and use of a syringe to administer Lantus or Detemir insulin.

Despite their relatively peakless activity, both Lantus and Detemir work well to control the Dawn Phenomenon. Their more consistent activity from day to day solves blood sugar management problems for some that would otherwise require an insulin pump.

Because of Detemir's structure which allows it to bind to the protein albumin in the blood, it is weaker than other insulins. In one study, users required 2.4 times as much Detemir on average compared to the NPH insulin which it replaced.[54] When Detemir is first started, two injections a day are required for three days before it reaches full activity. During this time, much of its initial peaking activity flattens out so that its action eventually appears very similar to that of Lantus.

Like Humalog and Novolog analogs, Lantus and Detemir are structurally different from human insulin. On very rare occasions, an immune or allergic response may occur. Symptoms of insulin allergy can range from a mild local itching to a severe allergic reaction with swelling of the tongue and inability to breath. Emergency medical treatment may be required, especially if early warning signs are ignored. Fortunately, allergic reactions with these insulins are quite rare.

> ## 9.10 How They Work
>
> ### Lantus
>
> Lantus is dissolved in the insulin bottle at an acid pH of 4. Once injected, it comes out of solution in the neutral pH of the body to form microprecipitates. These microprecipitates cause small amounts of insulin to be steadily released over several hours. The result is a relatively constant release of insulin over the next 18 to 26 hours.
>
> When mixed with another insulin with a neutral pH, Lantus will come out of solution and form microprecipitates in the syringe or bottle, rather than under the skin. Because of this, Lantus cannot be mixed with other insulins.
>
> ### Detemir
>
> Detemir is a modified insulin molecule to which fatty acids are able to attach. This modified structure allows Detemir to bind to albumin, a common protein found in the blood and fat cells. This results in a slow, steady release, but also causes it to have only about one fourth the potency of other insulins. Detemir has a fairly consistent action from day to day but may vary in activity from person to person.

What To Do If You Forget A Dose

What you do after forgetting a dose depends on when you remember. If 90 minutes or less have passed since you were supposed to take an injection, you can take the same basal and bolus dose that you would have taken before the meal. Your blood sugar will likely be higher than normal on the next blood sugar test, but it should eventually correct on its own if the dose was appropriate.

If an hour and a half to four hours have passed before you realize a dose was forgotten, the food from the meal has already been digested, so only the high blood sugar needs to be addressed. Measure your blood sugar, subtract your premeal target (a postmeal target is not used because no bolus insulin is active), and take a correction bolus for the difference. Do NOT take any insulin to cover the carbs that were eaten, but use the correction bolus to lower the high blood sugar which the uncovered carbs have caused. The basal insulin dose will usually be the same, although a slight reduction may be required to avoid a buildup of basal insulin later as it overlaps the next basal insulin dose. If it has been over 4 hours, again correct the high reading, but the basal dose will likely need to be reduced to avoid a larger buildup of basal insulin later.

Variable Insulin Absorption

The activity of older basal insulins can vary as much as 25 percent from one day to the next.[52] For instance, a 40-unit injection may have an effect equal to 35 units one day and 45 units the next. When cloudy long-acting insulins are injected under the skin, their uptake and activity are less consistent than today's rapid or flat-profile analog insulins, but even newer insulins are not immune from this effect. Figure 9.11 shows one extreme case of variable activity when a person's insulin action was measured on four different days.

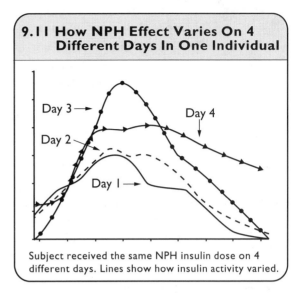

9.11 How NPH Effect Varies On 4 Different Days In One Individual

Day 3 →   Day 4

Day 2 →

Day 1 →

Subject received the same NPH insulin dose on 4 different days. Lines show how insulin activity varied.

As a rule, variability in basal insulin action increases from Detemir to Lantus, to Lente and NPH, and then to the greatest variability with Ultralente. When peaking activity is considered, the least peaking is seen with Lantus and increases from Detemir to Ultralente to Lente to NPH.

However, keep in mind that individuals vary greatly in how they will interact with a particular insulin. A basal insulin should always be tested to determine its true activity using the basal test shown in Chapter 11.

The effect of any insulin, including basal, is more likely to vary when:

1. injections are given near a muscle area before someone begins to exercise,
2. the skin is warmed by hot weather,
3. an injection site is massaged or rubbed, or
4. a hot bath or sauna is taken.

What To Do About Insulin Variability

One way to smooth out the peaking action of older basal insulins and reduce their variability is to give smaller injections more often. NPH, Lente, or UL can be split into three or four small doses through the day. Small overlapping doses that are given more often minimize peaking and variability. One advantage of Detemir and Lantus insulins and of

9.12 Causes For Variable Insulin Absorption

- Insulin dose
- Site of injection
- Depth of injection (IM vs SC)
- Exercise
- Local heat/massage
- Mixing insulins
- Poor resuspension of NPH, L, or UL
- Smoking

IM - intramuscular, SC - subcutaneous

Novolog and Humalog is that they offer more consistent activity from day to day compared to older insulins.

Contributing to the consistent action of Lantus and Detemir is that they are clear insulins that are already in solution. Lente, NPH, and Ultralente all have to be mixed carefully prior to use. Mixing involves turning and rolling the bottle or insulin pen at least 20 times prior to use.

Unfortunately, most users do not do this enough to resuspend the mixture. In one study of insulin pen users, who were carefully instructed to mix the NPH insulin in their pens at least 20 times before each use, only one of 11 people rolled the pen more than 10 times.

The researchers checked to see how much insulin was actually coming out of the pens and found that the insulin being delivered varied from 5% to 210% of its intended concentration. Few were receiving doses any where close to the dose intended.[53] Clear insulins, like Lantus, Detemir, Humalog, Novolog and Regular do not suffer from this type of inaccuracy. Of the mixed insulins available, only Novo Nordisk's 70/30 insulin, which is a clear combination of rapid and slower forms of Novolog, does not require mixing prior to use.

Cautions About Temperature And Storage

Any insulin can become degraded when exposed to excessive heat or freezing. Some users have reported that Humalog may deteriorate faster in hot weather than Regular or Novolog. When Humalog does go bad, it may do so quickly, so the blood sugar may be fine one day and high the next.

If any insulin does not appear to be having its expected effect, check for particles in the bottle. These are usually seen as one or two large floaters in the insulin, or as several small crystals in solution or on the sides of the bottle. Humalog may also acquire a slightly yellowish color when inactivated. If you have any doubts about the potency of an insulin, always try a fresh bottle to see if this improves the situation.

> ### 9.13 Beware Of Heat With Lantus
>
> High heat can cause any long-acting insulin under the skin to be more quickly absorbed, creating sudden, severe low blood sugars. Lantus' structure makes it especially prone to heat-related lows. Do NOT take very hot showers or baths, or a hot sauna when using this insulin!

One special caution with Lantus is the effect of excessive heat. Taking a very hot shower, bath, or sauna can cause a severe low blood sugar when the heat activates Lantus deposits under the skin. Activating these deposits can cause a large surge in insulin activity and severe hypoglycemia.

Lente insulin is also heat sensitive but in a different way. In research, when a bottle of Lente was kept at room temperature rather than refrigerated and then mixed with Regular insulin, the peak in insulin activity from this combination changed dramatically. The peak in insulin activity was 10% lower and was delayed by almost three hours (peaks at 6 hours rather than 3.2 hours), with a longer period of action.[55] No change in activity was found when Regular was mixed with NPH. It is not clear if Humalog or Novolog react in the same way when mixed with Lente.

How To Start Insulin

How soon after diagnosis a person needs to start insulin depends on what type of diabetes they have, psychological factors such as stress following diagnosis, and practical factors such as how much time is available for teaching. When the decision has been made to start insulin, the amount of insulin and the number of injections required will depend on factors such as how much internal insulin production remains, convenience, and stability of lifestyle.

Type I

In Type 1 diabetes, insulin is started immediately after diagnosis, but the regimen will vary. When an adult or the parents of a child who is starting on insulin has previous experience with diabetes, the person may go directly to a basal/bolus approach with four injections a day.

A simpler approach is often used at first until the passage of stress and hyperglycemia allow the person to learn better ways of delivering insulin, carb counting, and monitoring. One way to quickly start is to take fixed doses of a premixed insulin (70/30 or 75/25) twice a day before breakfast and dinner with an insulin pen. With this approach, the morning dose is usually larger, such as two thirds of the TDD, with the other third taken before dinner.

If sufficient internal insulin production and a relatively steady lifestyle allow this to work, it is continued. More often, erratic blood sugar control makes it apparent that more frequent injections with a rapid insulin dose that is matched to

Table 9.14 The Starting Insulin Dose Table For Type I Adults

This table is a guide for beginning insulin therapy in Type I diabetes. The first line shows the smaller total daily insulin doses required by weight when a diagnosis is made early in someone who feels relatively well. The TDDs on the second line may work for moderately high blood sugars with ketones but no ketoacidosis. The last line shows the much higher TDDs required for a person with high blood sugars in ketoacidosis. Ketoacidosis requires rapid and aggressive use of insulin in a hospital.

Fitness and Stress	100 lbs (45 kg) TDD units	120 lbs (55 kg) TDD units	140 lbs (64 kg) TDD units	160 lbs (73 kg) TDD units	180 lbs (82 kg) TDD units	200 lbs (91 kg) TDD units
Early Diagnosis	13-18	16-22	19-26	22-29	25-33	27-36
Mod. BG + Ketosis	20-26	24-32	29-37	33-42	37-48	41-53
DKA or Ketoacidosis	50-90	60-108	70-126	80-144	90-162	100-180

Table 9.15 The Starting Insulin Dose Table For Type 1 Children

Starting total daily insulin doses will be lower in children who feel well, have minimal blood sugar elevation, minimal ketosis, and minimal symptoms, as shown on the first line. TDDs on the second and third lines show the change in TDD before and after puberty with moderately high blood sugars but no ketoacidosis. Very high starting TDDs are required in those who have high blood sugars, marked symptoms, a recent illness, or are in ketoacidosis, as shown on the last line. Presence of ketoacidosis requires rapid and aggressive use of insulin in a hospital.

	40 lbs (18 kg) TDD units	60 lbs (27 kg) TDD units	80 lbs (36 kg) TDD units	100 lbs (45 kg) TDD units	120 lbs (55 kg) TDD units
Before Puberty	4-18	5-27	7-36	9-45	11-54
During Puberty	5-27	8-41	11-55	14-68	16-81
After Puberty	5-22	8-33	11-44	14-55	16-65
DKA	20-36	30-54	40-72	50-90	60-108

the carb in each meal is required, and the person has the visible proof of their own monitoring to show this. With progress in education and dietary consultation, more appropriate insulin dosing regimens can be devised.

Table 9.14 shows TDDs by weight for someone who is diagnosed relatively early in the course of their diabetes on line one, someone who is mildly ketotic on the second, and, finally, someone who is in full ketoacidosis on the last line. Table 9.15 shows typical dose requirements for children and teens with Type 1.

Type 1.5

Those who have Type 1.5 diabetes are usually over the age of 25, slender, and do not have an apple shape or the excess weight that is typical of Type 2 diabetes. Because they are often diagnosed early while they retain internal insulin production, oral medications alone may control the blood sugar for one to five years or longer. When insulin becomes required, the doses on the first line of Table 9.14 are usually adequate. If the need for insulin or the rise in blood sugar progresses rapidly, the person may actually have Type 1 and insulin doses would be increased appropriately.

How insulin is started in Type 1.5 is determined by blood sugar patterns and residual insulin production. A single injection of a flat basal insulin, combined with one or more oral agents may provide optimal control. Again, the pattern of the blood sugar will reveal how many injections and which types of insulin are required.

Table 9.16 The Starting Insulin Dose Table For Type 2 Adults

This table is a guide for beginning insulin therapy in insulin-resistant Type 2 diabetes. The first line shows the smaller total daily insulin doses required by weight when a diagnosis is made early in someone who feels relatively well. The TDDs on the second line are a good place to start when blood sugars are often above 300 mg/dl.

Fitness and Stress	140 lbs (64 kg) TDD units	160 lbs (73 kg) TDD units	180 lbs (82 kg) TDD units	200 lbs (91 kg) TDD units	220 lbs (100 kg) TDD units	240 lbs (109 kg) TDD units
Mild Symptoms/BGs	6-16	7-18	8-20	9-23	10-25	12-30
Mod. Symptoms/BGs	20-31	22-38	24-45	27-51	30-57	35-64

Type 2

When someone is largely insulin resistant as in Type 2 diabetes, the reasons for starting insulin will vary. Short-term use of insulin may be needed to overcome a cycle of high blood sugar readings caused by glucose toxicity, to lower high blood sugars caused by an illness, or to counteract high readings associated with the stress of surgery.

The more common reason for starting insulin is when it is needed long-term because oral medications are no longer able to provide optimal control. When the blood sugar can no longer be controlled with diet, exercise, and medications, a relative or absolute insulin deficiency exists in addition to insulin resistance.

People with Type 2 diabetes usually have an apple figure or excess weight. Someone with Type 2 diabetes and these characteristics typically may start with a single injection of a basal insulin. Using Table 9.16 as a reference for various weights:

1. Start with 10 units of basal insulin, either before dinner or at bedtime.
2. Check the blood sugar before dinner, at bedtime, and before breakfast.
3. Raise the starting dose of 10 units every 4th day by:
    a. 4 units if the breakfast reading is still over 180 mg/dl (10 mmol)
    b. 2 units if the breakfast reading is still over 140 mg/dl (7.7 mmol), or
    c. 1 unit if the breakfast reading is still over 120 mg/dl (6.6 mmol).

A simple approach provides a rapid and safe way to lower high blood sugars, but pay attention to the pattern of the readings. For instance, if the bedtime reading is still around 200 mg/dl (11.1 mmol) after the breakfast reading has reached 100 mg/dl (5.6 mmol), this once a day injection approach will not be adequate.

The choice of insulins depends largely on the blood sugar pattern. Try NPH at bedtime if the breakfast reading is the only elevated blood sugar. If readings are high at breakfast and at other times during the day, try Lantus or Detemir at dinner or bedtime. If the bedtime and breakfast readings are both high, a mixed insulin like 70/30 before dinner may be a good choice.

9.11 Why Is Insulin So Important?

Cells communicate with each other through messengers called hormones that travel through the blood. Insulin, derived from the Latin word for island, was the first and one of the most important hormones to be identified.

Insulin is produced, stored, and released by beta cells in the pancreas, an organ that weighs about half a pound and sits behind the stomach. Insulin circulates in the blood and attaches to receptors on the outer wall of cells, that are involved in the storage and delivery of energy.

Insulin is a very small protein that is formed from a longer protein called proinsulin. After proinsulin is created, it is folded and clipped into two separate chains of similar size. These two chains are linked together by three double sulfur bridges. This folding, cutting, and relinking process gives insulin a characteristic shape that enables it to bind to specific receptors on the outer cell wall.

Once attached to cell receptors, insulin triggers a cascade of biologic effects inside the cell. Paths in the cell wall are activated to move glucose from the bloodstream into the cell. In normal circumstances, a rise in the insulin level after a meal allows glucose from the meal to enter cells. When fuel is needed later, the insulin level falls to allow free fatty acids and stored glucose to be released as fuel.

When the insulin level falls too far in diabetes, glucose rises to very high levels, insulin resistance increases, insulin-dependent cells begin to starve, and less and less energy is available. As this happens, triglycerides and free fatty acids rise in the blood as the body attempts to correct the glucose imbalance by mobilizing large amounts of fat for fuel. This results in excessive ketone production.

Extremely high blood sugars, usually above 700 mg/dl (38.9 mmol), can kill, but the damage in diabetes is more often a slow accumulation over years of ongoing higher-than-normal blood sugars. Like a slow poison, high glucose levels cause widespread organ and tissue damage over time. Low blood sugars also create problems that range from those that are mildly annoying to very serious ones. Any disruption in insulin availability or effectiveness can create widespread long-term damage to organs and tissues, as well as immediate symptoms that reduce the quality of life.

For those using insulin, the critical question becomes how much insulin to take and when to take it so that the blood sugar remains relatively normal without serious lows or highs. The best solution comes from imitating normal insulin delivery.

Once the breakfast reading is less than 120 mg/dl, if the lunch and dinner readings are in a good range, a single injection is all that is needed. If control is still not adequate, a second injection of NPH or Detemir can be added before breakfast. If the blood sugar rises more than 40 to 50 mg/dl (2.2 to 2.8 mmol) at one to two hours after meals, consider using a rapid insulin like Humalog or Novolog before meals, or a rapid insulin releasing medication like Starlix or Prandin, or a starch blocker like Precose or Glyset. See Chapter 27 for more information.

Great control comes from testing and resetting your insulin doses whenever the need arises. The need to adjust doses is easily identified by blood sugar readings outside your target range. Neglecting to adjust can result in months or years of poor control, discouragement, and an increased risk of complications that could be avoided.

How much insulin you require on an average day is your total daily insulin dose (TDD). An accurate TDD is the most important number to work from for great readings. It is like true north on your diabetes compass. Once you've determined your TDD, you can closely estimate the basal doses, carb boluses, and correction boluses you require from it. This chapter shows how this is done, but any new insulin doses must be verified by your health care team before you use them, and must be tested for accuracy before you rely on them.

If you are currently having control problems, recalculate your doses as shown in this chapter. If your control problem is not severe, you may also try to refine your current doses using pattern analysis, as shown in Chapters 17 and 18.

In this chapter we'll show you

- How to determine an accurate TDD
- How to closely estimate basal and bolus doses from your TDD

Work first to achieve reasonable control on typical days. Once these insulin doses work, it becomes easier to make adjustments for days that vary from your routine. Your TDD should stay relatively steady from day to day, after allowing for variations in carb intake, activity, weight, stress, or season. Sudden deviations, like preparing to run a marathon, monthly menses for women, or tilling dirt for a spring garden may necessitate a rapid change in your TDD. Once you know your "standard" TDD, these adjustments become easier.

Determine Your Ideal Doses

To determine the doses that will keep your blood sugar as normal as possible, test and set your basal and bolus doses in the five steps described in this chapter. Steps

1 and 2, where an accurate TDD is determined are the most important ones. From this new TDD, starting basal and bolus doses are determined in steps 3 through 5.

How to test these basal and bolus doses is covered in Chapters 11, 12, and 13. You may want to review the Insulin Dose Checklist on page 18 or read the entire book for a good understanding of what you will be doing before you return to this chapter and start the procedure of testing and setting your ideal doses.

To Find Your Correct Insulin Doses:

1. Determine Your Current TDD

Your current TDD (basal doses plus carb and some of the correction boluses for the entire day) provides an excellent guide from which you can make adjustments to avoid frequent highs or lows. An accurate history of your insulin doses is needed to determine your current TDD. If you are not doing so already, start recording all the insulin doses you take each day. Add up your daily doses of bolus and basal insulin and average these over at least the last five to seven days. Then fill in the blanks in Go Figure 10.1a to determine your current TDD.

Include correction boluses in your current TDD that are used to correct high readings, unless these correction boluses are causing your blood sugar to drop too low. A good way

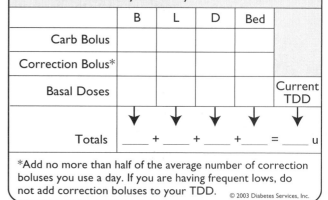

Go Figure 10.1a: Insulin Dose Calculations

① **Determine Your Current TDD**

Fill in the table below with your average basal doses, carb boluses, and and some of the correction boluses from the last few days to find your current TDD.

	B	L	D	Bed	
Carb Bolus					
Correction Bolus*					
Basal Doses					Current TDD
Totals	___ +	___ +	___ +	___ =	___ u

*Add no more than half of the average number of correction boluses you use a day. If you are having frequent lows, do not add correction boluses to your TDD.   © 2003 Diabetes Services, Inc.

to account for correction boluses is to add up all correction bolus units of insulin you have given during the last week and divide this total by 7. Take this average of the correction units you use each day and add about half this average to your TDD to estimate how many units you may need to add to your usual basal and bolus doses.

For example, if someone averages 50 units in his usual basal and bolus doses, but finds that he is using an average of 8 additional units a day for correction boluses over the last week, he will need to add about 4 units to his basal or carb bolus doses each day to keep the blood sugar under control. A conservative estimate for his new TDD would be 54 units per day.

However, if a person has been averaging 16 units of supplemental insulin a day to cover high readings, he might still add only 4 or 5 units to his TDD for safety, realizing that another increase will likely be needed within a few days.

The insulin currently used in correction boluses would not be added into your TDD if you are having frequent lows or if many of the highs you are treating are caused by overtreating lows. When correction boluses are often required only to correct highs caused by the overtreatment of lows, these correction boluses should not be added into the TDD. Instead, the TDD will first need be lowered to prevent low blood sugars.

2. Determine Your New TDD

If your current TDD provides optimal control, there is no reason to change it. Raise or lower your current TDD only if you are having frequent high or low readings. When control problems occur, modifying your current TDD provides a good starting point to calculate a new TDD and new basal and bolus doses. Go Figure 10.1b provides an easy way to increase or decrease your TDD when this is needed. If you are having frequent mild lows, use Go Figure 10.1b to reduce your TDD by 5%, then recalculate your bolus and basal doses. For frequent or severe lows, you will want to reduce your TDD by 10% or more. Similarly, if you are having occasional highs, increase your TDD by 5%, or increase by 10% if highs are frequent or severe.

Discuss how much to adjust your TDD with your physician and monitor more frequently following any change in insulin

Go Figure 10.1b: Insulin Dose Calc

(2) **Determine Your New TDD**

Does your current TDD work well, or does it need to be lowered or raised? If you are having frequent low blood sugars, reduce your TDD by 5% or 10%. If most of your readings are over 150 mg/dl, raise your current TDD by 5% or 10%.

10% Less	5% Less	Current TDD	5% More	10% More
18.0 u	19.0 u	20.0 u	21.0 u	22.0 u
22.5 u	23.8 u	25.0 u	26.3 u	27.5 u
27.0 u	28.5 u	30.0 u	31.5 u	33.0 u
31.5 u	33.3 u	35.0 u	36.8 u	38.5 u
36.0 u	38.1 u	40.0 u	42.0 u	44.0 u
40.5 u	42.9 u	45.0 u	47.3 u	49.5 u
45.0 u	47.6 u	50.0 u	52.5 u	55.0 u
50.5 u	52.4 u	55.0 u	57.8 u	60.5 u
54.0 u	57.1 u	60.0 u	63.0 u	66.0 u
58.5 u	61.9 u	65.0 u	68.3 u	71.5 u
63.5 u	66.7 u	70.0 u	73.5 u	77.0 u
67.5 u	71.4 u	75.0 u	78.8 u	82.5 u
72.0 u	76.2 u	80.0 u	84.0 u	88.0 u
76.5 u	81.0 u	85.0 u	89.3 u	93.5 u
81.0 u	85.7 u	90.0 u	94.5 u	99.0 u
85.5 u	90.5 u	95.0 u	99.8 u	104.5 u
90.0 u	95.0 u	100.0 u	105.0 u	110.0 u

My new TDD is _____ units

If your current control involves frequent lows or highs, you may need to adjust your current doses by more than 5 or 10%. Discuss this with your physician and adjust appropriately.

doses. Enter your new TDD at the bottom of Go Figure 10.1b. Once your current or a new TDD is selected, it can be distributed into appropriate basal doses, carb boluses, and correction boluses using the three steps in Go Figure 10.1c.

For a discussion of things that change your TDD, see Chapter 15.

3. Balance Your Basals And Boluses

For most people, the total basal and bolus doses used in a day will each make up about 50% of their TDD. Most people on insulin find their basal insulin works best when it makes up 45% to 65% of their TDD. Bolus doses make up the other 35% to 55%. It helps to periodically add up your basal and bolus doses to ensure that your basal/bolus balance is being maintained.

Once you determine an accurate TDD, 50% of your modified TDD is a good starting point for your basal doses. Use step 3 in Go Figure 10.1c to balance your basals and boluses by multiplying your modified TDD by 0.50. This gives you the number of units you will use each day in your basal insulin doses.

A slightly lower basal percentage may work better for those who use Lantus insulin and those who are more physically fit or eat a high carb diet. A higher basal percentage is often preferred for teens, those who have insulin resistance, and those trying to lower postmeal spiking of their blood sugar. Different ways to distribute your basal insulin are covered in Chapter 11.

4. Calculate Your Carb Factor

Next, you want to determine your carb factor, which is how many grams of carb are covered by one unit of Humalog or Novolog insulin. As shown in step 4 in Go Figure 10.1c, your carb factor is calculated by dividing 500 by your modified TDD. (Alternate methods to calculate the carb factor, including the 2.8 Rule, are discussed in Chapter 12.) Your carb factor may differ slightly at each meal of the day, but this difference is usually small. Your total carb boluses make up about 50% (35% to 55%) of your TDD.

Balancing carbohydrates in meals and snacks with precise boluses allows you to vary the number of carbs you eat without losing control of your blood sugar. To accurately match carbs with insulin, you will want to learn carb counting as shown in Chapter 8. How to test your carb factor and determine your carb boluses is outlined in detail in Chapter 12.

An alternate method that requires a consistent number of carbs at each meal and snack is also provided in step 4. For this method, half of your new TDD can be divided into three equal doses for the three meals of the day, or into 15% of your TDD for breakfast, 15% for lunch, and 20% for dinner, if this fits how you distribute your carbs through the day. Although this method is not as flexible and does require carb counting, it eliminates the need to use a carb factor. This may work for those who have a relatively set lifestyle and for people with Type 2 diabetes in reasonable control.

5. Calculate Your Correction Factor

When you encounter a high blood sugar, you want to bring it back to your target quickly and safely. Your correction factor is how many points your blood sugar usually drops on each unit of Humalog or Novolog insulin. You can closely estimate your correction factor by dividing your new TDD into 1600, 1700, 1800, 2000, or 2200 as shown in step 5. 1800 is an acceptable place for most people to start, 1600 and 1700 are more aggressive and give more insulin, while 2000 or 2200 provide less insulin. How to test your correction factor is covered in Chapter 13.

Once you know your correction factor, you can set up a

Go Figure 10.1c: Insulin Dose Calculations

③ Balance Your Basals And Boluses

Calculate your daily basal dose by multiplying your new or current TDD from Step 2 by 50% (ie, 0.50).*

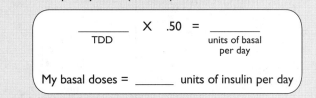

_____ X .50 = _____
TDD   units of basal
                       per day

My basal doses = _____ units of insulin per day

*Basal doses usually make up 45% to 65% (0.45 to 0.65) of the TDD

④ Calculate Your Carb Factor

Use the 500 Rule to determine your carb factor.

500 ÷ _____ = _____ grams of carb covered by 1 unit
       TDD

OR calculate fixed boluses by dividing half your new TDD into 3 equal meal doses, or by multiplying your TDD by 15% for breakfast, 15% for lunch, and 20% for dinner. Each gives half of your TDD as carb boluses.

My new TDD

Breakfast _____ units		_____ X .15 = _____ units
Lunch _____ units	or	_____ X .15 = _____ units
Dinner _____ units		_____ X .20 = _____ units

⑤ Calculate Your Correction Factor

Calculate your correction factor by using the 1800* Rule. Divide 1800 by your TDD

Example: 1800 ÷ 30 units = 60 mg/dl

$\dfrac{1800^*}{TDD}$ ÷ _____ units = _____ mg/dl per unit

1 unit of insulin will decrease my blood glucose by _____ mg/dl.

*The numbers 1600, 1800, 1700, 2000 and 2200 can also be used here. The larger this number, the safer or smaller a correction bolus becomes.

© 2003 Diabetes Services, Inc.

personalized table to safely lower high blood sugars with extra Humalog or Novolog. Under normal circumstances when control is acceptable, correction boluses will make up less than 10% of your TDD.

These five steps enable you to set your doses for great control and to reset them when your control has deteriorated or your life changes. Table 10.2 provides sample daily basal dose amounts, carb factors and correction factors for different TDDs. Simply find your current TDD if your control is reasonable or a modified TDD in the left column in Table 10.2 and find a close approximation for your insulin doses on that line. Be sure to take the time to test your basal and bolus doses as shown in the next few chapters. You will find that using insulin well can provide more stable control than you ever thought possible.

10.2 Table Of TDDs, Basal And Bolus Doses

For this TDD =	Day's Basal (50% of TDD)	Carb Bolus 1u covers this many carbs:	Corr. Bolus 1u lowers blood sugar:
16 units	8.0 units	31 grams	112 mg/dl
18 units	9.0 units	28 grams	100 mg/dl
20 units	10.0 units	25 grams	90 mg/dl
22 units	11.0 units	23 grams	82 mg/dl
24 units	12.0 units	21 grams	75 mg/dl
26 units	13.0 units	19 grams	69 mg/dl
28 units	14.0 units	18 grams	64 mg/dl
30 units	15.0 units	17 grams	60 mg/dl
32 units	16.0 units	15 grams	56 mg/dl
36 units	18.0 units	14 grams	50 mg/dl
40 units	20.0 units	12 grams	45 mg/dl
44 units	22.0 units	11 grams	41 mg/dl
48 units	24.0 units	10 grams	38 mg/dl
52 units	26.0 units	10 grams	35 mg/dl
56 units	28.0 units	9 grams	32 mg/dl
60 units	30.0 units	8 grams	30 mg/dl
65 units	32.5 units	8 grams	28 mg/dl
70 units	35.0 units	7 grams	26 mg/dl
75 units	37.5 units	7 grams	24 mg/dl
80 units	40.0 units	6 grams	22 mg/dl
90 units	45.0 units	6 grams	20 mg/dl
100 units	50.0 units	5 grams	18 mg/dl

Approximate basal and bolus doses for someone who receives 50% of their TDD in their basal doses.

© 2003 Diabetes Services, Inc.

Example 10.3 Frank Determines His TDD And Starting Doses

Franks weighs 160 pounds and is moderately active. He takes 7 Humalog and 32 NPH before breakfast, and 9 Humalog and 12 NPH before dinner. On these doses, however, Frank has been having frequent lows and cannot skip meals without going low. He uses the 5 steps in Go Figure 10.1 to calculate a new TDD and insulin doses.

(1) In step 1 (Go Figure 10.1a), Frank adds up his doses to obtain his current TDD of 60 units.

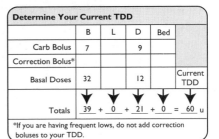

Determine Your Current TDD				
	B	L	D	Bed
Carb Bolus	7		9	
Correction Bolus*				
Basal Doses	32		12	Current TDD
Totals	39 +	0 +	21 +	0 = 60 u

*If you are having frequent lows, do not add correction boluses to your TDD.

(2) In step 2, because of his frequent lows, Frank reduces his current TDD by 10% to get 54 units as his new TDD.

10% Less	5% Less	**Current TDD**	5% More	10% More
54.0 u	57.1u	60.0u	63.0u	66.0u

(3) Using his new TDD in step 3, Frank finds his new basal dose per day will be 27 units of insulin. His doctor suggests that he take this as 27 units of Lantus before breakfast to avoid night lows.

$$\underline{54} \times .50 = \underline{27}$$
TDD — units of basal per day

My basal doses = ____27____ units of insulin per day

(4) In step 4, Frank uses the 500 rule to determine that his new carb factor will be 1 unit for every 9.3 grams of carb. Because of his frequent lows, he decides to try **1H for every 10 grams of carb** to reduce the size of his meal boluses that he will now take before breakfast, lunch, and dinner.

$$500 \div \underline{54} = \underline{9.3} \text{ grams of carb}$$
TDD — per 1 unit

(5) In step 5, he uses the 1800 rule to determine his new correction factor. This calculation suggests that his blood sugar will fall 33.3 mg/dl per unit. He decides to use **1H for every 35 mg/dl** above his premeal target of 100 mg/dl.

$$\underline{1800^*} \div \underline{54} \text{ units} = \underline{33.3} \text{ mg/dl per unit}$$
TDD

1 unit of insulin will decrease my blood glucose by __33.3__ mg/dl.

How Do My Weight, Fitness, And Stress Level Affect My TDD?

Your weight and your levels of fitness and stress affect how much insulin you need a day. In Table 10.4, compare your current or new TDD to the average TDDs for different levels of fitness and stress to get some idea of how your current insulin doses measure up.

10.4 The Insulin Dose Table

Your type of diabetes, weight, levels of fitness and stress, and special conditions provide a good guide to how much insulin you need a day. Compare your current or new TDD to the average TDDs below for your profile.

Fitness and Stress	100 lbs (45 kg) TDD units	120 lbs (55 kg) TDD units	140 lbs (64 kg) TDD units	160 lbs (73 kg) TDD units	180 lbs (82 kg) TDD units	200 lbs (91 kg) TDD units
New Start Type 2*	5-11	6-14	6-16	7-18	8-20	9-23
New Start Type 1*	13-18	16-22	19-26	22-29	25-33	27-36
Physically fit	20	24	29	33	37	41
Moderately active	26	32	37	42	48	53
Sedentary or an adolescent	31	38	45	51	57	64
Moderate stress or 2nd trimester preg.	36	43	51	58	66	73
Greater stress or 3rd trimester preg.	40	49	57	65	74	82
Severe stress	45	55	64	73	82	91
Infection, DKA, or steroid medication	50-90	60-108	70-126	80-144	90-162	100-180

After the new start values, the rest of the grid is primarily for Type 1's. Those with Type 1.5 or Type 2 diabetes may require more or less insulin than these estimates because the table cannot account for insulin resistance nor internal insulin production.

*These starting insulin doses are designed to be safe doses for beginning insulin therapy. A person may need much higher starting doses if they have been experiencing very high blood sugars, have an infection, or are an adolescent.

Adapted from: L. Jovanovic: Insulin Analogs. Program AACE annual meeting. Chicago. May 5, 2002
Diabetes and Exercise: N.S. Pierce. Br J Sports Med: 161-173, 1999.

For instance, if you are moderately active and weigh 160 lbs., your TDD should be close to 42 units a day. But if you use only 20 units a day, you are either very sensitive to insulin, are still producing some insulin of your own, or are not taking enough insulin to keep your blood sugar down. On the other hand, if you use 60 units a day, you may be resistant to insulin or your doses may be set too high.

If your weight is well above your

Go Figure 10.5: Control Numbers You Want To Know

Using insulin to control your blood sugar is based on knowing these essential numbers. You and your doctor will want to determine each number to make your control program easy and effective. Write your numbers here as a convenient record.

1. My TDD or total daily insulin dose = _____ units

2. My basal insulin = L, N, UL, Lantus, given as

   _____ units at _____ am/pm

   _____ units at _____ am/pm

   _____ units at _____ am/pm

3. The percentage of my TDD given as basal = _____ %

4. My carb factor = 1 unit per _____ grams of carb.

5. My correction factor = 1 unit to drop _____ mg/dl or mmol

6. 1 gram of carb raises my blood sugar _____ mg/dl or mmol

7. Unused bolus rule: 25% of a bolus will be used each hour

© 2003 Diabetes Services, Inc.

---

ideal weight, you eat a high fat diet, exercise only at your desk, have been in poor control for some time, or produce hormones that counteract insulin's action, you will require more insulin than typical in your TDD. For instance, teenagers have high hormone levels that aid growth and they require far more insulin until this five or six year growth phase passes. If you are thin, exercise regularly, and eat a healthy diet, you are likely to need less insulin than average.

The key is to always take the amount of insulin that keeps the blood sugar relatively normal. Keep in mind that any change in weight or activity may require a change in your TDD and would be indicated by your blood sugar starting to go low or high on a regular basis. See Chapter 15 for a list of typical things that require a change in your TDD. Your physician and health care team's familiarity with how these factors affect your individual care can allow them to make a more refined estimate of your actual insulin requirement. When in doubt, always ask for their advice.

Take Small Steps Or Change Everything At Once?

Whether you need to change the number of injections, types of insulin, or just the insulin doses depends on what your current control problem is and how severe it is. For instance, if you are currently experiencing a lot of highs or lows, your

TDD is likely the first thing that needs to be changed. Once your new TDD provides more reasonable control, small dose adjustments can be made to fine tune your readings.

If you currently use two injections of a premixed insulin each day before breakfast and before dinner and your control has been very poor, should you change from two injections to three or four injections,

use different doses, use different insulins, or remain on the two injections with minor adjustments in your doses? Everyone will make different choices here based on the severity of the control problem, their lifestyle, how variable meals and activities need to be, and on how willing they are to experiment with their doses with their health care team's assistance.

As you get closer to ideal blood readings, changes in insulin doses begin to be smaller. With your physician's approval, you can start to adjust your TDD in small increments. Reducing or raising one dose by 0.5, 1, or 2 units is a good place to start, rather than by a full 5% or 10% of your TDD. Your insulin adjustments will be based on the patterns in your readings.

For example, if you are waking up during the night or in the morning with readings in the 60's, you might reduce your basal insulin at bedtime by 1 unit or even a half unit. Always start with the smallest change in your TDD or doses that seems likely to improve your readings. Ask your doctor for assistance to speed your path to better control.

Any time that you change your insulin doses, test every two hours during the daytime hours and at least once in the middle of the night for a few days. You may not discover your best doses until you've tested and adjusted your doses several times with the help of your physician and health care team.

How Much To Change Your Doses Depends On

- The frequency of highs and lows
- How well your current doses work
- The need for additional flexibility in your lifestyle
- Whether you retain internal insulin production. Two injections a day and sometimes one may work for someone who retains a considerable amount of insulin production.

10.7 Suggestions For People On Less Than 30 Units A Day

Exact doses are especially important for those who have a low TDD. When someone uses a total of 30 units of insulin a day or less, her blood sugar may drop 70 to 140 mg/dl on each unit of bolus insulin. A half unit difference in a dose can create a difference of 35 to 70 mg/dl (2.0 to 3.8 mmol) in the next reading!

Suggestions for those who use small doses:

* Switch to 25 unit Terumo or 30 unit BD syringes which have half unit markings on the barrel. They allow accurate half unit or even quarter unit delivery. Novo-Nordisk sells an insulin pen, called Novopen Junior®, which also has precise half unit delivery.
* Stay away from whole unit boluses unless it is truly what you need. Closely guesstimate each dose to the nearest fraction of a unit.
* Use insulins which have less variability and a more consistent action profile, such as Lantus, Humalog and Novolog.
* Use frequent injections. Smaller doses given more often lessens the surges in insulin activity that can be encountered with larger doses.
* Consider an insulin pump. Pumps deliver doses as small as 0.05 units with accuracy. The ability to set basals and boluses precisely with a pump helps stabilize blood sugars in those who require small doses.

© 2003 Diabetes Services, Inc.

* Ability to frequently communicate with your physician or nurse educator until your new doses are worked out
* The experience of your physician with different insulin approaches
* Your willingness to do the testing and recording required

Will Frequent Injections Change My TDD?

Over time, people with Type 1 diabetes often end up on insulin doses that are too high. The TDD often needs to be reduced as insulin doses are better matched to need through the use of frequent injections or when the carb intake or carb factor are determined more correctly. When someone starts to have frequent or severe low blood sugars, the current doses need to be reduced.

Growing teens with high hormones and people with insulin resistance may find their previous TDD of 90 units a day needs to be rapidly dropped to 50 or 60 units a day after they start injecting more often and tailoring their doses to their need more precisely. Others may find no reduction at all is needed. A person who was having frequent highs on two injections a day may get better control on four injections with the same TDD when the insulin is distributed through the day based on real need.

Watch For Lows When You Change Insulin Doses

As you and your doctor work out better ways to deliver your insulin, your blood sugars may at first become more stable with fewer ups and downs. As soon as your readings look great and everything is going well, you may start to have low blood sugars. As you transition from mostly high readings or from frequent ups and downs which raise stress hormone levels and make you less sensitive to insulin, a sudden calming of your readings makes your insulin work better. Improved diet and increased activity may also accompany the improved insulin doses.

Better readings may be followed quickly by a series of lows. Do not stop your program at this point because of the lows. Instead, reduce your insulin doses to a lower and more appropriate level. Your insulin doses may need to be reduced a time or two within the first few days.

As insulin is matched to need, you have a new ability to maintain nearly normal blood sugars. Do not overdo this by setting your targets too low. Your goal is to stay between 70 to 120 mg/dl (3.9 to 6.7 mmol) before meals and lower than 140 to 180 mg/dl (7.8 to 10 mmol) after meals at least 75% of the time or between the ranges your health provider and you agree on. Set realistic goals, pace yourself, and celebrate small steps as you move toward a normal range.

During any transition to better control, check your blood

> ### 10.8 Insulin Storage Tips
>
> - Always keep insulin out of direct sunlight
> - Keep insulin refrigerated or cooled at all times, but no cooler than 36 degrees Fahrenheit
> - If your prescription is shipped by mail or via UPS when outside temperatures may go above 80 degrees Fahrenheit, demand that it be cooled during shipment
> - Never leave insulin in a car in freezing or hot weather
> - If you have an unexpected high, don't automatically assume it's your fault! It could be bad insulin.

sugar at least 7 times a day and anytime you think you may be going low. If you have access to a continuous monitoring device, use it. As your physician and health care team give you more responsibility in adjusting your basal doses, carb and correction boluses, make these adjustments only after adequate testing. Adjust your insulin doses gradually as recommended by your physician and health care team.

Dopeler effect: The tendency of stupid ideas to seem smarter when they come at you rapidly.

Washington Post's Style Invitational

Basal Insulin

Insulin has many important functions. These include helping glucose enter certain cells, regulating the production and release of fat as fuel, and assisting the entrance into cells of some amino acids that create enzymes and structural proteins. Insulin must be available in the blood at all times to accomplish these important tasks. About half of your total daily insulin dose (TDD) is required to cover these needs.[56]

The first goal in mimicking the pancreas is to deliver a steady flow of basal insulin around the clock. When basal insulin doses are set correctly, the blood sugar will remain almost level while fasting. A good target for basal doses is to have the blood sugar fall no more than 30 mg/dl (1.7 mmol) and rise no more than 15 mg/dl (0.6 mmol) during eight hours of sleep or daytime fasting. This target has become easier to achieve with today's new basal insulins which have flatter action profiles and less day to day variability.

Basal doses should be tested before testing carb boluses. The correct basal doses provide a stable base from which carbs may be eaten at any time and covered with matching carb boluses.

This chapter discusses

- Basal doses as a percentage of TDD
- How to set and test basal doses
- Suggestions on when to take basal doses

What Percentage Of Your TDD Should Be Basal Insulin?

About half of the normal body's total daily insulin production is needed to provide basal insulin coverage. For many people control is smoother when 50% to 60% of the TDD is given as basal insulin. Growing teens who have high levels of growth hormone and individuals who are insulin resistant often need more than 60% of their TDD as basal insulin. Those who are physically fit and sensitive to insulin may do well with 40% to 45% of their TDD as basal.

Using a slightly higher percentage of basal insulin often provides better control. When some basal insulin is used to balance some of the carbs in meals, less carb bolus insulin is required. Although it is counter-intuitive, using less carb insulin and more basal insulin can help reduce the spike in blood sugar that is often seen between meals. Basal doses must be chosen carefully so the blood sugar drops slightly but does not plummet when a meal is skipped.

When Lantus (glargine) or Detemir are taken before breakfast, the dose can be gradually increased until a good balance is found with the breakfast, lunch, and dinner bolus doses. When using extra basal insulin (usually more than 55% of the TDD), more care is required when a meal is eaten late or skipped, or extra activity is engaged in. Fast carbs should always be available to raise the blood sugar quickly if a low occurs. If lows are mild and occasional, this is usually offset by the improved control. A basal dose should never cause frequent or severe hypoglycemia.

Clinicians usually suggest starting with 50% of the TDD as basal insulin and adjusting upward or downward as needed. This helps avoid unexpected lows if the TDD is inaccurate.

Most users find that their Lantus dose makes up 45% to 55% of their TDD. When Lantus or Detemir are given at breakfast, the percentage can often be raised to 60% or 65% of the TDD while daytime lows can be avoided by reducing the breakfast and lunch boluses. If lows do occur, they are more likely to happen during waking hours.

How To Test Basal Insulin Doses

In basal tests, your goal is to find how much basal insulin is needed to keep your blood sugar relatively flat, that is to fall or rise only slightly when no food is eaten.

Correct basal doses let you:

- skip meals without encountering lows or highs
- eat meals later than usual without worrying about a low blood sugar
- use boluses to cover carbs precisely and lower high blood sugars safely

To start testing your basal insulin doses, you want to make sure that stress, exercise and your last bolus are not affecting your blood sugar. Testing basal doses is easier with use of Humalog or Novolog insulin for boluses because basal testing can begin four hours after the last bolus. With Regular, it is necessary to wait 5 to 6 hours after the last bolus before starting a basal test.

No matter which insulin you use, set and test your basal doses before starting to test your boluses so you do not confuse which dose is creating the problem. For instance, if you often have high readings after lunch, you might mistakenly assume you need more Novolog to cover your lunch carbs, but the afternoon rise may actually be caused by a breakfast dose of NPH or Lente that is too small. A test of your basal during the morning and early afternoon hours may uncover that your blood sugar is rising and you will know your morning basal dose is the real culprit.

When switching from another basal insulin to Lantus or Detemir, be conservative by choosing a dose that is:

• equal to 40% of your current TDD, or

• 20% less than your current total daily basal dose.

Starting doses might be lowered more than this if you have been recently experiencing frequent lows, or they might not be lowered as much if you have been having many recent high readings.

Whenever you or your doctor change a basal dose, use the basal tests in this chapter to ensure that the new dose is accurate. After you change to a new dose, it typically takes 24 to 36 hours following a change in a dose of Lantus, Lente or NPH, and 36 to 48 hours following a change in a Detemir or Ultralente dose before testing can begin. For convenience, you may want to switch to new basal doses on a Friday evening or Saturday morning when you have more time to do

11.2 Basal Doses As Various Percents of TDD			
When your	**And your basal is:**		
TDD =	**45% of TDD**	**55% of TDD**	**65% of TDD**
	Your basal dose equals this many units/day		
16 u	7.2 u	8.8 u	10.4 u
18 u	8.1 u	9.9 u	11.7 u
20 u	9.0 u	11.0 u	13.0 u
22 u	9.9 u	12.1 u	14.3 u
24 u	10.8 u	13.2 u	15.6 u
26 u	11.7 u	14.3 u	16.9 u
28 u	12.6 u	15.4 u	18.2 u
30 u	13.5 u	16.5 u	19.5 u
32 u	14.4 u	17.6 u	20.8 u
36 u	16.2 u	19.8 u	23.4 u
40 u	18.0 u	22.0 u	26.0 u
44 u	19.8 u	24.2 u	28.6 u
48 u	21.6 u	26.4 u	31.2 u
52 u	23.4 u	28.6 u	33.8 u
56 u	25.2 u	30.8 u	36.4 u
60 u	27.0 u	33.0 u	39.0 u
65 u	29.3 u	35.8 u	42.3 u
70 u	31.5 u	38.5 u	45.2 u
75 u	33.8 u	41.3 u	48.8 u
80 u	36.0 u	44.0 u	52.0 u
90 u	40.5 u	49.5 u	58.5 u
100 u	45.0 u	55.0 u	65.0 u

11.3 Basal Tests And Timing

Overnight basal test
Eat your dinner and take a carb bolus at least 3 ¹/₂ hrs before bed. Start the test at bedtime when your blood sugar is 100 to150* mg/dl (5.6 to 8.3 mmol). Take a test at bedtime, the middle of the night, and when you awake.

1st half-day basal test
On waking, start the test when your blood sugar is 100 to 150* mg/dl (5.6 to 8.3 mmol). Skip breakfast and eat a late lunch. Take a test every 1 to 2 hours.

2nd half-day basal test
Start when your last bolus and eating was at least 3 ¹/₂ hrs ago, and your blood sugar is 100 to150* mg/dl (5.6 to 8.3 mmol). Take a test every 1 to 2 hours.

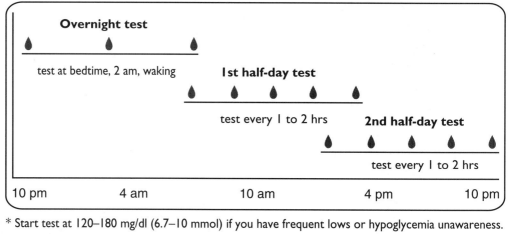

* Start test at 120–180 mg/dl (6.7–10 mmol) if you have frequent lows or hypoglycemia unawareness.

© 2003 Diabetes Services, Inc.

testing. If your activity level on weekends is significantly different from weekdays, however, weekday testing will need to be done to get precise weekday basal doses.

Figure 11.3 provides an overview of the timing for basal tests. How to test your basal insulin doses is shown in Go Figures 11.5, 11.7, and 11.8.

Basal testing is divided into three eight hour periods: overnight, first half of the daytime hours, and second half of the daytime hours. Testing usually begins with the overnight basal which allows sounder sleep and enables you to wake up with reasonable readings. This can be followed with a test during the first half or the second half of the day.

If your current control is not adequate, use these tests to determine whether your basal insulin is the source of the problem. Remember that the goal in your basal tests is to find doses that cause the blood sugar to fall or rise only slightly when no food is eaten.

Test The Overnight Basal

Overnight basal tests are usually done before daytime basal tests. Activities that affect the blood sugar, like exercise and eating, are suspended during the night so this test is usually the most convenient. Having an accurate overnight basal is important because control of your waking blood sugar is usually the most important aspect of your overall control. Repeat the overnight basal test until desirable results are obtained on two or more days using the same dose.

> ### 11.4 An Accurate Overnight Basal Dose Lets You:
>
> • Go to bed with a normal blood sugar, eat little or no bedtime snack and wake up with a normal blood sugar in the morning, assuming you have no bolus insulin still active at bedtime and your day was not unusually active.
>
> • Correct a high blood sugar at bedtime and wake up with a normal reading in the morning.
>
> • Rest peacefully.
>
> You, your spouse, parents, children, friends, roommates, and physician/health care team will all sleep better knowing you're unlikely to have an insulin reaction during the night.

Make a copy of Go Figure 11.5 and fill in your test results. Once you fill out the graph, go to Table 11.6 to interpret your results and to learn how to adjust your basal insulin dose.

Test The Overnight Basal

• Start your test near bedtime at least 4 hours after you last ate and after your last dose of Humalog or Novolog insulin.

• Begin the test when your bedtime reading is between 100 and 150 mg/dl (5.6 to 8.3 mmol) or between 120 to 180 mg/dl (6.7 to 10 mmol) if you have hypoglycemia unawareness. If you are afraid to go to bed within these ranges, your overnight basal insulin may need to be lowered before starting the test. The starting range should allow room for the blood sugar to fall during the night without causing a low blood sugar.

• Do not conduct an overnight test if you had a low blood sugar, major emotional stress, or strenuous exercise that day. Hypoglycemia and excessive stress cause the release of stress hormones that can raise blood sugar levels for several hours. Strenuous exercise has the opposite effect.

• If your bedtime blood sugar is between 70 and 100 mg/dl (3.9 to 5.6 mmol), you may consume 15 to 20 grams of glucose tabs or other quick carbs to raise your blood sugar. Retest in 30 minutes and then start the night test once your blood sugar is in your target range.

• Do not eat anything before going to bed (except glucose tablets as noted above) and do not take any Humalog or Novolog insulin. Test your blood sugar around 2 a.m. to ensure that the blood sugar is not dropping or rising in the middle of the night.

- If you go below 70 mg/dl (3.9 mmol) at any point, stop the test and eat 15 grams of carb. Reduce the evening basal dose by 0.5 to 2 units and wait 48 hours before retesting.

After completing the test, look at your test results. The goal for the overnight basal test is to drop no more than 30 mg/dl (1.1 mmol) and rise no more than 15 mg/dl (0.8 mmol) from the bedtime reading at any point during the night. If your blood sugar meets these goals, the evening basal dose is keeping the blood sugar level overnight. Repeat the test once or twice to verify it.

If the dose you are testing does not work, raise or lower the dose by a half to three units as shown in Go Figure 11.6. Wait 48 hours and retest until you find a dose that keeps your blood sugar relatively flat. Larger dose changes may be required if you find a dramatic rise or fall in your readings. Always check with your physician or nurse educator to discuss your results and any questions you have about your doses, how to interpret your readings, or whether a change in your dose is needed.

An ideal overnight basal dose keeps the blood sugar from rising more than 15 mg/dl (0.8 mmol) and falling more than 30 mg/dl (1.7 mmol) overnight.

Test The Day Basal

Daytime basal testing is split into two 8 hour tests done on different days. Testing in two segments requires that you skip only one meal and eat another meal earlier or later on the day of the test. Repeat each test until the daytime basal dose is shown to work on two separate days during the period of the day being tested.

Skipping a meal is required to test each of the daytime basal doses. Some people may object to going a few hours without food, because "I've always been told to eat when I take any insulin." This is true when the insulin is a carb bolus but not for basal insulin, which is ideally set up so it allows meals to be skipped. The human body is amazingly adaptive and will survive a short fast. The beauty of correctly set basal insulin doses is that you are able to delay or skip meals without worrying about your readings going out of control.

A few hours of fasting is a small price to pay for a correctly set basal dose since this is usually the most important step toward having normal blood sugar readings. If you are concerned about having a low blood sugar during a test of your basal insulin dose, you can check your blood sugar more often during the test or consult with your physician/health care team about using a lower dose for your tests. If the test with a lower dose is successful, you will want to continue using this lower dose.

If you take two or more doses of basal insulin and one dose is significantly changed due to your testing, you will need to retest the other dose(s) during the time each one is active. After changing one dose, wait a day or two for this dose to equilibrate before retesting the dose that precedes it or follows it.

During testing, keep in mind the time at which your basal insulin dose will peak in activity (See Table 9.4). Test your blood sugar more often during this peak period to avoid a low blood sugar.

Go Figure 11.5: Test The Overnight Basal Dose

Steps:

Start testing when your bedtime blood sugar is 100 to 150 mg/dl (5.6 - 8.3 mmol) at least 4 hrs after your last carb or correction bolus. Take your usual evening basal insulin dose, but eat no bedtime snack

1. Test your blood sugar every two hours if you wish, but be sure to test 4 and 8 hours from the beginning. Write your results in the spaces below. Determine the rise or fall in your blood sugar from the bedtime reading to those taken 4 and 8 hours later.

2. Plot the change in your blood sugar on the graph below. Your goal is to rise no more than 15 mg/dl and fall no more than 30 mg/dl. Once you plot your readings on the graph, look to the right to see which area of the graph described by the letter matches your readings. Then refer to Table 11.6 for information on how to adjust your basal insulin dose.

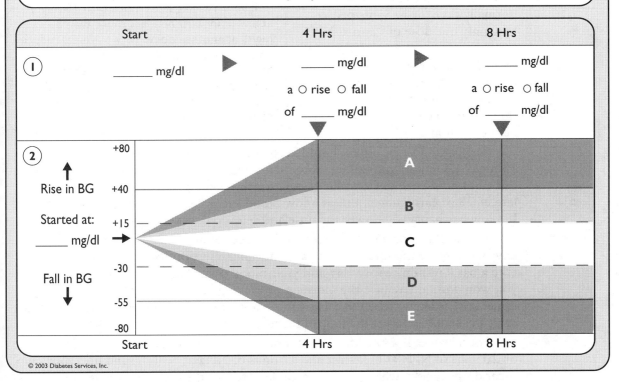

© 2003 Diabetes Services, Inc.

"*Normal is a setting on a dryer.*"

Anon.

Basal Test For The First Half Of The Day

Start this test when you wake up with a blood sugar between 100 and 150 mg/dl (5.6 to 8.3 mmol) or between 120 and 180 mg/dl (6.7 to 10 mmol) if you have hypoglycemia unawareness.

The basal test for the first half of the day determines the action of the basal dose given the previous night along with the basal dose given that morning. Take your morning dose of Lantus, NPH, Lente or UL as usual, but skip breakfast and the carb bolus you normally take for it. Some people take only one dose of Lantus, NPH, or Lente in the evening, so the first half-day basal test is testing just this evening dose. Test your blood sugar every two hours or at any time you think it may be high or low over the next eight hours.

> ### 11.6 Suggested Basal Changes
>
> Adjust your evening or morning basal dose by the following amount if your results consistently rise or fall and show up in the specified area of the basal test charts.
>
> A. Increase basal by 1 to 3 units
>
> B. Increase basal by 0.5 to 2 units
>
> C. Basal is OK
>
> D. Reduce basal by 0.5 to 2 units
>
> E. Reduce basal by 1 to 3 units
>
> If your reading rises more than 15 mg/dl at any point but then falls more than 30 mg/dl at another point, or vice versa, reduce your basal dose to eliminate the low reading first. If the blood sugar still rises after the low is eliminated, change the timing of the basal doses or the type of basal insulin to eliminate the rise.

The basal dose or doses should keep your blood sugar from rising more than 15 mg/dl (.8 mmol) and falling more than 30 mg/dl (1.7 mmol) at any point during this eight hour period. Continue fasting for this eight hour period and then have a late lunch or early dinner, unless a low blood sugar has already required you to eat. If a low has happened, lower the dose and retest on another day.

Repeat this morning basal test until you get desirable results on two separate days when using the same evening and morning injections of basal insulin. If you take a basal insulin twice a day and your blood sugar falls too far during this test, you would usually reduce the morning or evening basal dose that is larger. The larger dose is likely to be the cause for the low blood sugar unless the timing indicates the major action at the time of the fall.

For instance, if a breakfast NPH dose is usually than the evening dose, if you are on 20 units of NPH at breakfast and 12 units of NPH at bedtime and find your blood sugar drops rapidly when you skip breakfast, reduce the evening dose. It is relatively large compared to the morning dose, and will be much more active during the breakfast hours than the morning dose, which is just beginning its action. However, if the evening dose of NPH is only 5 units, with 35 units at breakfast, the evening dose is unusually small compared to the morning dose. The morning insulin will be the one that needs to be changed even though its action has just begun.

Go Figure 11.7: Test Your Basal For The First Half Of The Day

Steps:

Start testing when your breakfast blood sugar is 100 to 150 mg/dl (5.6 - 8.3 mmol) at least 4 hours after your last bolus insulin. Take only your morning basal insulin dose, skip breakfast, and plan to have a late lunch.

1. Test your blood sugar every two hours. Write your results in the spaces below. Determine the rise or fall in your blood sugar from the breakfast reading to those taken at each two hour interval.

2. Plot the change in your blood sugar on the graph below. Your goal is to rise no more than 15 mg/dl and fall no more than 30 mg/dl. Once you plot your readings on the graph, look to see which area of the graph described by the letter matches most of your readings. Then refer to Table 11.6 for information on how to adjust your basal insulin dose.

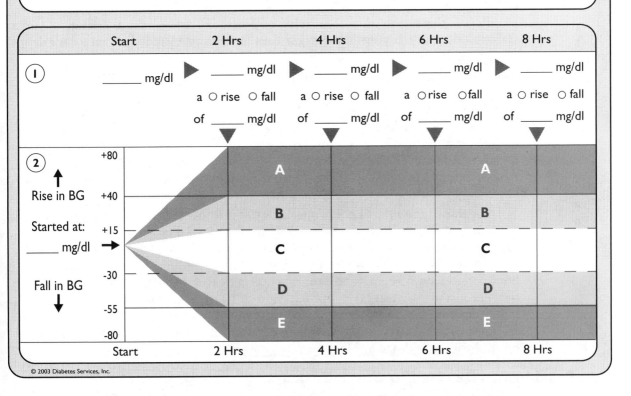

If you take only one basal insulin in the evening and the blood sugar rises during the first half-day test, you will need to raise the evening dose. If this higher dose causes a low in the middle of the night, you will need to lower the evening dose to avoid a low and add another dose of basal insulin at breakfast. If your blood sugar rises during the test, you would usually increase the smaller of the two basal doses.

133

Also consider taking the
original dose of Lantus in the
morning instead of night. If
Lantus is producing a small peak,
it is better to have it during the
daytime. The morning dose may
control the nighttime blood sugar
without a low because it is not
peaking at night.

Basal Test For The Second Half Of The Day

On another day, do the test for the second part of the day. Start this test about nine hours before you usually go to bed. This starts three and one-half hours after an early lunch has been eaten and covered with a bolus. It ends near bedtime. Skip any afternoon snacks and eat dinner around bedtime if you desire.

Repeat this test until your morning or previous evening's basal dose gives you a stable blood sugar. If your blood sugar rises more than 15 mg/dl (.8 mmol) or drops more than 30 mg/dl (1.7 mmol), you know that the basal insulin dose is not correctly set and you need to adjust your morning dose. Occasionally you may need to adjust your previous evening basal dose.

If the blood sugar rises during this test, add or increase NPH or Lente at breakfast. If you make any changes, you will need to test the new dose with a first half-day test. If the dose of Lantus taken the previous evening seems to last less than 24 hours, and the blood sugar starts rising in the afternoon, consider splitting the Lantus into two injections, taking one in the evening and one in the morning. Test any changes you make in your basal rate.

For those who inject Lantus once a day, it is important to see whether it remains active for a full 24 hours. If it is active for only 18 hours, your blood sugar may begin to rise about four hours before you usually give your injection and stay high for two hours after you have given it. See Figure 9.8 on page 104. This six hour period would be an important time to check to see that your blood sugar stays flat. For instance, if you take your injection at 10 p.m., skip dinner and test your blood sugar hourly from about 6 p.m. until midnight to ensure you are getting a full 24 hours of action from your Lantus. If not, consider breaking it into two doses-- one at bedtime and one at breakfast.

Can Basal Insulin Be Used To Cover Carbs?

This depends. Ideally, you want to mimic a normal pancreas which delivers relatively steady amounts of basal insulin around the clock, but adds quick boluses of insulin to cover food. Lantus has a flat, day-long profile that mimics the background release, so it makes a poor choice for covering carbs. However, intermediate insulins like Lente and NPH have a peaking action that can be used to cover eating

Go Figure 11.9: Test Your Basal For The Second Half Of The Day

Steps:

Start testing when your lunch blood sugar is 100 to 150 mg/dl (5.6 - 8.3 mmol) at least 4 hours after your last carb or correction bolus. Eat breakfast and take your usual insulin that morning, but skip lunch and your lunch bolus, and plan to have a late dinner.

1. Test your blood sugar every two hours. Write your results in the spaces below. Determine the rise or fall in your blood sugar from the early afternoon reading to those taken at each two hour interval.

2. Plot the change in your blood sugar on the graph below. Your goal is to rise no more than 15 mg/dl and fall no more than 30 mg/dl. Once you plot your readings on the graph, look to the right to see which area of the graph described by the letter matches most of your readings. Then refer to Table 11.6 for information on how to adjust your basal insulin dose.

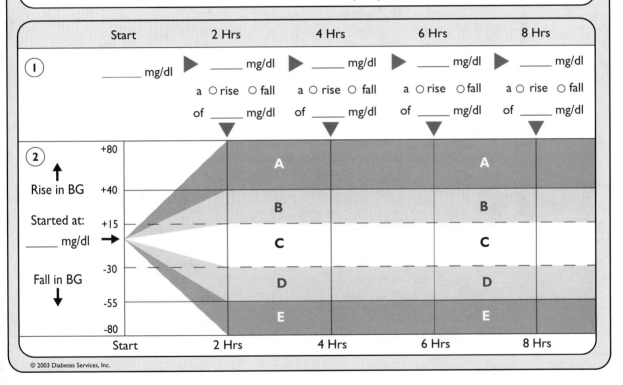

© 2003 Diabetes Services, Inc.

that occurs when they peak. For instance, Lente or NPH given before breakfast may cover lunch with no extra bolus injection. For those who eat a consistent lunch at the same time each day, this may work well.

Tips On Testing Basal Doses

- Always select your basal doses and other doses with the help of your physician or health care team.

11.10 Basal Testing With A Continuous Monitor

A continuous blood sugar monitor allows you to quickly see whether your basal insulin keeps your blood sugar level. Overnight tests can be revealing and expose low blood sugars in the middle of the night that you were not aware of. For daytime testing, skip a meal and watch your blood sugar on the monitor. If your blood sugar rises or falls, discuss with your physician how much to raise or lower your basal dose, whether the basal doses need to be taken at a different time, or whether another basal insulin may work better for you.

- Test and set your nighttime basal dose first to allow yourself to sleep 8 hours and wake up with a normal blood sugar without a low.

- During tests, monitor more often if you suspect your blood sugar may drop.

- If eating, activity, or stress are different on weekends, you may require different basal doses for the weekend.

- Add up your basal insulin doses periodically to make sure they make up an appropriate percentage (usually 45% to 65%) of your TDD.

- If your blood sugar drops below 70 mg/dl (3.9 mmol) during a basal test, have some carbs and end the test. Discuss lowering your basal dose with your physician or health care team. If the drop is rapid, a greater reduction in your basal dose will be needed. If the drop is slow, a smaller reduction may be sufficient.

- If your blood sugar rises above 240 mg/dl (13.3 mmol), take a correction bolus and end the test. Discuss raising your basal dose with your physician or health care team. If your blood sugar rises rapidly, a larger increase may be needed. If the rise occurs slowly, a small increase may be sufficient.

- Change your basal insulin doses by 1 or 2 units unless frequent high or low blood sugars indicate that larger changes are needed.

- A fast carb snack may be needed when the bedtime blood sugar is less than 100 mg/dl (5.6 mmol).

"One hundred thousand lemmings can't be wrong."

graffito

Jamie

Jamie was diagnosed with Type 1 diabetes six months ago and was recently referred to a diabetes clinic while still on one injection a day before breakfast of 40 units of 75/25 insulin (75% NPH and 25% Humalog). His blood sugars are usually high before breakfast and lower before dinner, but his readings vary from 30 to 450 mg/dl (1.7 to 25 mmol). His doctor suggests more frequent injections and mixing his own insulin rather than using one with a fixed ratio. Jamie decides he is willing to try two injections a day.

His doctor placed him on 4 Humalog plus 28 NPH before breakfast and 5 Humalog plus 3 NPH before dinner. With this, his TDD remained the same at 40 units a day, but his control improved considerably. After this improvement, Jamie was willing to try three injections a day. Per his doctor's suggestion, he began using 4 H plus 18 NPH before breakfast, 4 H before lunch, and 6 H plus 4 NPH before dinner for a TDD of 36 units.

With this change, the size of the morning basal insulin pool under the skin drops from 28 units to 18 units. The total daily insulin dose also drops from 40 units to 36 units. Lowering the total insulin dose and spreading the basal insulin more evenly

11.11 Jamie's Dose Changes

	Brkfst	Lunch	Dinner	Bed	TDD	% Basal
Original dose	40 75/25				40 u	75%
1st Option	4H/28N		(5H/3N)		40 u	78%
2nd Option	4H/18N	4H	(6H/4N)		36 u	61%
3rd Option	4H/12N	4H/3N	(6H/3N)	(4N)	36 u	61%
4th Option	(6H)	5H	(7H)	(18 Lantus)	36 u	50%

results in more stable blood sugars with less insulin.

If he were willing to give four injections, Jamie's basal insulin doses could be redistributed to give smaller doses in each injection. For example, 4 H plus 12 NPH before breakfast, 4 H plus 3 NPH before lunch, 6 H plus 3 NPH before dinner and 4 NPH at bedtime could be tried. Although this requires an extra injection, giving the 36 total units in this way helps smooth out insulin action and stabilize the blood sugar. With Lantus, Jamie might take 6 H before breakfast, 5 H before lunch, 7 H before dinner, and 18 Lantus at bedtime (36 total units).

Did Jamie's control improve after he changed to more injections of insulin spread through the day? Yes, his A1c went from 10.5% on one injection to 7.5% on three injections (2nd option). If he were willing to go to option 3 or 4, his A1c might drop to 7% or even 6.5%, values recommended by the ADA and ACE, the professional organizations of endocrinologists.

Correct Basal Doses

Your basal insulin doses are too high if:

- you sometimes wake up during the night or early in the morning with a low blood sugar
- your blood sugar drops when you skip a meal
- you have frequent lows during the day

Your basal insulin doses are too low if:

- your blood sugar rises when you skip a meal
- you have frequent high blood sugars
- you need frequent correction boluses to bring down high blood sugars

An ideal daily level of basal insulin keeps your blood sugar level or allows it to fall no more than 30 mg/dl (1.7 mmol) or rise no more than 15 mg/dl (.8 mmol) during an eight-hour test period.

With experience, you will be testing and making changes as needed. Be sure to consult with your physician if you are uncertain what your test results mean.

Never change your dose based on one test unless this dose proves to be seriously incorrect. Never assume a dose is correct after one test. Test at least twice to confirm.

Quick Check: Do your basal insulin doses make up 45% to 65% of your TDD?

"If you tell the truth you don't have to remember anything."
Mark Twain

The 500 Rule For Carb Boluses

CHAPTER 12

"How much insulin do I take to cover a bagel, a plate of pasta, or a bowl of fruit?" Being able to answer questions like these accurately determines half your control each day.

For an accurate carb bolus, you want to first determine how many grams of carbohydrate one unit of insulin covers for you. This is your insulin-to-carb ratio or your carb factor. Once you know this, you can count the grams of carb in the food you want to eat and divide by your carb factor to find how many units of bolus insulin are needed to cover the carbs. This allows flexibility in your food choices because any number of carbs can be covered with a matching dose of insulin.

The formula used to determine your carb factor is based on your TDD. As with basal doses, an accurate carb factor can be determined only after you've calculated an accurate TDD for yourself.

This chapter shows:

- How to cover carbs
- Finding your carb factor
- Testing your carb factor
- How to time carb boluses to match different types of carbs and conditions

Most people find that they need one unit of insulin for somewhere between 6 and 20 grams of carbohydrate. Those using a small total daily dose of insulin each day will use a higher carb factor at one end of this range, while those who require a large TDD will use a lower number at the other end of this range for their carb factor. Some people will fall outside this 6 to 20 range. For example, someone who is thin or physically active may need only one unit of Novolog or Humalog for every 25 grams of carbohydrate. A growing teen, on the other hand, may need one unit for every 4 or 5 grams. Someone who has Type 2 diabetes and severe insulin resistance may require one unit for every 2 grams.

Some sources use a general rule and say that one unit of insulin covers 15 grams of carbohydrate because this is easier than doing the math to find a personal factor. But for most people, a carb factor of 15 is not going to be precise enough to provide optimal control and will give some people too much insulin and others too little. A personal carb factor is much more effective and is easy to determine as this chapter will show.

Carb Coverage

The amount of carbohydrate eaten in a meal or snack considered together with your TDD will determine the carb bolus needed to cover these carbs. The more carbohydrate in a meal, the larger the carb bolus that will be needed. Also the higher your TDD, the larger the carb bolus needed to cover a specific amount of carbohydrate.

The rapid insulins, Humalog and Novolog, provide the best match for most carbs. These analog insulins begin working in 10 to 15 minutes, peak in about an hour, and are gone in about four hours. The action time of these insulins is a close match for most meals. Glucose from the digestion of carbs in a meal begins to reach the blood stream in 10 minutes and rises to a peak in about an hour.

When carb amounts are not too large, Novolog or Humalog can be given shortly before eating and keep the blood sugar reasonably well controlled afterward. For meals that contain large amounts of carbs or foods that have a high glycemic index, the carb bolus can be taken 20 or 30 minutes before eating to reduce the blood sugar spiking that may occur an hour or two later when all that carb hits the blood stream.

Regular insulin has a slower onset and longer action time than Humalog and Novolog. It starts in 20 minutes, has a more gradual peak at two to three hours, and keeps working for five to six hours. Due to Regular's slower action time, high blood sugar readings will often be seen an hour or two after eating before Regular begins to work. Regular continues to lower the blood sugar for three or more hours beyond the time when most meals have been digested, causing a low blood sugar several hours after the food is eaten. When used before the evening meal, Regular is a frequent cause of lows in the middle of the night.

Regular needs to be given at least 30 to 60 minutes before meals to avoid spikes in the blood sugar at one to two hours after eating. With its slower onset and longer duration of action, Regular may provide better control for someone whose digestion is slow. Slowed digestion is characteristic of gastroparesis, a complication of diabetes that delays digestion because of nerve damage in the digestive tract. But most other people find that Humalog or Novolog works better for them.

Your carb coverage is correct when your blood sugar starts at your target before a meal and ends up within 40 mg/dl (2.2 mmol) 2 hours later and within 30 mg/dl (1.7 mmol) of your starting value 3 1/2 to 4 hours later with Humalog or Novolog or 5 to 6 hours later with Regular.

Finding Your Carb Factor

The 500 Rule[57] provides a reasonable first estimate for determining your own carb factor when using Humalog or Novolog insulin.

The 500 Rule:

To estimate your carb factor, divide 500 by your current TDD.

Example

If someone's TDD = 25 units

500 / 25 = 20, or a 1 unit carb bolus will cover about 20 grams of carbohydrate.

The carb factor obtained from the 500 Rule helps to set accurate carb boluses and keep your postmeal readings well controlled. This rule is not precise enough on its own, however. Once a carb factor is selected with the 500 Rule, its accuracy must be validated using the test in Go Figure 12.2.

The 500 Rule will be most accurate for those who make no insulin of their own and receive 50% to 60% of their TDD as basal insulin. The 500 Rule works best for those who are using a basal/bolus approach. For others, such as those who use two injections a day with the morning basal insulin covering carbs at lunch, the 500 Rule works only as a rough guide for matching carbohydrate.

With Type 2 diabetes, there is usually internal insulin production that cannot be accounted for when determining the TDD. This makes it harder to know an individual's exact TDD (injected plus internally produced insulin). In Type 2, the

12.1 Use The 500 Rule To Determine Your Carb Factor

The 500 Rule estimates your carb factor or how many grams of carbohydrate are covered by one unit of Humalog or Novolog insulin.	The **500** Rule*	
	If Your TDD is:	**Your Carb Factor is:**
The number of grams of carb covered by one unit of rapid insulin equals 500 divided by your average total daily insulin dose (TDD). Once you know your carb factor, count the carbs in your meal, divide by your carb factor, and the resulting bolus should cover these carbs.	15 units	33 grams
	20	25
	25	20
	30	17
	35	14
	40	13
For example, someone who uses 50 units of insulin a day will need one unit for every 10 grams of carbohydrate (500/50 units = 10). If they have two slices of bread with 15 grams each, these 30 grams of carbs can be covered by 3 units of Humalog or Novolog.	45	11
	50	10
	55	9
	60	8
	70	7
	80	6
This rule is most accurate for those who use a basal/bolus insulin approach after having accurately determined their TDD.	90	5
	100	5
© 2003 Diabetes Services, Inc.	*500 ÷ TDD = # of grams of carb covered by 1 unit	

500 Rule may underestimate insulin requirements. This underestimate is safe since it will give carb boluses that are slightly lower than those actually needed. Again, testing the carb factor provides the best guide.

Testing Your Carb Factor

Test your carb boluses and carb factor after your basal doses have been set and adjusted to keep your blood sugar flat when you are not eating. Once you estimate your carb factor from Table 12.1, use Go Figure 12.2 to test your carb factor to make sure it is correct. Until your carb factor has been tested, be as consistent as possible in the number of carbs you eat and in the timing of your meals. Once you have determined that your carb factor is accurate, you can be more confident in varying the timing and quantities of the food you eat.

Test your carb bolus when:

- you have not had a low blood sugar or symptoms of one in the last 8 hours
- your blood sugar before a meal is between 70 and 150 mg/dl (3.9 to 8.3 mmol)
- you can count the exact carb content in your meal

Once you know the grams of carb you will eat, divide this total by your carb factor to get the size of your meal bolus. For instance, if you use a unit of insulin for every 10 grams of carb and you plan to eat 70 grams, you would take 7 units.

With Novolog or Humalog, take the bolus 15 minutes before the meal or 30 minutes with Regular. Test your blood sugar at hourly intervals after the meal or more often if you suspect you may go low. Your blood sugar should rise 40 to 80 mg/dl (2.2 to 4.4 mmol) above your starting blood sugar at one or two hours after the meal. If your blood sugar at one hour has risen less than 40 mg/dl, your carb bolus may have been too large, so begin testing more often to avoid a low.

If your blood sugar at one hour is above 240 mg/dl (13.3 mmol), your carb factor was too high giving you a carb bolus that was too small. End the test and lower the high blood sugar with a correction bolus.

To lower the high reading, use 180 mg/dl (10 mmol) as your 2-hour postmeal target unless your physician has recommended a different one. Subtract 180 from the current reading and use a correction bolus for this difference. For instance, if your reading is 270 mg/dl (15 mmol), 270 minus 180 equals 90 mg/dl (5 mmol), so you would use a correction bolus to lower your blood sugar 90 mg/dl. (See Chapter 13 for how to determine your correction factor.) Test hourly until you return to normal.

When your carb factor is correct, your blood sugar will return to within 30 mg/dl (1.7 mmol) of your starting blood sugar after 3.5 to 4 hours with Humalog or Novolog, or after 5 to 6 hours with Regular. Once your carb factor appears to be correct for one test, repeat the test to verify that it is correct.

If your blood sugar often goes low after meals when you use a particular carb factor, your carb factor should be increased to reduce the amount of insulin you receive. If lows occur only an hour or two after a carb bolus is given, a larger

Go Figure 12.2: Test Your Carb Factor

Steps:

Start test when blood sugar is 70 to 150 mg/dl (3.9 to 8.3 mmol), and you have had no boluses or food in the last 3 ½ hours.

1. Enter how many grams of carbohydrate you will eat.

2. Enter your carb factor from Go Figure 7.4

3. Divide the grams of carb you will eat by your carb factor to get your carb bolus for this meal. Take your carb bolus and eat as planned.

4. Check your blood sugar each hour to see if this carb factor works.*

5. Does your carb factor work?

   *Check more often if blood sugar is dropping. Stop test if > 240 mg/dl (15mmol) or < 65 mg/dl (3.6 mmol).

(1) Carbs in this meal

_____ grams of carb

(2) Your carb factor

1 unit for every _____ grams of carb

(3) Divide your carb grams by your carb factor

$$\frac{\text{_____}}{\text{grams of carb}} \div \frac{\text{_____}}{\text{carb factor}} = \frac{\text{_____}}{\text{carb bolus}} \text{ units}$$

(4) Check your blood sugars

Starting BG = _____ mg/dl

1 hr BG = _____ mg/dl

2 hr BG = _____ mg/dl

3 hr BG = _____ mg/dl

3.5 hr BG = _____ mg/dl

(5) Does your carb factor work?

After 3.5 hours, are you within 30 mg/dl (1.7 mmol) of your starting blood sugar?

No

My BG fell over 30 mg/dl below my start

↓

Retest - use a larger carb number, ie: if it was 1 u/12 grams, use 1 u/ 13 grams

Yes

No

My BG rose over 30 mg/dl above my start

↓

Retest - use a smaller carb number, ie: if it was 1 u/12 grams, use 1 u/ 11 grams

Your carb factor is correct.
Test again to verify.

increase in your carb factor will be needed. If lows occurs three or four hours after the dose is given, a small increase in your carb factor will be needed. See Table 12.4, the Zero To 60 Carb Bolus Guide.

For instance, if a low occurs an hour or two after you eat and you are using 1 unit for each 12 grams of carb, next time use 1 unit for each 14 or 15 grams. This gives you less insulin for the same amount of carbohydrate. However, if the low blood sugar happens 3 hours after the last carb bolus with Humalog or Novolog, try adding 1 to the carb number, so that instead of 1 unit for each 12 grams, you now give 1 unit for each 13 grams.

If a high blood sugar occurs during testing, increase the amount of Humalog or Novolog you take for a meal. Be cautious when increasing your carb bolus. Subtract 1 from your carb factor, so that instead of 1 unit for each 12 grams of carb, you would use 1 unit for each 11 grams of carb. Test this new carb factor before reducing it further.

Some people find that 1 unit of insulin may cover fewer grams of carbohydrate at breakfast than at other meals. This may occur because insulin sensitivity is often lower at breakfast following the normal rise in growth hormone, cortisol, and free fatty acids during the early morning hours. You may find you need to use one carb factor for breakfast and another for lunch, dinner, and any snacks eaten later in the day. The carb factor might only differ by 1 but using the right carb factor will simplify your management significantly. However, if you need a lot more insulin for carbs at breakfast, you may want to retest your overnight basal dose to check whether your evening basal dose needs to be raised. You might also require a higher carb factor (smaller boluses) for meals later in the day if your activity level is greater at these times.

If you use Regular insulin for carb boluses, a different reason may be at play causing your carb boluses to be smaller for meals later in the day. Doses of Regular given for breakfast and lunch overlap during the afternoon and evening hours due to Regular's long action time.[58] Less Regular is needed for lunch and dinner to cover the same number of carbs because you have residual Regular insulin still working from previous boluses. Using a rapid insulin reduces or eliminates the problem caused by Regular's overlapping action and makes management easier.

Determining The Carb Factor With The 2.8 Rule[59]

Dr. Paul Davidson, originator of the 1500 Rule, which is used to determine correction factors for Regular insulin, and the more recent 1716 Rule[57] used for Humalog and Novolog, has developed an alternative method for determining the carb factor. Dr. Davidson's carb rule is:

Weight (lbs) X 2.8 / TDD = the Carb Factor

We have concerns about using the 2.8 Rule with people who weigh less than 150 pounds, however. As weight drops, the 2.8 Rule begins to give larger boluses for carbs than the 500 Rule. For instance, for someone who weighs 100 lbs. and has a TDD of 25 units per day:

500 Rule: *500 / 25* units = 1 unit for every 20 grams of carb

2.8 Rule: *100 X 2.8 / 25* units = 1 unit for every 11.2 grams of carb

So, for 60 grams of carb, the 500 Rule advises trying 3 units, while the 2.8 Rule would advise trying 5.4 units for the same number of carbs. We believe the 2.8 Rule will provide carb boluses that are too large for individuals whose weight is low.

As weight rises above 200 pounds, the 2.8 Rule begins to give less insulin for the same TDD than the 500 Rule. Whereas the 500 would continue to give 1 unit for every 20 grams for a 200 pound person whose TDD is 25 units, the 2.8 Rule would give 1 unit for every 22.4 grams. At 300 pounds, it would be 1 for 20 versus 1 for 33.6. Again, testing is the best way to determine your own carb factor, but until a better rule comes along, stay with the 500 Rule if you weigh less than 200 lbs.

Another Way To Set The Carb Factor

Another way to determine your carb factor is to add up all the carbs you eat in a typical day and how many units you take for carb boluses. If you do this for three days, you will have a close estimate of your carb factor, provided your control at the time is reasonable. For instance, if you typically eat 300 grams of carb a day and use 30 units of Novolog before meals to cover them, your carb factor would be:

300 grams / 30 units = 10 grams per unit or 1 unit for every 10 grams of carb

Some people prefer to eat a set amount of carbs at each meal or snack and take fixed carb boluses to cover them. This can be easier and works well for people who have routine meals and snacks each day. If 50% of your TDD is used as basal insulin, the other 50% can be divided into the total grams of carb you eat each day to determine what your boluses are likely to be.

For instance, if your TDD is 50 units, and you eat 300 grams of carbs each day, about half of the 50 units, or 25 units, would be used to cover carbs.

300 grams / 25 units = 12 grams per unit or 1 unit for every 12 grams of carb

If you always eat 72 grams of carb for dinner, you can take 72/12 or 6 units as your carb bolus everyday for dinner. Before you rely on this factor, it would need to be tested with any adjustments made as required. Once testing has been done, you can follow your meal plan and take set boluses for these meals.

When To Reduce A Carb Bolus

When first using a carb factor to determine carb boluses, you may want to subtract 10 or so grams of carbohydrate from your total in each meal until you can test the accuracy of your carb factor. This lowers your carb boluses and your risk of a low blood sugar until you are certain that your carb factor is correct.

Carb boluses can also be reduced by increasing your carb factor. If your TDD is 38 units a day, your carb factor would be one unit for every 13 grams of carb (500 / 38 equals 13.2 grams per unit). Increase the number you use as your carb factor to 14 or 15 grams to reduce the size of your carb bolus and your risk for lows.

Another time to reduce a carb factor is when you are going to exercise after eating. For instance, if you plan to engage in two or three hours of activity after a meal, you might take 1 unit for every 20 to 26 grams of carb for that meal, rather than 1 unit for 13 grams. Chapters 23 and 24 on exercise describe ways to adjust bolus and basal doses for activity.

Boluses for bedtime snacks are often reduced to prevent night lows. An easy

> ## 12.3 If Your Carb Factor Doesn't Work
>
> If your carb factor usually works, but you experience a high or low reading after a particular meal, consider:
>
> - Did you count the carbs carefully?
> - Did you take your insulin the usual number of minutes before eating?
> - Do the carbs in this meal have an unusually high or low glycemic index?
> - Did the meal contain more fat or protein than usual that may have slowed the digestion of the carbs or caused a delayed rise in your reading?
> - Was your activity level more or less than usual?
> - Did you have a recent insulin reaction?

way to reduce the bedtime snack bolus is to cut the carb bolus in half. For example, rather than taking 3 units, take 1.5 units at bedtime. (Half units can be guesstimated on your syringe.) Correction boluses for bedtime highs can be reduced in the same way.

A carb bolus may be reduced or skipped entirely:

- when extra carbs are eaten to raise a low blood sugar
- when extra carbs are eaten to cover increased activity
- if you experience nausea or vomiting and are unsure if you can keep carbs down.

For instance, if your blood sugar is 50 mg/dl (2.8 mmol) before a meal, you would need to eat enough free carbs to raise your blood sugar to normal. Free carbs are carbs that you do not take any bolus for because they are used to raise your blood sugar. Since one gram of carbohydrate raises your blood sugar about 4 mg/dl, the 15 grams of carb you need to raise your blood sugar to 110 would not require any bolus insulin. Once your blood sugar level has been raised, you can eat your meal and take a carb bolus to cover the carbs in the meal itself.

Carb Bolus Timing

Although using the correct carb factor is the most important way to cover food well, the timing of your carb bolus will also affect your postmeal reading. Carb boluses are often given when a meal is ready to eat, but they work best when given at least 15 to 20 minutes before eating. Of course, bolusing 20 minutes before a meal should only be done when your blood sugar is in a safe range and you are certain you will eat on time. When the timing of a meal is uncertain, it may be better to not bolus ahead. This may cause a postmeal high but that is preferable to a serious low.

When a blood sugar is high before a meal, it helps to take your carb bolus plus your correction bolus early enough to lower your blood sugar before you begin to eat. Postmeal readings are better when you bring your blood sugar below 150 mg/dl (8.3 mmol) before you begin to eat. This may mean taking a short walk before you eat or delaying the meal for a half hour.

Set an alarm, if necessary, so you do not delay your eating any longer than planned. In general, delayed eating is the most common cause of severe hypoglycemia. Recheck your blood sugar a half hour after the bolus, and again an hour and a half or two hours after eating. For safety, you may prefer to take only the correction bolus, wait a while for a partial drop in your blood sugar and then give the carb bolus right before eating.

When you eat out at an unfamiliar restaurant, you may not know when the meal will begin or what its carb content will be. It is best to not give a full carb bolus until you see the food on your plate. You might want to lead the meal with a partial dose, perhaps half of the total carb bolus you estimate you will need for the meal. Take a second injection of the remainder of the carb bolus after the food arrives and its true carb content can be more accurately determined. Splitting the carb bolus into two injections allows the blood insulin level to rise by the time eating starts, while reducing the risk of a low blood sugar from excess insulin. A few fast-acting carbs in your purse or pocket will help in case your blood sugar drops more than expected before the meal is served.

Although most carb-rich foods are digested and turned into glucose within an hour or two of eating, certain carbs that digest more slowly may need to be matched with carb boluses that are delivered over a longer period of time. Foods with the same amount of carbohydrate but different ratings on the glycemic index may require that carb boluses be adjusted. For instance, 50 grams of carbohydrate from kidney beans (low glycemic index) is unlikely to require as much insulin as 50 grams of

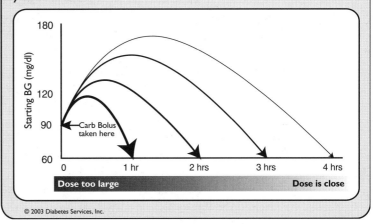

12.4 The Zero to 60 Guide For Carb Boluses

When your blood sugar goes low after a carb bolus, keep the Zero to 60 Guide in mind. After taking a carb bolus at time zero, how long it takes to reach 60 mg/dl (3.3 mmol) tells you how excessive your bolus was. If you are below 60 mg/dl an hour later, your bolus was far too large, but if you reach 60 mg/dl 3 $\frac{1}{2}$ or 4 hours later, your carb bolus was close to what you needed.

© 2003 Diabetes Services, Inc.

carbohydrate from cold cereal (high glycemic index). Some meals are also slower, such as a brunch where food is eaten in small amounts over several hours. For those who take several injections a day to cover carbs or highs, using an insulin pen can be very helpful.

Matching Insulin To Gastroparesis

Matching insulin to gastroparesis, a condition in which damage has occurred to the nerves that control digestion, often requires a slower acting insulin to better match indigestion as the condition develops. The effect of gastroparesis on digestion can be unpredictable because the delays or reductions in food absorption occur at different times depending on the foods and individual involved.

With gastroparesis, Regular insulin may be preferred over Humalog or Novolog because of its slower action. Some people with gastroparesis find they do better when they eat small meals several times a day and cover them with small doses of Regular taken through the day. The blood sugar can be checked two hours after the meal and corrected with Novolog or Humalog if it is excessively high. It is risky to take all the insulin before the meal because the slowed digestion is likely to cause a low shortly after eating. Keep fast carbs handy to treat possible lows.

Several medications are available that improve digestion and aid in the treatment of gastroparesis. Taking acidophilus capsules for a week each month to restore normal intestinal bacteria and eating carbs that rank low on the glycemic index also can be very helpful with this condition. Discuss these options with your physician/health care team and experiment to find what works best for you.

Jeremy

Jeremy is 26 and works at a UPS counter. He has Type 1 and takes 6H/23N before breakfast and 5H/7N at dinner. A large local distributor mails their orders out on Monday, Wednesday, and Friday, so Jeremy works harder in the sorting area handling packages on these days. On Tuesday and Thursday he works at the front counter with customers checking the packages in.

12.5 How Should Jeremy Change His Doses?		
	Breakfast	**Dinner**
Original	6H/23N	5H/7N
M/W/F Dose		
S/T/T/S Dose		

He is having problems with his pre-dinner readings, which are often low on Monday, Wednesday and Friday, but usually on Tuesday and Thursday are around 200 mg/dl .

How would you change Jeremy's doses? Place your recommendations in the boxes above for Monday, Wednesday, and Friday when he tends to go low before dinner, and for the rest of the week when he tends to be high at dinner.

(Suggested answer at the end of chapter)

12.5 Testing Your Carb Factor With A Continuous Monitor

Continuous monitoring makes it easier to test your carb factor. You can see immediately the effect that carbs have on your blood sugars when readings are displayed several times each hour for the full three and a half hours that a carb bolus works. You may assume that since you've been taught to test 2 hours after a meal, this will be your lowest number for the next hour or so, but that is not true. A bolus of Regular takes 5 to 6 hours to finish its job, and Humalog or Novolog take 3 to 4 hours.

Food takes 1 to 3 hours to digest. If you react to highs at 2 hours by giving more insulin immediately, you can drop seriously low a short time later. With practice, continuous monitoring lets you more accurately judge the impact of a bolus at any time, avoid low blood sugars, and respond more quickly to a high reading postmeal.

A continuous monitor allows you to quickly identify foods that have a low or high glycemic index so that you can match them with appropriate bolus changes. You also can experiment by changing the timing of your bolus before a meal to get the least rise in your blood sugar after you eat.

You can even run your own experiments to see if foods enter your bloodstream in the fashion predicted by their ranking in the glycemic index in this book. When your carb factor is correct, a carb bolus of Humalog or Novolog will take your blood sugar from a starting value of 100 mg/dl (5.5 mmol) back to approximately 100 mg/dl 3.5 hours later. If the carb factor is correct the second reading should vary no more than 30 mg/dl (1.7 mmol) from the original one. This works only if you test one food at a time.

Continuous monitoring lets you tailor carb boluses to different meals. It also allows you to identify specific food effects more easily. You can see whether certain fatty foods, such as potato chips or meat pizzas, cause your blood sugar to rise for several hours.

Tips On Carb Coverage

- Test your carb factor (how many carbs are covered by one unit of insulin) only after you have correctly set and tested your basal insulin.

- The carb bolus for a meal is determined by the carb factor and the number of grams of carbs the meal contains. After determining the carb bolus, adjustments to the bolus can be made for the current blood sugar reading and any planned activity.

- Count or estimate the carbs in all meals and snacks to match them correctly with carb boluses.

- The correct carb factor returns the blood sugar to within 40 mg/dl (2.2 mmol) of the original blood sugar 2 hours after eating and within 30 mg/dl (1.7 mmol) 3.5 hours after eating when using Humalog or Novolog or after 5 hours using Regular.

Your carb factor may be too high: when your premeal blood sugar starts in a normal range but goes high afterward and does not return to normal four hours later. Try lowering your carb factor number, i.e., change from 1 unit for every 16 grams to 1 unit for every 15 or 14. This increases the amount of insulin in your carb boluses. (Check your basal insulin dose also, as too little basal will cause the same problem.)

12.6 How Jeremy Changed His Doses		
	Breakfast	**Dinner**
Original	6H/23N	5H/7N
M/W/F Dose	(5H/21N)	5H/7N
S/T/T/S Dose	(6H/25N)	5H/7N

Your carb factor may be too low: when your premeal blood sugar starts in a normal range before meals but goes low one to four hours later. Here, raise your carb factor, i.e., change from 1 unit for every 16 grams to 1 unit for every 17 or 18. This reduces the amount of insulin in your carb boluses. (Check your basal insulin dose also, as too much basal will cause the same problem.)

Quick Check:

Do your carb boluses make up 40% to 50% of your TDD?

Murphy's Law For Carb Boluses (per Joanne Scott, RN, CDE)

When your blood sugar is low at a restaurant, you will be the last served. When your blood sugar is high, the first.

"For fast-acting relief, try slowing down."
Lilly Tomlin

The 1800 Rule
For Correction Boluses

After setting your basal doses and carb boluses, determining your correction boluses is the last piece of your control puzzle. When your blood sugar goes unexpectedly high, a correction bolus can be used to bring it down. To use the right amount of correction bolus for a high blood sugar, you first determine your correction factor. Your correction factor tells you how far your blood sugar will drop on each unit of bolus insulin. Once you know this, you can bring most high blood sugars back to target safely. Bringing a high down safely will take more time than you might like, but patience prevents lows caused when too much insulin is taken in frustration.

This chapter shows:

- How to determine your correction factor (how far your blood sugar drops on each unit of insulin), using the 1800 Rule
- How to test your correction factor
- How to set up a personalized correction scale
- When to combine bolus and meal bolus
- How to handle frequent high readings
- How to reduce your correction bolus

Setting up your correction boluses can be done only after your basal doses have been tested for accuracy. If your basal doses are set too high, using a correction bolus may lead to lows, while basal doses that are too low will make it appear that correction boluses are not the right amount to bring high readings down as expected.

When you first start on any new insulin doses, you want to be extra cautious. After taking a correction bolus, test your blood sugar each hour for 4 hours. Watch the trend in your readings and gradually you can make changes to avoid a low or a continuing high reading. Use Go Figure 13.3 to test the accuracy of a correction factor and Go Figure 13.4 to pick up the trend in a blood sugar that is dropping after a correction bolus.

A continuous monitoring device can be a great aid for reducing the number of high readings and the number of correction boluses, especially if it has a screen that allows you to see the recent trend in your readings to detect unexpected rises as well as falls. When you encounter a test result you don't expect, this screen can tell you whether your blood sugar is stable or going higher or lower. This can give you insight into the situation and help you determine the action you need to take to prevent a problem that may be pending.

An alarm on the continuous monitor will also warn when your blood sugar rises above a selected upper limit or drops below a certain lower limit. When a carb bolus is too small and is followed by a rapid rise in the blood sugar, a correction bolus can be taken as soon as the high is detected, taking into account the residual carb bolus insulin still left to act. The monitor then can be used to ensure that a low does not occur as the correction bolus takes effect.

13.1 The 1800 Rule* for mg/dl	
If your TDD is:	**Your Correction Factor is:**
15 units	120 mg/dl
20	90
25	72
30	60
35	51
40	45
45	40
50	36
55	33
60	30
70	26
80	23
90	20
100	18

*1800 divided by TDD = how far your BG will fall in mg/dl.

© 2003 Diabetes Services, Inc.

How To Determine Your Correction Factor

How many points your blood sugar will drop per unit of bolus insulin depends on your TDD. For instance, someone who uses 30 units of total insulin per day will find that she drops farther per unit, around 60 mg/dl (4.2 mmol) than someone who uses 100 units of insulin per day. The second person will find that his blood sugar drops only about 18 points (1 mmol) per unit of Humalog or Novolog. To lower the same high blood sugar, he will require a bolus three times as large as the first person.

The original rule by which point drops per unit were estimated was the 1500 Rule for Regular insulin developed by Paul Davidson, M.D. in Atlanta, Georgia.[60, 61] He created this rule based on his clinical experience with people with diabetes. We found that the number 1800[62] works better for Humalog and Novolog for most people than the original 1500 Rule. Recently, Dr. Davidson surveyed a large number of people on insulin pumps treated in his clinic who were in good control. He found that the number 1716 was the average for his patients and revised his rule to a 1700 Rule. We prefer 1800 because it works and gives a slightly smaller correction bolus when treating high readings.

Numbers between 1600 and 2200 can be used to determine the correction factor. The number 1800 should work when the TDD is set correctly and the basal insulin makes up 50% of the TDD in someone with Type 1 diabetes. A number smaller than 1800 will work better when basal insulin doses make up less than 50% of the TDD, while a number higher than 1800 works better for those whose basal doses make up more than 50% of their TDD. Also recheck your TDD and basal percentage to make sure they are correctly set.

The 1800 Rule:

- estimates the point drop in mg/dl per unit of Humalog or Novolog
- gives the point drop or correction factor by dividing 1800 by your TDD (total daily dose of insulin)
- 1800/TDD = point drop per unit of Novolog or Humalog (see Table 13.1)

This number provides an estimate for how many mg/dl or points your blood sugar will drop when you give one unit of Novolog or Humalog to counteract a high blood sugar.

Example:

Jack's TDD = 45 units

1800 / 45 u/day = a 40 mg/dl drop per unit of Novolog or Humalog

40 is Jack's correction factor

The accuracy of your correction factor, however, is only as good as the accuracy of your TDD. Once estimated, the correction factor must always be tested for accuracy. Table 10.2 provides a convenient way to estimate your carb and correction factors once your TDD has been determined. If the values from this table do not seem to work, reexamine whether your TDD is correct.

The 1800 Rule allows you to set up an accurate personal correction table or sliding scale to lower unwanted highs. For instance, in the example above Jack's blood sugar drops about 40 mg/dl (2.2 mmol) per unit. If his blood sugar before a meal is 260 mg/dl (14.4 mmol) and his premeal target blood sugar is 100 mg/dl (5.6 mmol), a 160 point drop (8.9 mmol) is desired. 160 points divided by 40 points per unit equals 4 units, so he takes a 4 unit correction bolus.

If his blood sugar falls to 100 mg/dl (5.6 mmol) 3.5 to 4 hours later, Jack knows that his correction factor is right. For convenience, Jack can then set up a personalized high blood sugar scale with various high readings along with how large a correction bolus will be needed to return his blood sugar to target. See Table 13.5 for a sample correction scale.

For those who use millimoles, the 1800 Rule can be conveniently replaced by the 100 Rule for millimoles in Table 13.2.

You can also determine your correction factor from your own experience. On three or four occasions, do not eat for 3.5 hours after you take a correction bolus. After 3.5 hours, divide how many mg/dl you drop by the number of units you took to correct the high reading. After checking in this way on several occasions and throwing out any result where you went too low, take the average of these results and use it as a correction factor unless these results vary greatly.

How To Test Your Correction Factor

The 1800 Rule gives you an estimated correction factor but you must test it for accuracy. Select premeal and postmeal blood sugar targets along with your correction factor with your physician's help, and then set up your personalized correction table. Keep in mind that a blood sugar target 2 hours after a meal will always be higher than your premeal target. For instance, targets of 100 mg/dl (5.6 mmol) before eating and 150 mg/dl (8.3 mmol) two hours after eating would be reasonable for many people.

Use Go Figure 13.3 to test your correction boluses and find out if your correction factor is working for you. Use these simple rules:

- With your physician's help, select a premeal target, usually between 90 mg/dl (5 mmol) and 140 mg/dl (7.8 mmol).
- If you use Humalog or Novolog, start your test whenever your blood sugar is above 200 mg/dl (11.1 mmol), provided it has been at least 3.5 hours since the last bolus was given, and at least 2 hours since food was eaten.
- Once you start the test, do not eat for 3.5 hours until the test is complete, unless, of course, your blood sugar goes low.
- Test your blood sugar often, at least once an hour, to catch and treat any low blood sugar that might occur.
- Repeat the test until a correction factor is found that brings your blood sugar to within 30 mg/dl (1.7 mmol) of your target on two consecutive tests without a low blood sugar.

With Regular insulin, the test can be started when a blood sugar is above 200 mg/dl (11.1 mmol) but at least 5 hours have passed since the last bolus was given. The test will be successful when the blood sugar is within 30 mg/dl 5 hours later with no low blood sugar and no eating.

If your correction factor for lowering your blood sugar to target differs significantly from the amount predicted in Table 13.1, your TDD may be incorrect or your basal insulin dose may be incorrect and need retesting. A good clue that your TDD is correct is that you rarely need to use a correction bolus and you have few low blood sugars.

13.2 The 100 Rule* for mmol	
TDD: Total Daily Insulin Dose	Correction Factor: 1 Unit Lowers BG by
15 units	6.7 mmol
20	5.0
25	4.0
30	3.3
35	2.9
40	2.5
45	2.2
50	2.0
55	1.8
60	1.7
70	1.4
80	1.3
90	1.1
100	1.0

*100 divided by TDD = how far your BG will fall in mmol

© 2003 Diabetes Services, Inc.

Go Figure 13.3: Test Your Correction Factor

Steps:

Start test when blood sugar is over 200 mg/dl (11.1 mmol) and you can wait 3.5 hours to eat.

1. Determine how many mg/dl (mmol) to drop by subtracting your target blood sugar from your current blood sugar.

2. Enter your correction factor from Table 14.1

3. Divide the mg/dl (mmol) you want to drop by your correction factor to get your correction bolus.

4. Take this correction bolus unless it seems to be wrong. Check your blood sugar each hour to see how it works.*

5. Does your correction factor work?

*Check more often if dropping quickly. Stop the test if your blood sugar does not come down or goes low.

(1) Determine how far you are above target:

_____ − _____ = _____ mg/dl
current BG   target BG   above target

(2) Your Correction factor

1u drops your BG _____ mg/dl

(3) Divide desired drop by your correction factor

_____ ÷ _____ = _____ units
mg/dl to drop   cor. factor   cor. bolus

(4) Check your blood sugars

Starting BG = _____ mg/dl

1 hr BG = _____ mg/dl

2 hr BG = _____ mg/dl

3 hr BG = _____ mg/dl

3.5 hr BG = _____ mg/dl

(5) Does your correction factor work?

After 3.5 hours, are you within 30 mg/dl (1.7 mmol) of your target?

No

I'm more than 30 mg/dl below my target or I went low

Eat fast carbs to raise your BG
Retest using a larger correction factor.
i.e, if it was 1u/40 mg/dl use 1 u/45 mg/dl

Yes

No

I'm more than 30 mg/dl above my target or I went high

Take extra correction bolus as needed.
Retest using a smaller correction factor.
i.e, if it was 1u/40 mg/dl, use 1 u/35 mg/dl

Your correction factor works.
Test again to verify.

To alert yourself to a rapid fall in blood sugar when a correction bolus is so large that it might result in a low, graph your blood sugar results each hour on Go Figure 13.4. If your blood sugar appears to be falling into the dark gray area, your bolus was too large and you will need to eat soon. If your blood sugar is headed into the light gray area, your correction bolus may be slightly too high and a snack may be needed. If you are headed toward the target area, the bolus appears to be correct.

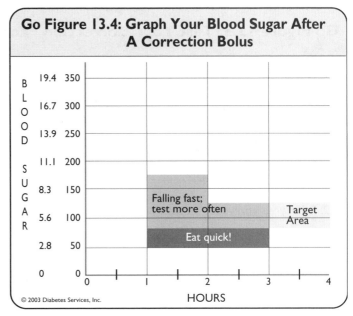

Go Figure 13.4: Graph Your Blood Sugar After A Correction Bolus

Falling fast; test more often

Eat quick!

Target Area

HOURS

© 2003 Diabetes Services, Inc.

Remember: BG targets after a meal are always higher than before a meal

Set Up Your Correction Scale To Lower High Readings

Once you have tested your correction factor and found it to be accurate, you can set up your own correction bolus scale for highs that occur before and after meals and at bedtime.

A sample correction bolus table is shown in Table 13.5. This person weighs 120 pounds and is in excellent control on 30 units of insulin a day, with 50% of her TDD as basal insulin. The scale was created after referring to Table 13.1 to determine that this person's blood sugar was likely to drop about 60 points per unit. This correction factor was tested twice to make sure it worked. With her physician's help, she selected her target blood sugar as 100 mg/dl (5.6 mmol) before meals and 160 mg/dl (10 mmol) two hours after meals. The correction table shows how much Humalog in half unit increments to take for a high blood sugar that occurs either before or after meals or at bedtime.

The size of the bolus you need to bring a high blood sugar down to target is determined by:

- How high your blood sugar is at the time
- What your selected target blood sugar is for that time of day (before or after a meal, bedtime, etc.)
- How many points your blood sugar drops per unit of insulin (correction factor)
- Whether any other bolus insulin is still active

Using Table 13.5 as an example, make your own personalized Correction Bolus Scale in Go Figure 13.6. Use Table 13.5 as an example, and Tables 13.7 and 13.9 to help you fill the values for your own correction factor. The most important thing to know is your correction factor. Once your basal doses have been correctly determined, your correction factor should be relatively consistent from meal to meal and from day to day. Your blood sugar target will vary, depending on when the blood sugar is measured relative to meals, bedtime, and prior boluses. For example, a target blood sugar of 90 to 120 mg/dl (5.0 to 6.7 mmol) might be ideal before meals, but would be too low two hours after eating and possibly too low at bedtime for someone who lives alone.

If the blood sugar is high at bedtime, a good rule of thumb for preventing nighttime lows is to take the correction bolus in the last column of Table 13.6 called "2 hours after meals and at bedtime" on

13.5 Sample Correction Bolus Scale

My blood sugar drops	My blood sugar targets are
__60__ mg/dl per unit of Humalog or Novolog	__100__ mg/dl before meals and __160__ mg/dl 2 hrs after meals

When my blood sugar is:	I will correct by giving:	
	before meals	2 hrs after meals or at bedtime
less than __130__ mg/dl*	no extra	no extra
__130__ to __159__ mg/dl	+0.5 units	no extra
__160__ to __189__ mg/dl	+1.0 units	no extra
__190__ to __219__ mg/dl	+1.5 units	+0.5 units
__220__ to __249__ mg/dl	+2.0 units	+1.0 units
__250__ to __279__ mg/dl	+2.5 units	+1.5 units
__280__ to __309__ mg/dl	+3.0 units	+2.0 units
__310__ to __339__ mg/dl	+3.5 units	+2.5 units
__340__ to __369__ mg/dl	+4.0 units	+3.0 units

* Though 100 mg/dl is the target, 130 mg/dl is used here because it is hard to give less than 0.5 units as a bolus.
© 2003 Diabetes Services, Inc.

your correction scale. A reduction in the correction bolus at bedtime helps eliminate night lows and provides for safer sleeping. Of course, if the morning blood sugar is always high after you have reduced your bedtime correction bolus, you can try increasing the bedtime correction bolus by a small amount. Set an alarm to test at 2 a.m. to avoid a possible low.

Do not use the 1800 Rule to lower a high blood sugar:

- before discussing it with your physician
- if your high readings often come down on their own
- if you are having frequent or severe low blood sugars
- when the extra insulin of a correction bolus is not needed
- if correction boluses don't work for you
- if it's only two hours after your meal and you took your carb bolus late

Correction boluses from your correction bolus scale should work in most circumstances, except when more insulin is required as outlined in Text Aid 13.8, or when a smaller bolus is required because of exercise or extra physical activity. If your high blood sugars come down to your target on their own without a correction bolus, you would not need to start using one to lower highs. If your high blood sugars come down on their own, you may have some insulin production of your own, or your insulin doses are set too high.

Go Figure 13.6: My Correction Bolus Scale

Find your correction factor in Table 13.1 and set up a personalized correction bolus scale below using different targets for your blood sugar before and after meals. Sample targets might be 100 mg/dl (5.6 mmol) before meals and 180 mg/dl (10 mmol) two hours after meals.

My blood sugar drops _____ mg/dl per unit of Humalog or Novolog	My blood sugar targets are _____ mg/dl before meals and _____ mg/dl 2 hrs after meals

When my blood sugar is:	**I will correct by giving:**	
	before meals	**2 hrs after meals or at bedtime**
less than _____ mg/dl* ▶	no extra	no extra
_____ to _____ mg/dl	+ ___ units	no extra
_____ to _____ mg/dl	+ ___ units	no extra
_____ to _____ mg/dl	+ ___ units	+ ___ units
_____ to _____ mg/dl ▶	+ ___ units	+ ___ units
_____ to _____ mg/dl	+ ___ units	+ ___ units
_____ to _____ mg/dl	+ ___ units	+ ___ units
_____ to _____ mg/dl ▶	+ ___ units	+ ___ units
_____ to _____ mg/dl	+ ___ units	+ ___ units

* This is your before meal blood sugar target.   © 2003 Diabetes Services, Inc.

When To Combine A Correction Bolus And Meal Bolus

When a high reading occurs before a meal, a convenient way to bring it down quickly is to combine and inject your correction bolus and your carb bolus for the meal, but then wait to eat if possible until your blood sugar is below 150 mg/dl. This reduces the time you spend at an elevated reading, but does require that you do not delay eating too long and let your blood sugar go low.

Experience provided by keeping complete records becomes a great guide for knowing when to add a correction bolus between meals. If you forgot a meal bolus before eating but take it just after eating, you can probably ignore a blood sugar of 200 or 300 mg/dl (11.1 to 16.7 mmol) one or two hours later because the blood sugar is likely to return to target as the delayed bolus begins to take effect. You also might skip a correction bolus when a blood sugar is 200 or 300 mg/dl (11 mmol or 16.6 mmol) two hours after a meal if it was higher than this before the meal and you have already given a correction bolus. For instance, if your reading is 250 mg/dl (13.9

mmol) two hours after a meal but it had been 350 mg/dl (19.4 mmol) before the meal when you took a correction bolus, your blood sugar is already beginning to drop because of your correction bolus.

Following a meal, the blood sugar normally rises 40 to 60 mg/dl (2.2 mmol to 3.3 mmol). In this example, it has already fallen 100 mg/dl (5.6 mmol) for an actual drop of at least 140 mg/dl (7.8 mmol) in just two hours. The drop of 140 is 100 from the 350 to 250 and 40 because ordinarily the blood sugar would be about 40 higher. No additional insulin is likely to be needed in this situation despite the still-elevated reading. The Unused Bolus Rule, covered in the next chapter, would be helpful to use in a situation like this where boluses overlap.

In most circumstances, when a blood sugar of 200 or 300 mg/dl (11 mmol or 16.6 mmol) occurs

13.7 Correction Boluses For Highs

Add this many units to the meal dose ↓	If your blood sugar drops this many mg/dl per unit of Humalog or Novolog:				
	150	120	100	80	60
	And your before meal blood sugar is:				
0.5	175	160	150	140	130
1.0	250	220	200	180	160
1.5	325	280	250	220	190
2.0	400*	340	300	260	220
2.5	475*	400*	350	300	250
3.0		460*	400*	340	280
3.5			450*	380	310
4.0			500*	420*	340
4.5				460*	370
5.0				500*	400*

* If there is not a clear reason for your blood sugar to be this high, call your physician.

13.8 A Postmeal Situation To Be Careful About

Suppose you entirely forget your carb bolus for a meal and when you check your blood sugar two hours later, you find it is very high. In this situation, many people would take their forgotten carb bolus and also take a correction bolus to bring down the high blood sugar.

Do not do this! Although your blood sugar is high because the carb bolus was forgotten, the carbs from the meal have already been digested and no insulin is needed to cover them. Only a correction bolus in needed at this point to bring down the high blood sugar created by the uncovered carbs.

However, because no carb bolus was taken, you would use your premeal target blood sugar to calculate the correction bolus and not your higher postmeal target. For instance, if Michelle forgets her carb bolus for the 60 grams of carbohydrate she ate at lunch and her reading two hours later is 340 mg/dl, she would subtract her premeal target of 100 mg/dl from 340, and divide these 240 mg/dl by her correction factor to obtain the correction bolus she needs.

two to three hours after a meal, the blood sugar will not return to normal unless a correction bolus is taken. It is important to know what your own blood sugar does in this situation at different times of the day and to have an individualized correction bolus table to guide you in taking the correct dose. As with all insulin doses, get personal guidance from your physician/health care team to ensure that your correction boluses are accurate.

What About Frequent Highs?

Correction boluses are intended to be used to correct an occasional high blood sugar. If correction boluses are needed every day or several times a day, this suggests that your TDD may be too low. In children, a rise in the need for insulin may be caused by growth or the surge of hormones that occurs during puberty. Both adults and children will require extra insulin when weight is increased, activity is reduced, or stress is increased. Whatever the reason, if the need for correction boluses become frequent, your TDD will need to be raised to regain control. Chapter 15 suggests guidelines for when and how much your TDD should be changed.

In your charts or logbook, look for the time or times of the day when you are giving correction boluses. If high readings occur throughout the day, split the increase in your TDD evenly between your basal doses and carb boluses. If highs typically occur before breakfast, the night basal will likely be the dose that needs to be raised. If dinner readings are usually the culprit, try raising the basal insulin at work in the afternoon or increase the carb bolus at lunch.

13.9 Correction Boluses For Highs

Add this many units to the meal dose ↓	If your blood sugar drops this many mg/dl per unit of Humalog or Novolog:					
	50	40	30	25	20	10
	And your before meal blood sugar is:					
1.0	150	140	130	125	120	110
2.0	200	180	160	150	140	120
3.0	250	220	190	175	160	130
4.0	300	260	220	200	180	140
5.0	350	300	250	225	200	150
6.0	400*	340	280	250	220	160
7.0	450*	380	310	275	240	170
8.0	500*	420*	340	300	260	180
9.0		460*	370	325	280	190
10.0		500*	400*	350	300	200
12.0				400*	340	220
14.0				450*	380	240

* If there is not a clear reason for your blood sugar to be this high, call your physician.

If you find that you need to frequently use a correction bolus to lower high readings caused by overtreating lows, reducing your TDD will be more appropriate than raising it, because excess insulin is the source for the lows. Once these lows are eliminated, many highs will disappear as well with less need for correction boluses.

> ## 13.10 Cautions About Treating High Readings
>
> When correcting high blood sugars, always take into account other recent boluses that may still be working. If you have insulin still active from a recent bolus, take this unused bolus insulin into account when you determine a correction bolus by using the Unused Bolus Rule found in Chapter 14.
>
> When your meter reads above 360 mg/dl (20 mmol), its accuracy becomes more and more suspect. If your actual blood sugar is 400 mg/dl (28.6 mmol), even the best meters can be no more accurate than somewhere between 360 (20.0 mmol) and 440 mg/dl (31.4 mmol). Be careful when giving correction boluses for very high blood sugars because your meter is not as accurate at these high readings.

How To Reduce Correction Boluses

When first using a correction factor, add 5 or 10 mg/dl (0.3 to 0.5 mmol) to your calculated factor for safety. For example, if you calculate your correction factor as 40 or one unit of rapid insulin should lower your blood sugar by 40 mg/dl (2.2 mmol), try using 45 or 50 at first to reduce the size of your correction boluses. If this causes your blood sugar to remains higher than your target, then you can try using the original correction number of 40. It is better to err at first on the side of safety. As you use a correction factor more frequently, you will be able to reach your target more easily and establish your correction boluses more accurately.

> ## 13.11 The Zero to 60 Guide For Correction Boluses
>
> When your blood sugar goes low after a correction bolus, keep the Zero to 60 Guide in mind. After taking a bolus at time zero, the time it takes to reach 60 mg/dl (3.3 mmol) tells you how excessive your bolus was. If you are below 60 mg/dl an hour later, your bolus was far too large, but if you reach 60 mg/dl 3 1/2 or 4 hours later, your correction bolus was close to what you needed.
>
>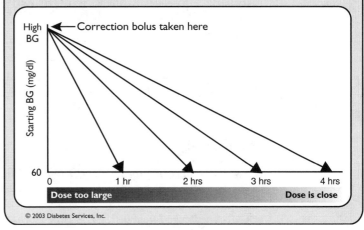
>
> © 2003 Diabetes Services, Inc.

Correction Dose Tips

• A properly set correction bolus allows you to bring down high blood sugars to within 30 mg/dl (1.7 mmol) of your target blood sugar after four hours with Novolog or Humalog insulins or after six hours with Regular.

• The mg/dl or mmol that your blood sugar drops per unit of insulin will generally be stable at breakfast, lunch and dinner. If your correction factor varies at different times of the day, retest your basal doses to be sure they are correctly set.

13.12 What If Your Blood Sugar Doesn't Come Down?

Not all high blood sugars are equal. For instance, in the presence of a bacterial infection, much more insulin than usual is needed to bring down a high blood sugar.

If your correction factor normally works well but now is not working as expected, consider these possible causes:

• you forgot to take your last carb bolus
• you forgot your last basal dose
• your basal doses or TDD needs to be raised
• your blood sugar has been high for several hours
• your meter reading is somewhere over 360 mg/dl (20 mmol) but your blood sugar may actually be much higher due to loss of meter accuracy when the blood sugar is very high
• you are in ketosis
• you are experiencing physical or emotional stress
• you have a bacterial infection
• your insulin is bad

• Factors such as an extremely high blood sugar, ketoacidosis, infection, increased weight, or less activity can reduce how many points the blood sugar will drop per unit and cause more insulin to be needed to bring down a high blood sugar.

• Loss of weight or increase in activity lowers your TDD and causes your blood sugar to fall farther per unit of insulin.

• When an unexpected high blood sugar occurs, think about what may be causing it to rise. If illness, pain, or bad insulin is causing the problem, you may require a larger correction bolus.

• If your high blood sugars often do not drop to your target, you may need a larger TDD and smaller correction factor.

• If your high blood sugars frequently drop below your target, you may need a smaller TDD and larger correction factor. Recalculate your TDD and raise both your basal insulin and carb boluses appropriately.

• Use extra caution when correcting a high blood sugar near bedtime. Consider reducing the correction bolus to half its normal amount.

Your correction factor should bring down a high blood sugar to target over 3 1/2 to 4 hours with Humalog or Novolog insulin.

Quick Check: Do your correction boluses make up less than 10% of your TDD?

The Unused Bolus Rule

CHAPTER
14

A great advantage of frequent injections is giving small, precise doses of insulin at any time that a need arises. In doing this, however, injections can begin to overlap in their action. For example, a carb bolus can be given for dinner, another for an unplanned dessert, and then a correction bolus for a high blood sugar that follows. This can create confusion about how much residual bolus insulin remains active when the next injection is given.

Determining how much insulin from earlier boluses is still working can tell you if a correction bolus is really needed. Remember that Humalog and Novolog continue to lower the blood sugar for about four hours after an injection, and Regular does so for about six hours. Allowing for this long action can prevent overdosing and the unnecessary low blood sugar that follows.

When another bolus is needed within four hours of the last bolus, any unused bolus insulin must be taken into account. When several boluses have been given during the evening hours, it is especially important to interpret the bedtime blood sugar in light of how much insulin is remaining. A normal blood sugar at bedtime may be dangerous if you have a large residual dose still left to work. You may need a bedtime snack larger than usual. A high reading at bedtime will require no correction bolus if there is sufficient residual insulin still working to bring it down.

This chapter explains:

- The unused bolus rule
- How to determine the amount of insulin or carbohydrate needed in situations where recent injections are still active
- How to use the unused bolus tables
- How to use the unused bolus rule with the correction scale

What Is The Unused Bolus Rule?

The Unused Bolus Rule[63] helps when you have a high blood sugar and you need to decide whether more insulin or more carbohydrate is needed. Keep in mind that you should never assume you need more insulin simply because your blood sugar is high at the moment. Always determine how much unused bolus insulin remains to work before taking more. If your blood sugar is currently normal, you may need to decide if carbohydrate is required because your blood sugar will drop lower if you have unused bolus insulin still at work.

The Unused Bolus Rule:

- shows how much insulin from recent boluses remains to work,
- provides a good estimate for how much additional insulin may be needed to lower a high blood sugar, and
- warns when carbs may be needed soon despite a current normal or high blood sugar because there is an excess of bolus insulin still active.

The Unused Bolus Rule For Humalog And Novolog:

25% of any bolus is used each hour after it is given

Humalog and Novolog start working about 15 minutes after they are given, peak in activity in one and a half to two hours, and are no longer lowering the blood sugar after four hours.

The Unused Bolus Rule For Regular:

16% of any bolus is used each hour after it is given

Regular insulin starts working a half hour after the injection, peaks two to three hours later, and stops dropping the blood sugar after six hours.

Determine Unused Bolus Insulin

Table 14.1 for Humalog and Novolog and Table 14.2 for Regular provide an easy way to determine how much unused bolus insulin remains at hourly intervals after a carb or correction bolus. Be sure to discuss the use of these tables with your physician. Once you take a bolus, testing your blood sugar over the next few hours is the best way to determine its effect, since a variety of factors can influence your blood sugar.

With Novolog or Humalog insulin, it is wise to avoid taking correction boluses more often than

14.1 Unused Bolus - Humalog/Novolog

Insulin acticity that remains at 1, 2, 3, and 4 hours after a carb or correction bolus of Humalog or Novolog insulin.

Original Bolus Amount	Units Of Humalog Left After:			
	1 hr	2 hrs	3 hrs	4 hrs
1 unit	0.75	0.50	0.25	0
2 units	1.50	1.00	0.50	0
3 units	2.25	1.50	0.75	0
4 units	3.00	2.00	1.00	0
5 units	3.75	2.50	1.25	0
6 units	4.50	3.00	1.50	0
7 units	5.25	3.50	1.75	0
8 units	6.00	4.00	2.00	0
9 units	6.75	4.50	2.25	0
10 units	7.50	5.00	2.50	0

every two hours. At least two hours are required to get a good idea of what the last bolus is doing. If you feel you have to take carb or correction boluses less than two hours apart, check your blood sugar more often to keep track of how the unused bolus insulin is working. If you see you are reaching normal too quickly, you know a low blood sugar is likely to follow.

A blood sugar taken only an hour after a bolus may provide some information about that bolus, but it is best to wait at least two hours to get a better idea of what it is doing (three hours for Regular). When extra insulin is taken too soon after a meal, it is easy to misjudge how much is needed. This can cause an excess accumulation of insulin, complicate your unused insulin calculations, and make hypoglycemia more likely.

14.2 Unused Bolus - Regular

Insulin activity that remains at 1, 2, 3, 4, 5, and 6 hours after a carb or correction bolus of Regular Insulin.

Original Bolus Amount	Units Of Regular Left After:					
	1 hr	2 hrs	3 hrs	4 hrs	5 hrs	6 hrs
1 unit	0.8	0.7	0.5	0.3	0.2	0
2 units	1.7	1.3	1.0	0.7	0.3	0
3 units	2.5	2.0	1.5	1.0	0.5	0
4 units	3.3	2.7	2.0	1.3	0.7	0
5 units	4.2	3.3	2.5	1.7	0.8	0
6 units	5.0	4.0	3.0	2.0	1.0	0
7 units	5.8	4.7	3.5	2.3	1.2	0
8 units	6.7	5.3	4.0	2.7	1.3	0
9 units	7.5	6.0	4.5	3.0	1.5	0
10 units	8.3	6.7	5.0	3.3	1.7	0

In certain circumstances, such as when giving a correction bolus at bedtime, taking less than the full coverage recommended by your correction factor for a high blood sugar may be desired. Anyone who has hypoglycemia unawareness, a history of frequent lows, lives alone, or for any other reason wants to lessen the risk of a low caused by correcting a high blood sugar will want to reduce the correction bolus. This can be done by raising the correction factor by 10, 20, or 30 mg/dl (0.5, 1.0 or 1.5 mmol) to lessen the amount of insulin that will be given. Another simple way to do this is to calculate the correction bolus using your correction factor, and then reducing the dose by 1 or 2 units, or simply cutting the dose in half.

The Unused Bolus Rule And The Correction Scale

When you estimate how much bolus insulin may be needed to lower a high blood sugar two hours after a meal using the correction scale from Chapter 13 and the unused bolus rule described in this chapter, discrepancies between the two doses are likely to occur.

Randall

Randall's blood sugar meter reads "High", meaning that he is somewhere above the maximum of 450 mg/dl (25 mmol) on his meter. He realizes that he forgot to cover several slices of pizza with an injection. A blood test for ketones on his Precision Xtra meter shows that none are present. Randall's TDD is 45 units a day, so his correction factor is 1 unit of Humalog for every 40 mg/dl (2.2 mmol) above his target blood sugar of 100 mg/dl (5.6 mmol). Because he never took a bolus for his pizza.he will use his premeal target of 100 mg/dl rather than his post-meal target of 150 mg/dl. A premeal target is always used when there is no bolus insulin that is active.

Unsure of his exact blood sugar, he takes 9 units of Humalog to bring down the high reading approximately 360 mg/dl (40 x 9). Two hours later, he rechecks his blood sugar and finds it is now 380 mg/dl (21.1 mmol). Does he need to take another correction bolus?

Using Table 14.1, he finds that of the 9 units he took, 50 percent is now gone after 2 hours, leaving 50% or 4.5 units of insulin still to work. Knowing his blood sugar drops 40 points per unit, he estimates that this 4.5 units of unused bolus insulin will lower his blood sugar:

4.5 units times 40 mg/dl per unit = 180 mg/dl (10 mmol) left to drop

From his current blood sugar of 380 mg/dl (21.1 mmol), Randall should come down another 180 mg/dl. This means his blood sugar will be near 200 mg/dl (11.1 mmol) in another hour and a half when the last of the 9 unit bolus is used up.

This tells him he will need another correction bolus to finish correcting his high blood sugar. To reach a target of 100 mg/dl by dropping the additional 100 mg/dl (5.6 mmol) from his current reading, he will need:

100 mg/dl left to fall ÷ 40 points per unit = 2.5 more units of insulin

Randall can now make an informed decision. If he has at least 3 hours until bedtime, he could take 2 or 2.5 units (visually estimating the half unit) as a safe choice. If it is closer to bedtime, he could use 1 or 1.5 units. This would get him close to his target, while lessening the risk of a nighttime low.

The unused bolus rule tends to be more conservative than the correction factor and scale. The correction factor and scale only look at how high the blood sugar is and how much insulin it takes to drop it to target and assume that no insulin from previous boluses is still active. On the other hand, the unused bolus rule considers how much residual insulin remains to work, so it will usually provide a lower estimate for the amount of additional insulin that is needed. It is purposely conservative to lessen the risk of hypoglycemia caused when a high blood sugar is chased with too much insulin.

If there is a conflict between a correction bolus recommended by the unused bolus rule and another recommended by the difference between your target and actual blood sugar two hours after a meal, decide on a dose only after weighing all the factors that may be affecting your blood sugar. If in doubt, always use the smaller estimated bolus. The unused bolus rule will usually recommend a smaller correction bolus than the postmeal correction scale. A slightly high reading is preferred over a debilitating low.

Tips On The Unused Bolus Rule

- Be conservative when giving extra insulin, especially before bedtime. Take less insulin than usual if you are not going to be awake four hours later. If you must go to sleep, set an alarm so you can test your blood sugar again at least three hours after the last bolus of the day was given.
- Try not to take carb and correction boluses more often than every two hours unless there is a clear reason to do so. It takes at least two hours to get an indication of the effect of the last bolus.
- Always determine how much unused bolus is still active when you test two hours after you eat. What appears to be a high reading may resolve itself before the next meal once the residual insulin has acted.
- If the unused bolus rule and your postmeal correction scale give different estimates for how much insulin you should take, use the one that recommends the smaller bolus.

The unused bolus rule is accurate only if you use a basal and bolus approach to your insulin doses, and your TDD, basals, and carb and correction boluses have been accurately set.

"There's a deception to every rule."
Hal Lee Luyah

Loren

Loren goes out for breakfast at a new restaurant. After ordering pancakes and fruit, she checks and finds that her blood sugar is normal. She delays taking her carb bolus until the food arrives in order to better estimate how many carbohydrates it contains. When her plate arrives, she estimates 100 grams of carbohydrate and takes 9 units of Humalog to cover them. (Her TDD is 45 units, and she uses 1 H for each 11 carb grams.)

Two hours later she rechecks her blood sugar to find it is now 200 mg/dl (11.1 mmol). She knows her blood sugar drops 40 points per unit of Humalog. Does she need to do anything to correct her high blood sugar? To find out, let's determine how many of the 9 units she took for breakfast are still lowering her blood sugar. After 2 hours, 60% of the 9 units are gone (30 percent times 2 hours), leaving 40% of the meal bolus remaining to work. Table 15.1 shows that 9 units times 0.4 equals 3.6 units remaining to work.

Loren multiplies 3.6 units times her drop of 40 mg/dl (2.2 mmol) per unit to find that she is likely to drop another 144 points. By the time her breakfast bolus is finished, her blood sugar should be 200 minus 144 mg/dl or 56 mg/dl (3.1 mmol).

This tells Loren that her high blood sugar will likely come down without any additional insulin, and that she may need to eat additional carbohydrate to avoid a low blood sugar before lunch. She decides to recheck her blood sugar 60 minutes later to clarify whether this is happening.

Loren has encountered a common problem when eating out. Because she was unsure how many carbs would be on her breakfast plate and exactly when the food would be served, she delayed her injection until the food arrived. This caused her postmeal blood sugar to rise higher than her desired target of 140 to 150 mg/dl (7.8 to 8.3 mmol) two hours after the meal. The carb-rich breakfast and the delay in her bolus raised her blood sugar even though she had taken an adequate or slightly excessive bolus for it.

One way to handle high-carb restaurant meals is to lead the meal by taking half of the estimated bolus a half hour before the meal. The rest of the dose can be taken after the meal arrives and the true carb count is known. Keep glucose tablets handy in case you overestimate the carbs in the meal or eating is delayed.

"Beware of the young doctor and the old barber."
Benjamin Franklin

When Your TDD Needs To Change

Any time you experience control problems that are not remedied by small changes in your carbs or carb boluses, recheck your TDD or total daily dose of insulin. As your life changes, your TDD may need to change as well.

The most reliable sign that your TDD needs to be changed is that you are having frequent high or low blood sugars. A consistent pattern of frequent highs or lows or both tells you that your TDD needs to be adjusted.

This chapter explains:

- When to consider a change in your TDD
- Some of the common and not so common reasons for needing to change your TDD

As soon as your control becomes a problem, look carefully for what may be causing it. If you have been guessing at the carbs in your meals, your control will improve with a simple reckoning of your carbs and calculating the appropriate carb boluses to cover them. If you require correction boluses for high blood sugar several times a day or are gaining weight because you are eating often to correct low readings, your TDD needs to be adjusted.

Try to determine first whether your primary problem is too many highs or too many lows. If you are almost always high, your TDD likely needs to go up. Keep in mind, however, that frequent highs may be a result of overeating to correct frequent lows or of eating excess carbs in an attempt to avoid lows. Under these circumstances, raising your TDD would only worsen the problem. Instead, a lower TDD may be needed to solve the basic problem of too many lows.

Your TDD needs to be raised when many highs are occurring and lowered when frequent lows begin. Generally, the TDD is adjusted by 5% to 10% at a time. For example, if you rarely experience lows but often have readings in the upper 100's and low 200's, a 5% increase in your TDD is appropriate. However, if your readings are more often in the 200's and 300's, a 10% increase may be needed. If you have concerns that a 10% increase is too large, simply increase your TDD by 5% and give this a few days to see how your blood sugar responds. If your readings are still high after 3 to 7 days, increase by another 5%.

Frequent lows almost always indicate that your TDD needs to be lowered. A good way to solve this problem is to determine your current TDD and reduce it by 10% using Go Figure 10.1b.

Once you know your new TDD, go back to Go Figure 10.1c, and recalculate your bolus and basal insulin doses using the new TDD. Be sure to test your new basal insulin doses and bolus insulin doses before relying on them completely.

Keep in mind that rapid and massive changes in your insulin doses and TDD may occasionally be needed. For instance, if you develop a bacterial pneumonia, your blood sugar will rise rapidly, and you will need to double or even triple your TDD in the space of a few days. Once an antibiotic has been started, insulin requirements will drop again to normal over a period of two to seven days. In this instance, where the blood sugar and insulin doses change rapidly because of other physical changes, raise the bolus insulin doses first and follow this in a day or two by raising the basal doses if the blood sugar remains high. See Table 10.4 for estimated TDD insulin doses dependant on your type of diabetes, weight, levels of fitness and stress, and special conditions.

Reasons To Adjust Your TDD

Many situations may make it necessary for you to change your TDD as well as your bolus and basal insulin doses. Some require that insulin doses be increased gradually over time, such as during a child's growth spurts or during a pregnancy. Others, like an infection or the use of a steroid prescription, may require an immediate and large increase in TDD. Some situations that affect your TDD may be very gradual and not obvious. A few of the more common situations are discussed here.

A change in activity

Physical activity and physical fitness have a great impact on your sensitivity to insulin. A marathon runner, for example, may need only half as much insulin circulating in the blood as a person of the same weight who does not exercise. Less insulin is required as a result of a marked increase in sensitivity to insulin from physical training. Whenever someone moves to a higher fitness level, a reduction in TDD is required. See Table 10.4.

For example, if you work as a moderately active flight attendant but are starting a vacation bicycling for two weeks in Europe, lower your TDD. Plan on just the opposite if your vacation will be spent seeing plays in New York. If you previously worked as a framer on a construction crew but have been promoted to a desk job as a project cost estimator, the reduction in physical activity will increase your need for insulin unless you substitute more exercise for your reduced activity at work.

Weight change

Your bathroom scale serves as a clear gauge for adjusting your TDD. When you increase your weight, you need more insulin. If your weight drops, your TDD will need to be lowered.

The speed of the weight change mirrors how quickly to change your insulin. When swimsuit season is suddenly upon you, or you decide at the last moment to attend your high school reunion, or out-of-town relatives call to tell you they'll be visiting next month, weight-panic often sets in. Where did those extra pounds come from and how can they be shed quickly? You may reduce eating immediately in an effort to bring about a quick image change.

This type of weight loss is not recommended, but if you are determined to lose weight in this manner, be aware that your TDD will also need a rapid reduction and rebalancing. You may find you need to reduce your TDD by 10% to 30% if you suddenly restrict calorie intake. You will need to lower your basal doses and raise your carb factor with the reduced carb intake and increased sensitivity to insulin as your weight goes down.

How much weight is lost or gained is also important. A gradual weight change of 5 pounds or less may have little effect on your TDD, but if your weight change is more than 5 pounds, an adjustment in your TDD likely will be needed. See Table 10.4.

A change in weather, season, or altitude

With the warmer weather and longer days of spring and summer, people often need less insulin. Most people are more active during this time and eat less fat which allows insulin to work better. Also, more energy may be required for cooling the body in hot weather. Warm weather, along with a higher percentage of carb intake during the summer, often necessitates a lower TDD.

Just the opposite happens with the approach of winter. Most people need more insulin unless they are outside during very cold weather and use more energy by shivering to stay warm. In general, most people eat more fat when the weather is cold, and they exercise less. A higher TDD is often required.

At high altitudes, more energy is needed to breath and pump blood because the air is thinner. Until your body acclimates to the altitude change, which usually takes a few days, less TDD or more carbohydrate may be required. When you return to a lower altitude, more insulin or less carbs may be needed.

Menstrual periods

Many women find their blood sugar rises in the days just before their menstrual period begins and they require a substantial increase in basal dose and carb bolus coverage for the few days prior to their period. The extra insulin may lessen premenstrual symptoms as well as improve blood sugar control. The need for the increase may occur gradually over these days, but the need for insulin quickly returns to normal, usually on the first day of the period. Insulin doses then need to be abruptly lowered to their usual levels. Some women need rapid, large adjustments in their basal and bolus doses during these changes to avoid very high or very low blood sugars.

Illness

Illnesses place extra stress on the body and causes more resistance to insulin. A higher TDD with both higher bolus and basal doses is often needed to counteract the physical stress of illness. See Table 10.4. Especially stressful are bacterial infections like pneumonia, strep throat, an impacted wisdom tooth, a bladder infection, or a sinus infection. These infections can cause the need for insulin to double or triple due to stress combined with the release of inflammatory particles, like tumor necrosis factor and cytokines, that cause resistance to insulin. After an antibiotic has been started, however, any temporary increase in basal insulin or bolus insulin will need to be reduced quickly to prevent a low blood sugar.

Shorter viral illnesses, like a cold or flu, have a more varied and milder effect on the blood sugar. Control during short-term viral illnesses may be achieved by increasing carb boluses and using additional high blood sugar boluses as needed rather than by raising the basal dose. When you are ill, higher boluses may be needed for meals even though your intake of carbs is reduced. Illnesses that last several weeks, like hepatitis and mononucleosis, often require an increase in the basal dose. You will want to test your blood sugar frequently to determine how much extra insulin you require.

Illnesses that cause vomiting or diarrhea may mean you cannot eat. If this occurs, you do not need carb boluses, but you still need your basal insulin. Correct any highs as needed. Be sure to test your blood sugar more often or have someone else test it during any illness. If your blood sugar is high and has been for a while, test for ketones and be sure to drink plenty of liquids.

Always keep in mind that a severe illness can cause ketoacidosis, which has the same symptoms as bad insulin or skipping insulin doses. Always check blood sugar and ketone levels frequently whenever nausea or vomiting occur. Never fall asleep before getting assistance if you have ketones present in your urine or blood, and, of course, never fall asleep before checking. Vomiting and ketones in the blood or urine require a visit to the nearest emergency room immediately. Prepare for this now because you and your caregiver need to be ready to take action at once as soon as this occurs.

Stress

People and their blood sugars respond differently to stress. Mild emotions and excitement may lower the blood sugar. The activity and "nervous energy" that comes with it will often lower the blood sugar. However, moderate or higher levels of stress usually raise the blood sugar. Stress may not be obvious until it has already raised the blood sugar. When this happens, a correction bolus would be used to bring down the high blood sugar, similar to a high caused by excess carbs. Stress may also change eating patterns with either more or fewer carbs being eaten.

If you anticipate only a short period of stress, such as a day of tension-filled business meetings, check your blood sugar often and take extra Novolog or Huma-log if it goes high. If you are going through a long stressful period, such as having a

Amy

Amy has Type 1 diabetes and plays softball in a local league. Though small in size and with hits that rarely make it out of the infield, she is fast, has an accurate throw, and her teammates love her defiant attitude. She has played almost every game through the summer. When the softball season ended, she noticed her blood sugar readings began to climb. By late September, her daytime readings were 50 to 60 mg/dl (2.8 to 3.3 mmol) higher than they had been during the season.

The previous spring, her doctor had helped her reduce her doses and had mentioned that she would need to raise them again after the season ended. He had said that she could probably do this on her own when the time came and the increase in her doses would likely be only a couple of units.

Amy's doses during the summer were 1 unit of Humalog for every 28 grams of carbohydrate and, when she was high, 1 extra H for every 120 mg/dl (6.7 mmol) over her goal of 100 mg/dl (5.6 mmol) before meals. At bedtime, she takes 9 units of Lantus as her basal insulin. Though her insulin doses are small, she gives fractions of units by using a Terumo 25 unit syringe that has half-unit markings and by eyeballing her doses carefully.

Amy noticed in September that her blood sugar was rising about 30 mg/dl (1.7 mmol) overnight, so she knew that her dose of Lantus had to be raised. An increase from 9 units to 9.5 units seemed safe, so she did this first. After six days, her blood sugars were still rising slightly during the night, so she increased the Lantus 10 units at bedtime. Within four days, she could tell her overnight blood sugars were now staying relatively flat, but her blood sugars were still spiking after meals.

To reduce her after meal spikes, she lowered her carb number from 28 to 26 to increase her insulin dose slightly for each meal. This helped, but not enough. After another week she again lowered it, this time to 1 unit for every 25 grams of carb. Now two hours after meals she was closer to the target of 150 mg/dl that her doctor had suggested.

In a little over three weeks of gradual changes, Amy got her blood sugars back into control with a rise in her TDD of about 2 units (8.3 mmol). More importantly, she was able to do it on her own.

family member in the hospital, consider raising your TDD, especially your basal insulin, to help your control and coping skills. See Table 10.4. When possible, maintain or increase your exercise during periods of stress and resist changing your eating habits. This lessens the impact that stress would otherwise have.

Medications

Certain drugs will cause a mild rise in the blood sugar, while a few can greatly increase the need for insulin. The ones that raise the blood sugar the highest are steroids like prednisone and cortisone. These may be prescribed orally for poison ivy, for allergic reactions to medications, and for illnesses such as lupus, asthma, or arthritis. Use of a steroid will make your insulin need rise quickly and sharply. One of us with diabetes got a severe case of poison oak while clearing fire brush out of a field and required prednisone tablets for a few days. To control the high blood sugar reading caused by the prednisone, all insulin doses were increased. Bolus doses four to five times larger than normal were required to offset the effect of the prednisone. See Table 10.4.

Older steroid medications that are injected into a joint to treat arthritis or injury would usually increase insulin need for three to five days. However, newer injectable steroids are longer lasting and when placed into a joint can raise insulin requirements dramatically for one to three weeks. Oral steroids also increase insulin requirements during the time they are being used. When only a short course of steroid is required, such as for poison ivy, the dose of the medication is tapered off gradually over a few days with the need for extra insulin gradually disappearing some three to five days after the last pill is taken.

A physician who prescribes oral or injected steroids for medical problems may not be aware of how dramatically they can raise blood sugar levels. If you require steroids, make sure the physician prescribing them is aware of your diabetes so that your diabetes team can be notified. You can then work with your diabetes physician/health care team to make the insulin adjustments that will be needed.

Other medications will lower the blood sugar. For instance, antibiotics of the quinalone class, especially Tequin (gatifloxacin), can cause severe hypoglycemia when taken by someone using a sulfonylurea such as glyburide or glibenclamide to treat Type 2 diabetes.[64]

Thyroid disease

Thyroid disease occurs fairly often in people with Type 1 or Type 2 diabetes. It occurs with Type 2 because both thyroid disease and Type 2 diabetes become more common as we age. In fact, one out of every 10 women over the age of 65 has thyroid disease. It occurs with Type 1 diabetes because Type 1 and some forms of thyroid disease can both result from an autoimmune attack on hormone-producing glands.

Thyroid disease occurs gradually over a period of weeks or months. It may begin as a release of too much thyroid hormone, then gradually change to too little. The blood sugar may go higher with an overactive thyroid and lower with an underactive thyroid. Because thyroid disease occurs gradually, the reason for the loss of blood sugar control is often difficult to identify. If your blood sugar control seems to have changed and you have thyroid symptoms such as nervousness, tiredness, sleeping difficulties, or feeling hot or cold, have your thyroid checked.

If you have a low thyroid level and are placed on thyroid medication, you will probably need to raise your insulin doses slightly to regain control, especially if your insulin doses were previously adjusted downward as your thyroid became less active. If you have an overactive thyroid and take radioactive iodine or undergo surgery to knock out part of the excess thyroid production, you may need to lower your basal and bolus doses.

Gastroparesis

Gastroparesis, a partial paralysis of the intestine, involves damage to the nerves that control their wavelike motion. This disorder often delays the absorption of food after a meal. If people with gastroparesis give boluses in the usual way to cover meals, they often experience lows two to three hours afterwards because the food has not yet been absorbed. This is followed by a high blood sugar six or eight hours later as the food is finally absorbed and converted to glucose in the blood.

Gastroparesis does not change TDD as much as it may require changing the distribution and timing of basal insulin and carb boluses. A person with gastroparesis may benefit from a higher than normal daytime basal insulin dose, perhaps as high as 70% of the TDD. Higher basal doses from early morning through the late evening may counter slowly digesting carbs. With this strategy, carb boluses can be greatly reduced. To do this, increase the carb factor used to figure carb coverage.

If adjusting the doses in injections does not work well, someone with gastroparesis might consider switching to an insulin pump. A pump can give a different basal rate every hour if needed, and it can spread the delivery of carb boluses over several hours to match the delayed absorption of food seen with gastroparesis. An extended meal bolus delivered by a pump can be tailored to almost any situation.

Gastroparesis may be improved also by eating acidophilus culture, which some yogurt has, and by eating lower glycemic index foods so that the food is digested more dependably at the same time. Some medications developed for gastroparesis may help with some of the uneven digestion problems.

Keep in mind that most blood sugar problems have nothing to do with gastroparesis, even though this condition is not rare. Symptoms that suggest the presence of gastroparesis include a mild stomach pain, a feeling of fullness after eating or for prolonged periods, excessive gas, bloating, nausea, and vomiting.

Gastroparesis, a form of autonomic neuropathy, is almost always accompanied by other signs of damage to the autonomic nerves, such as loss of constriction of the pupils to light, loss of variability in the heart rate, and inability of the blood vessels to constrict when going from reclining in bed to standing. Signals which suggest that autonomic neuropathy is present include light-headedness when first standing up, a heart rate that does not rise appropriately when exercising, sweating after eating, and impotence.

Fortunately, simple tests can determine whether gastroparesis is a cause of blood sugar control problems. One method of detecting autonomic neuropathy involves lying down for a few minutes. The blood pressure is then checked and rechecked just after standing. A drop of more than 20 points in the upper blood pressure number or more than 10 points in the lower blood pressure number suggests autonomic neuropathy.

Another way to detect autonomic neuropathy involves a standard EKG test. If the QTc interval, which measures how long it takes the heart muscle to lose its electrical charge after a heart beat, is longer than 0.44 seconds, autonomic neuropathy is likely. Other tests are the heart rate variability seen after deep breathing (Valsalva maneuver) or the results from a 24-hour Holter monitor worn during daily activities.

Consult your physician if you believe gastroparesis may be contributing to control problems.

Summary

Whenever your control is not what you desire and your usual solutions don't seem to be working, always consider starting from the beginning. From your current records, try to determine a new TDD, then reset and test your basal doses, carb factor, and correction factor. Be patient and keep looking until you find an approach that helps your control. If you find you require repeated changes in your TDD for menses or changes in activity, you may want to consider an insulin pump. Today's pumps allow insulin dose adjustments to be made more easily. Most importantly, stay in close contact with your health care team, especially when things do not make sense to you. The next chapter shows how to use your records to improve control.

"You can pretend to be serious. You can't pretend to be witty."
Sacha Guitry

Use Records To Adjust Insulin

Using your records to improve control is fairly straightforward. After you test and record your blood sugars along with the things that affect them, you want to identify any problem patterns and learn how to change insulin doses and other factors to improve your control.

Reset and retest until your control is really improved. Consider different basal doses for daytime and overnight and different carb factors for breakfast, lunch and dinner. Make only one change at a time and see the effect for several days before moving on.

This chapter helps solve blood sugar problems by identifying:

- Your most important blood sugar problems
- When you want to adjust insulin doses
- Which insulin to change

Determine The Complexity Of The Problem

On the path to better control, you first want to decide the complexity of your patterns and in what order they need to be fixed. Simple problems take only a simple fix. For instance, high or low readings that occur at the same time of day present an obvious problem that can be solved with more or less insulin. Someone whose blood sugars are mildly elevated before breakfast, but has fine readings the rest of the day may need only a small increase in the overnight basal dose to correct the problem.

On the other hand, if someone's pattern is inconsistent, such as having three highs and three lows after breakfast in the same week, the problem and solution are more complex. Insulin doses, carb intake, and activity may all need to be examined. When several factors are involved, try to work on one at a time. An extremely variable blood sugar pattern may require changes in TDD, basal doses, and carb and correction boluses. Adjustments may involve changes in the timing and number of injections or in the type of insulin used. Focus first on the solution most likely to have an impact.

Some problems that initially appear complex, such as frequent lows followed by frequent highs in a person who injects four times a day, can usually be fixed with simple dose reductions and eating only enough carbs to raise a low. However, when control is erratic and the person is only on one or two injections a day, or has never learned carb counting, a number of changes are going to be needed. Education will lead these efforts. Know when to call for help.

Fix Emergencies First

Fix emergencies first. A severe low is one that causes you to have trouble thinking clearly. This may be a reading of 60 mg/dl (3.3 mmol) for one person and a reading of 30 mg/dl for another. After the severe low is corrected by eating fast carbs, you want to determine what caused the severe low so another one can be avoided. A severely high blood sugar, especially when accompanied by ketoacidosis, is another situation to be prepared for so that it can be remedied quickly and avoided afterward.

The most dangerous problem in the short term is severe low blood sugars. If you have a pattern of frequent low blood sugars and also one of high blood sugars, stop the lows first both to avoid danger and also because many of the highs may disappear once the lows are eliminated. Highs can be created by lows as a result of excess stress hormone release or by overtreating the low with too much carbohydrate. Stop the problem you are working on, whether lows or highs, by adjusting one or more insulin doses or by taking steps to correct other underlying causes.

Most very high blood sugars can be brought down with correction boluses, but it is important to keep in mind that illnesses create extra physical stress and may require one and a half to three times as much insulin to bring down the same high blood sugar. This extra insulin may be needed after basal doses and carb boluses have already been increased. Again analyze the situation for its cause to better prevent future highs.

16.2 Fix Emergencies First

A Problem Of	Is Caused By	And Can Be Fixed By
Frequent Lows	weight loss, extra activity, insulin doses too high	reducing insulin doses
Severe Lows	excess insulin, missed meal, delayed meal, increased activity	reducing insulin doses or correcting the situation that causes the low
Severe Highs	bad insulin, too little insulin, forgetting or skipping injections, infection, severe illness, steroids, other med. change	raising the insulin doses or better lifestyle choices

When an emergency occurs, decisions must be made quickly. Have a strategy in place before an emergency arises to ensure these decisions will be good ones. Having fast carbs available at all times is critical to properly handling lows. Controlling excessive eating impulses can help you bring yourself out of a low without going high. Better lifestyle choices may help you avoid extreme highs, while monitoring every couple of hours when you become ill can improve insulin doses and return numbers to normal more quickly.

Determine What Will Help You Avoid Lows And Highs

You probably have many clues about how well your control is doing. The A1c blood test provides a measure of your average blood sugar for the last 8 weeks. Many meters provide an average of your blood sugar readings for the last 7, 14, or 30 days. If you test only before meals and your meter says your average is 160 mg/dl (8.8 mmol), your insulin doses are probably not optimally adjusted. A premeal average closer to 100 or 120 mg/dl (5.5 or 6.6 mmol) without many lows is a realistic goal when you understand how to use insulin.

Whenever blood sugars are out of control, many people automatically assume, "It has to be what I ate." Common wisdom likes to blame poor control on what is eaten rather than on whether insulin doses are correctly matched to the carbs in food. Few

> ## 16.3 Common Causes For Lows
>
> - Delayed or skipped meal for which insulin was taken
> - Eating less food or less carbs than planned
> - Being more active
> - Excess Insulin

people think, "The main problem might really be my insulin dose," or "Is this the right dose to take at this time?" or "Maybe it would help if I took insulin at each meal and matched the dose to the number of carbs," or "If I'm high all the time, maybe I need more insulin in my total daily dose."

Sometimes food or the amount eaten is the major problem. If you are seriously overweight, you definitely want to consider the amount and type of food you are eating and how this may damage your control. If excess quantities are a problem, consider how to reduce them. If you are forced to eat to prevent lows, consider how to reduce your insulin doses. If you do not match carb boluses to carb counts, learn to count carbs and match the size of your premeal injection to the meal's carb content.

Many software programs are able to analyze the blood sugars downloaded from your meter to tell you what percentage of your premeal and postmeal readings fall within your selected target ranges. These percentages help identify the times of day your blood sugars tend to be too high or too low. Charts and logbooks can also be used to determine what percentage of your blood sugars fall within your target ranges using the instructions on page 65 in Chapter 6 on charting.

Another indicator for whether you need to change your food or insulin doses is the stability of your readings. If you have lots of ups and downs and your readings are outside of your ranges more than 25% of the time, then your insulin doses are not well matched to your needs. Friends, spouses and family members often are able to provide useful feedback about your control and whether your insulin doses are being matched to your need. They notice changes in your behavior that you may not be aware of, so seek their advice and listen carefully.

Adjust Insulin Doses For Better Control

When and why are adjustments in your insulin doses needed? Generally, they are needed whenever your blood sugar is not staying within your target range 75% of the time. This may show up as a pattern of frequent lows, or having to take frequent correction doses to bring down highs, or blood sugars that go up and down day after day in an erratic manner.

> ### 16.4 Common Causes For Highs
>
> * Too little insulin
> * Eating more carbs than usual
> * Being less active
> * Emotional or physical stress
> * An infection or other illness
> * Pain
> * A medication like prednisone that raises the blood sugar
> * Outdated or bad insulin

Having clear targets helps you to achieve better control. Set a target range for premeal and another desired range for your two hours postmeal readings. Select targets that are reasonable for you at each time of day. Perfection is not needed as you start. Rather, gradual progress is a better sign for long-term success. Your target ranges are likely to be broad at first. Pick starting ranges so that 50% to 70% of your current readings fall into this range.

Keep adjusting insulin doses, carbs, and activity until you meet your current target ranges 75% of the time. Once you are able to stay within your first target ranges about 75% of the time, set more ideal ranges for before and after meals. Keep your health care team informed of the progress you are making and how you are achieving your goals. Recognize also that few people can keep within an ideal range at all times.

Adjust Your Insulin Doses:

* when low blood sugars are frequent or severe
* at the first sign of hypoglycemia unawareness
* as soon as highs become frequent
* to stop morning highs caused by a Dawn Phenomenon
* when your A1c is above 6.5%
* to prevent, delay, or reverse complications
* for excellent control during pregnancy
* to match growth spurts in adolescence
* to reduce wide blood sugar swings, often called "brittle" diabetes
* to fine-tune doses for children and insulin-sensitive adults
* to better match erratic food absorption with gastroparesis
* to get better control and reduce insulin resistance in Type 2 diabetes

If you have any of these problems, go to Chapters 10 to 13 to read about how to find your correct TDD, basal doses, carb boluses, and correction boluses. To determine which part of this process you may need to work on, look at the checklist on page 18.

Decide Which Insulin Dose Needs To Change

When your blood sugar records suggest that your insulin doses are not correct, you want to decide whether the total amount of insulin you use each day is too low or too high, or whether your TDD may be correct but you have an imbalance between your basal and bolus doses. Does a carb bolus or a basal dose need to change? Changing from one type of insulin to another may provide a solution, or you may stay with the same insulins but change the doses or timing, such as taking Lantus at dinner rather than bedtime.

There is nothing sacred or unchangeable about your insulin doses. Your goal is to find doses that work for you, whatever they may be. The insulin you choose to adjust depends on when the problem occurs and the action times of your insulins.

As an example, let's say someone's pattern shows three lows at bedtime in one week, which suggests the Humalog taken for dinner may need to be reduced. Humalog's action time is 4 hours, so if blood sugar readings 2 hours after dinner are often normal or at the lower end of the postmeal target range, this suggests that the dinner Humalog dose is the one to reduce.

16.5 Which Insulin To Adjust	
For Highs Or Lows	**Adjust This Dose**
Before breakfast	Dinner or bedtime basal
After breakfast	Breakfast bolus
Before lunch	Breakfast bolus or basal
After lunch	Lunch bolus or breakfast basal
Before dinner	Lunch bolus or breakfast basal
After dinner	Dinner bolus or breakfast basal
Bedtime	Dinner bolus or breakfast basal
2 am	Dinner or bedtime basal

Be conservative when you change your insulin doses unless there is a clear reason to do otherwise. With basal insulin, change one dose by one or two units at a time and wait a few days to see what effect this change has before making another one. If you are sensitive to insulin, you may want to adjust by even less than one unit. Change one dose at a time because when more than one dose is changed and an improvement occurs, it becomes difficult to see which correction may have caused the improvement.

There are times, however, when more than one dose change needs to be made. If you go on a diet and suddenly reduce your calorie intake and lose weight, you may need to reduce all your insulin doses. If you increase your carb bolus before breakfast, you may also need to lower your breakfast basal insulin dose at the same time. As a rule, you can determine which insulin dose to adjust by noting when you took the insulin and its action time.

As continuous blood sugar monitoring becomes more common, data collection and analysis, especially trending and pattern analysis, will assume a bigger role in the approach to better control. Future meters will not only recall blood sugar readings when you test and store them, but also analyze the numbers in the context of the other information you provide. This will allow blood sugar corrections to be more easily made, such as your total daily dose of insulin and how many grams of carb you cover with one unit of insulin. Some PDA software programs already provide help with carb counting and setting up insulin doses to cover carbs. As meters and other tools give more meaningful advice about changes you can make to improve control, you and your doctor will be able to adjust your insulin doses more quickly and correctly.

You will learn more about recognizing your patterns and changing doses to improve them in Chapters 17 and 18. Remember to use your records to make these changes. When you collect good records, everything you need to spot problems and change your doses is there.

"What's on your mind if you will allow the overstatement?"
Fred Allen

Patterns
— Correct Low Blood Sugars First

Unwanted blood sugar patterns are any consistent repetition of high or low readings at the same time of day or in the same or similar circumstances. A typical desirable pattern is waking up every morning between 70 and 120 mg/dl (3.9 to 6.7 mmol), while a typical undesirable pattern is waking up almost every morning with a reading over 200 mg/dl (11.1 mmol). Blood sugar control can be greatly improved by identifying unwanted patterns and applying corrective actions to them.

This chapter presents:

- How to identify common blood sugar patterns
- How to identify common patterns of lows
- Ways to fix unwanted patterns of lows

An erratic lifestyle usually leads to erratic readings. Identifying problem patterns in your readings will be easier when your lifestyle is as consistent as you can make it. To start, reduce static in your lifestyle. Regularity in meal times, testing, exercise, and insulin doses helps you to tune out the static for clearer patterns on your charts.

A good record system or meter provides a way to associate your blood sugar readings with the food, exercise, stress, insulin injections or medications that affect them. Test often and write down your results. Using a system like the *Smart Charts* in *My Other Checkbook* or our *Enhanced Logbook* (see pages 322 and 323 for blank samples) makes the associations between cause and effect more apparent. Good records help you identify causes for blood sugar problems and aid in problem solving them. If you record essential details, your physician or nurse educator can assist you in spotting unwanted patterns. For extra help, show your records to a friend, your spouse, or a family member and ask if they can identify patterns in them.

People who visually process information will see patterns more quickly in a graphic record system like *Smart Charts*. Others, who think in a more numeric or analytic way, may see patterns best in a standard or enhanced logbook. Either approach works, so use the one that is easier for finding your patterns.

Determine Your Current Patterns

Recognizing your patterns lets you steer toward stability and health and avoid hypoglycemia and complications. Many people avoid looking at their readings because they want no reminder of how bad things are or they have little hope of changing what is happening. Ignorance may not exactly be bliss, but it seems a good choice to them. Unfortunately, this usually hastens the path to complications or increases the frequency and severity of hypoglycemia.

If you record and periodically review your blood sugars, you have probably already spotted certain patterns. Once you know the action times for your insulins (see Table 9.4 page 101), an adjustment in the amount of your insulin doses or being more aware in the timing of these doses is usually the best way to stop a pattern of consistently high or low blood readings.

A great way to identify when changes are needed in your insulin doses is to review your readings once a week. For instance, if you consistently get low before dinner, you can lower your breakfast basal dose, reduce your carb bolus for lunch if you take a bolus at that time, eat more carbs for lunch, or add a snack in the afternoon. The key to success is to identify problems quickly and make one correction at a time until you find a correction that works. Looking for patterns regularly allows this to happen and allows you to make changes that are based on a current analysis of your situation.

A regular review of your charts allows you to take action before problems become severe. Call for assistance when your readings fall outside your target ranges. This enables you to learn more quickly when and how to change your insulin doses. Having four or more readings above 180 mg/dl (10 mmol) before lunch within the last week may signal that it's time to call your doctor to discuss what options to consider. Usually the options are an adjustment of insulin or food.

But sometimes control problems are caused by the unusual situation. A sudden and severe worsening of your control may signal that you have an infection, that your new herbal weight-loss medication contains ma huang or ephedra, or that your insulin has lost potency. If a pattern occurs only under unusual conditions, other occasional happenings such as when low blood sugars are overtreated or when highs happen after eating at a particular restaurant, will also need to be treated only when these occur. Your solution will need to apply to these specific situations. Good records allow occasional problems like these to be remembered and corrected more easily.

Samples of common patterns for low blood sugars are shown in this chapter, while patterns for high readings are displayed in the next chapter. These patterns are ones you are likely to encounter in your charts or logbooks. Make your own lows and highs easier to spot by highlighting them in different colors or shapes.

Look for patterns similar to your own. Your own patterns may not stand out as clearly as the ones in these examples, but each provides a glimpse of what you may encounter and will assist you in spotting your patterns.

How To Correct Unwanted Patterns

Information about each sample pattern is illustrated by a one-day sample *Smart Chart* and by a logbook that covers several days. A discussion accompanies each pattern with options to correct it. Sample insulin dose changes to correct the problem pattern are included, along with other suggestions for how you can shift the pattern back toward desirable target ranges.

The logbook that is used in the examples displays only blood sugar results. This simple logbook is not one we would recommend, but patterns can be identified even with this crude tool. An enhanced logbook would include blood sugars, insulin doses, carb intake, exercise, and the time for each to help you find solutions. For instance, if your breakfast carbs vary from 30 grams to 90 grams but you always take 5 units of Novolog to cover them, it is easy to see why your lunch readings might be erratic. Simple logbooks do not allow you to record this detail, but an enhanced logbook has room for all of these.

The blood sugar ranges on the left of the charts are given in both mg/dl for the U.S. and in mmol for Canada, Europe, and other countries.

Normal Blood Sugar

Let's start pattern recognition with an easy one. The blood sugar pattern shown here shows the normal rise and fall in the blood sugar in someone with-

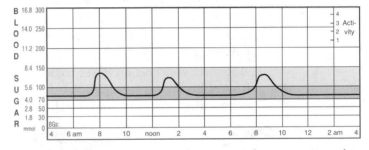

out diabetes. The blood sugar rises slightly after eating no matter what is eaten and the readings consistently remain in a normal range. If your readings already look like this graph, keep up the great work! Keeping a graph like this becomes its own reward.

Stop Lows First

Low blood sugar patterns are presented first because of their importance in improving control. Lows are the most dangerous short-term pattern, so it is best to stop them first. Recurring lows can lead to fuzzy thinking and hypoglycemia unawareness. Highs often follow lows because of overtreatment or excess stress hormone release, so as you stop lows you are also likely to reduce the number of highs.

Some patterns that involve lows occur often, while others tend to be random. Patterns of frequent lows, lows after eating, afternoon lows, and night lows occur often in records. Other patterns of low-to-high, high-to-low, and exercise-related lows occur at odd times, usually after a change in normal eating or exercise patterns.

A pattern of frequent or severe lows requires that one or more insulin doses be lowered. Early intervention can save a lot of trouble and, when done carefully, will not raise your A1c. It is always better to prevent lows rather than having to treat them. A consistently normal blood sugar with only a little time spent outside the target range is what the body needs.

Frequent Lows

Frequent lows, such as the ones shown in the *Smart Chart* to the right, are a common cause for variable readings, which are discussed in more detail in Chapter 19. The chart and the accompanying logbook below reveal a pattern in the lows caused when too much insulin is being given.

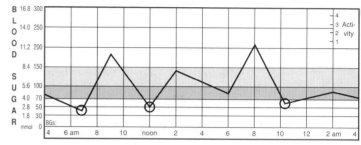

What To Do

- Use glucose tabs or fast carbs to treat all low blood sugars. Glucose tablets relieve symptoms fast and can be measured precisely to prevent overtreatment.

- Frequent lows are a sure sign of excess insulin. Lower your TDD by 5 to 10% as described in Chapter ___ or discuss how to reduce your doses with your physician right away.

- Review your insulin doses to determine where the excess insulin is coming from. Check your basal/bolus balance, and calculate new carb and correction factors after reducing your TDD.

Case Study

Frequent lows began to appear in Jeanine's logbook after she started a diet to lose 30 extra pounds. Prior to

Sugar	Breakfast		Lunch		Dinner		Night	
	Before	After	Before	After	Before	After	Bed	2 a.m.
Sun	(41)	163	(51)	147	90	196	(56)	92
Mon	(37)	186	89	121	(53)	203	128	132
Tues	63	119	(47)	174	66	163	(59)	177
Wed	94	131	63	110	(41)	237	184	139
Thurs	73	162	(38)	394	207	110	(48)	211
					72		65	70

starting the diet, she had taken set insulin doses before each meal and she continued to take the same doses even after she had reduced her food intake.

In her logbook shown here, notice what happens to her blood sugar from bedtime on Wednesday to Thursday morning. Her blood sugar at bedtime on Wednesday night was taken four hours after her dinner bolus, so no bolus insulin was still active. Her blood sugar falls from 184 mg/dl (10.2 mmol) at bedtime on Wednesday to 139 mg/dl (7.7 mmol) at 2 a.m. on Thursday and then to 73 mg/dl (4.1 mmol) at breakfast. Jeaninine's blood sugar dropped 111 mg/dl (6.2 mmol) overnight, well beyond the +15 to -30 mg/dl (+0.8 to -1.7 mmol) change that is preferred during the overnight period. This provided a clear picture of Jeanine's overnight basal dose, and the excessive drop shows that her night basal dose is too high.

When carb and calorie consumption are reduced at the start of a diet, there is an immediate need to lower carb boluses. After a few days of successful dieting, the basal doses will also need to be reduced.

Jeanine's Dose Change To Stop Frequent Lows						
	Brkfst	**Lunch**	**Dinner**	**Bed**	**TDD**	**% Basal**
Original dose	6H/10N	6H	6H	10N	38 u	53%
What she did	(5H/10N)	(5H)	(5H)	(8N)	33 u	55%

Prior to starting her diet, Jeanine had been taking set doses of insulin because her diet at that time was consistent. She had not told her doctor she was starting a diet, but when she finally called because of the lows, he suggested that she reduce all of her doses as shown above. He also referred her to a dietician to learn carb counting and start using a carb factor to cover the grams of carbs she eats, rather than taking set carb boluses. This allows her to adjust her carb boluses when her food intake changes. Doing a basal test periodically will reveal when basal doses need to change as well.

Lows After Eating

The pattern on this chart and in three others in the same week looks similar to the pattern just seen with frequent lows, but here the blood sugar does not drop

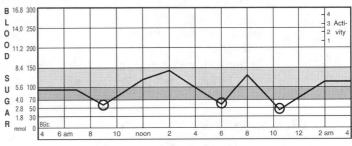

overnight. This suggests that the overnight basal dose is fine and that the real problem more likely has to do with the carb boluses.

What To Do

These lows occur after carb boluses are taken, suggesting that a rise in the carb factor is needed in order to lower the size of the carb boluses. The daytime basal dose does need to be checked to ensure it is not causing the problem with excess insulin.

Test the day basal and check that your basal/bolus balance is about 50% each. If the day basal test shows the blood sugar is dropping more than 30 mg/dl in a 5 hour period when you do not eat, lower the morning basal dose. If boluses make up more than half of your TDD, or if your basals and boluses are balanced, raise your carb factor to reduce your carb boluses. For instance, if you use 1H for every 16 grams, try 1H for every 17 or 18 grams. Also make sure you are counting grams of carb accurately. If you are uncertain about your carb counting, visit your dietician and bring with you a detailed three-day diet record to verify your carb counting.

Case Study

In Jeff's logbook, his blood sugar goes low either right after a meal or before the next meal. We will assume he has tested his day basal dose and proven it to be good. When a blood sugar goes low within a couple of hours of eating, the carb bolus is generally much too large. When the blood sugar does not go low until before the next meal, the carb bolus is slightly too large. Obviously,

Sugar	Breakfast		Lunch		Dinner		Night	
	Before	After	Before	After	Before	After	Bed	2 a.m.
Sun	97	(60)	123	146	(53)	129	(42)	110
Mon	89	71	95	123	(37)	121	103	99
Tues	89	152	(45)	207	111	(56)	106	101
Wed	78	144	84	(41)	214	98	65	122
Thurs	100	137	92	151	83	141	107	154
					70		95	110

Jeff's carb boluses are too large, but his lows might also be caused by not counting carbs accurately.

On Wednesday morning Jeff's blood sugar was 78 mg/dl (4.3 mmol), so he reduced his carb bolus from 5 units for 80 grams (80/5 or 1 unit of H for every 16 grams of carb) down to 4 units (80/4 or 1 unit of H for every 20 grams of carb). This bolus reduction was enough to avoid a low after breakfast that morning. On returning to his original carb factor of 1 to 16 at lunch, he went low Wednesday afternoon and again at bedtime. On Thursday morning, Jeff decided it would be better to use one unit of Humalog for every 20 grams for all his meals to reduce his carb boluses. He also reviewed his carb counting and set aside time to retest his daytime basal dose on the coming weekend.

Afternoon Lows

A low in the afternoon as shown on this chart occurred 4 out of 7 days this week for Jody. Afternoon lows are common for many people who are physi-

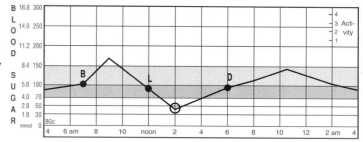

cally active at work or school. They may also be caused by an excess of insulin from the combination of the bolus dose given for lunch plus a morning basal dose that peaks in the afternoon. Another contributor can be the bedtime basal insulin dose if this dose is relatively large.

What To Do

To stop lows in the afternoon, one or more of the insulin doses that are active in the afternoon must be lowered.

Case Study

Sugar	Breakfast Before	Breakfast After	Lunch Before	Lunch After	Dinner Before	Dinner After	Night Bed	Night 2 a.m.
Sun	101	167	89	(43)	96	117	144	105
Mon	124	138	92	(51)	163	176	103	99
Tues	83	149	84	67	94	143	92	
Wed	88	241	143	103	(41)	139	107	93
Thurs	83	133	76	184	(52)	158	129	121
					78		115	100

Jody works days as a parts picker in an automobile parts distributor plant. As shown in her logbook to the right, she is having low blood sugars in the afternoons and before dinner. Jody's readings on Monday and Tuesday are typical of her problem with afternoon lows. On Wednesday morning, however, Jody stopped to eat breakfast at a local restaurant and apparently underestimated how many carbs were in her pancakes. Her blood sugar rose from 88 mg/dl (4.9 mmol) before breakfast to 241mg/dl (13.4 mmol) afterward. She did not take a correction bolus for this high reading, so she was still high at 143 mg/dl (7.9 mmol) before lunch.

Because of her afternoon lows, she decided she would not add a correction bolus for Wednesday's high lunch reading. Even though she took no correction bolus for lunch that day, her

Jody's Dose Change To Stop Afternoon Lows						
	Brkfst	**Lunch**	**Dinner**	**Bed**	**TDD**	**% Basal**
Original dose	6H/17N	6H	6H	10N	45 u	(60%)
1st Option	(6H/15N)	6H	6H	10N	43 u	(58%)
2nd Option	(6H/15N)	(5H)	6H	10N	42 u	(60%)

blood sugar again went low before dinner. The low occurred just before dinner rather than in the middle of the afternoon because she started higher at lunch.

To stop her afternoon lows, Jody's first option might be to take less morning basal insulin to reduce her insulin level during the afternoon. She lowered her breakfast NPH from 17 units to 15 units. When Jody continued to have some afternoon lows, she decided to also reduce her carb bolus at lunch by raising the carb factor she uses for her lunch carbs.

Low To High

Eating too much for a low blood sugar can lead to a high reading an hour or two later. If your blood sugar following a low often goes higher than 150 mg/dl (8.3 mmol), it is likely you are eating more than 20 grams of carb to treat these lows. Stress hormones released at the time of the low cause sweating and shaking, and can raise the blood sugar. Although stress hormones contribute to a rise in the blood sugar, they will usually not cause a rapid rise from 40 to 320 mg/dl (2.2 to 17.7 mmol) over a short period of time, as shown on the graph on the next page.

If a pattern of high readings often follows lows in your charts, you have the low to high pattern. Check your charts or logbook to see whether readings below 60 mg/dl (3.3 mmol) are followed by readings of 150 mg/dl (8.5 mmol) or higher. One gram of carbohydrate raises the blood sugar between three and five points for most adults, so only 15 to 20 grams of quick carbohydrate are needed to stop most lows. This is equivalent to a cup of milk plus one square graham cracker, 3 graham cracker squares, two-thirds of a medium banana, or 5 to 6 ounces of a regular soda.

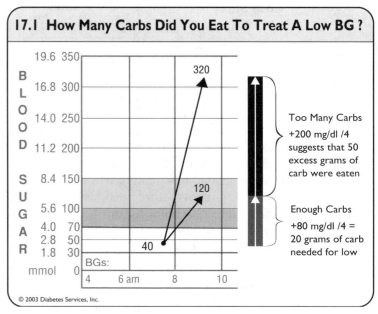

17.1 How Many Carbs Did You Eat To Treat A Low BG ?

Too Many Carbs
+200 mg/dl /4 suggests that 50 excess grams of carb were eaten

Enough Carbs
+80 mg/dl /4 = 20 grams of carb needed for low

© 2003 Diabetes Services, Inc.

When you consume 15 to 20 grams of quick carbs as soon as you recognize that your blood sugar is low, you will also lessen the amount of stress hormones released. The lower your blood sugar goes and the longer it stays there, the more stress hormones that will be released and the more shaking and sweating that will occur. Although excess stress hormone release does little to raise your blood sugar in the short term, it can cause the blood sugar to rise for six to ten hours afterward.

Fast carbs help you feel better faster and, when taken in the right amount, can eliminate subsequent highs. If you must eat more than 20 grams of carbohydrate to get your blood sugar to rise, this suggests that the insulin dose responsible for the low was excessive and needs to be lowered.

What To Do

Practice, patience. Even fast carbs require 10 or 20 minutes to have an effect. In most situations, you will need to eat no more than 20 grams of fast carbs, unless there is a clear reason to do otherwise. In about 20 minutes after you eat 20 grams of carb, brain function will improve and you can retest your blood sugar to determine whether you really need more carbs.

More than 20 grams may be needed if you injected a recent carb or correction bolus and you have unused bolus insulin still active, or if extra activity is the reason for the low. In situations like these, some complex carbohydrate plus protein can help keep your sugar from dropping again. If you will not be eating a meal within 30 minutes, you can ensure your blood sugar does not drop again by having a half sandwich or an equivalent amount of carbohydrate and protein.

Program yourself to use only glucose tablets or fast-acting carbs for lows. If you do overeat, calculate the total grams of carbohydrate you have eaten and subtract the amount needed to cover your low reading. Then take a carb bolus to cover most of the excess carbohydrate to avoid a subsequent high. Taking a carb bolus right after a low may seem strange, but it's exactly what's needed when you overeat. Test your blood sugar one, two, and three hours after taking this bolus.

17.2 How Much Does 1 Gram of Carbs Raise Your BG?	
If your weight is:	**1 gram will raise you about:**
50 lbs (23 kg)	8 mg/dl (0.44 mmol)
75 lbs (34 kg)	7 mg/dl (0.39 mmol)
90 lbs (41 kg)	6 mg/dl (0.33 mmol)
120 lbs (55 kg)	5 mg/dl (0.28 mmol)
160 lbs (73 kg)	4 mg/dl (0.22 mmol)
200 lbs (91 kg)	3 mg/dl (0.17 mmol)
© 2003 Diabetes Services, Inc.	

Once your blood sugar returns to normal, take some time to consider why the low happened and whether any changes are needed in your basal doses, your carb factor, or your correction factor so that the chance of encountering another low is reduced.

Case Study

Several times a week, Joe has been having readings that go from low to high. On Tuesday, Joe goes from high before lunch to low afterward back to high at dinner and then low again, and high at bedtime. Up and down patterns like these may be grouped together in some people's readings, especially in those who have become frustrated with their lack of control. It is somewhat common

Sugar	Breakfast		Lunch		Dinner		Night	
	Before	After	Before	After	Before	After	Bed	2 a.m.
Sun	193	287	212	127	(40)	320	273	142
Mon	132	125	(48)	219	171	152	107	91
Tues	84	73	216	(58)	248	(39)	211	71
Wed	(53)	347	227	184	132	63	188	142
Thurs	134	167	118	169	126	141	(53)	277

among those who feel physically or emotionally uncomfortable when their blood sugar rises above a certain number. Overtreating a high reading in this situation is not a good idea. Focus first on preventing highs, and if one does occur, prevent a subsequent low so that another rebound high becomes unlikely.

Joe discussed the situation he was encountering with his physician, who suggested that he start by lowering his TDD from 38 units to 35 units a day. Joe lowered his morning bolus insulin by one unit and raised his carb and correction factors to reduce the Novolog he was taking for both carbs and highs. On the way home from the doctor's office, he stopped at his pharmacy and bought a large bottle of glucose tablets to have available whenever he might go low. These steps helped to smooth out his blood sugar and he felt a lot better. His A1c dropped from 7.4% at the office visit to 6.6% four months later, much to his delight.

Overtreating Nighttime Lows

When the blood sugar goes low during the night, it is often followed by a high in the morning. It's hard to be rational when you wake in the middle of the night feeling the effects of stress hormones released by a low blood sugar. In this situation, your brain cells aren't getting enough fuel to think clearly, and the fear and confusion that accompany a low makes emptying the refrigerator seem quite rational. Overeating, however, only makes your blood sugar sky-high the following morning and for several hours into the day. The graph shows a low during the night and the high blood sugar before breakfast that follows when excess carbs are eaten during the night.

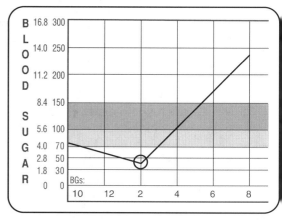

What To Do

First determine why the nighttime lows are happening. If they happen often, reduce the evening basal dose or the dinner carb bolus as necessary. If the low happens only after increased daytime activity, eating extra carbs at bedtime on active days may be the perfect solution. When nighttime hypoglycemia occurs only after a correction bolus is taken for a high blood sugar at bedtime, a smaller correction bolus at bedtime is needed.

Keep glucose tablets or fast-acting carbs at the bedside and use them routinely for all night lows. Even in the panic of a nighttime low, it is hard to overdose on glucose tablets. Once sufficient fast carbs are eaten, wait a few minutes for your appetite to ease. Then have a cup of milk or some cheese as insurance against another low.

Case Study

As can be seen in his logbook, Jared has been overtreating his night lows. He found he could stop the high breakfast readings by keeping glucose tablets on his

---

17.3 The Importance Of Overnight Control

The time period from dinner to waking is more than half of the day. By controlling blood sugars during this time, more than half your control can be taken care of. Night basal doses are easier to determine because there is no eating during this time. When you are able to go to bed and wake up with a normal reading, the rest of the day is easier to control. To rapidly improve your A1c, focus on covering dinner so you go to bed with a normal reading, then set your night basal dose so you stay there.

nightstand and using only three tablets.

Sugar	Breakfast		Lunch		Dinner		Night	
	Before	After	Before	After	Before	After	Bed	2 a.m.
Sun	185	341	188	162	76	142	96	37
Mon	284	289	204	187	123	163	132	53
Tues	259	323	225	156	98	138	105	89
Wed	102	291	198	182	143	189	116	46
Thurs	287	284	233	142	107	154	93	48

Jared wanted to stop the night lows, so he reduced his basal dose of NPH at dinner from 20 to 18 units. He also discussed with his doctor splitting his dinner basal dose and giving part at bedtime. This reduces the amount of insulin that will peak in the middle of the night. He can later give less basal insulin at dinner to again reduce the amount of insulin peaking in the middle of the night, as shown in the third option in the table. A fourth option is to eliminate the peak in NPH insulin entirely by replacing his three NPH insulin doses with one dose of Lantus insulin at bedtime.

Jared's Dose Changes For Night Lows						
	Brkfst	**Lunch**	**Dinner**	**Bed**	**TDD**	**% Basal**
Original dose	12H/20N	12H	12H/20N		76 u	53%
1st Option	12H/20N	12H	12H/18N		74 u	52%
2nd Option	12H/20N	12H	12H/10N	10H	76 u	53%
3rd Option	12H/20N	12H	12H/8N	10N	74 u	51%
4th Option	12H	12H	12H	36 Lantus	72 u	50%

Lows That Follow Highs

Plummeting from a high to a low blood sugar over a two to four hour period may be caused by a correction bolus that is too large, by boluses that overlap, or by taking too much insulin for a particular need. A high to low pattern is shown in the graph to the right. If this pattern is seen several times on your charts, this a problem you will want to address.

What To Do

Determine where the problem starts. Ask yourself what is causing your highs. If you are not counting carbs or are not counting them accurately, review carb counting. Recheck your carb factor and review how to match carbs with your carb boluses.

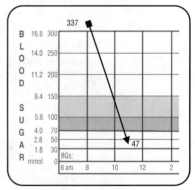

If you frequently go from highs to lows, the amount of insulin taken to correct these highs needs to be reduced. Even if it happens only occasionally, you want to be able to lower high readings safely. Calculate and retest your correction factor. When lows follow highs, the most likely cause is that the number used for your correction factor is too small making your correction boluses too large. Use less insulin in correction boluses by raising your correction factor. For instance, if your correction factor is 50, use 55 or 60 instead. Recalculate your correction factor to determine how many points you drop per unit using your current TDD and the 1800 Rule (Table 13.1).

Sugar	Breakfast		Lunch		Dinner		Night	
	Before	After	Before	After	Before	After	Bed	2 a.m.
Sun	96	127	82	337	(41)	168	129	128
Mon	137	179	138	162	107	171	141	125
Tues	119	284	(51)	117	84	136	91	84
Wed	73	121	87	148	121	345	(38)	167
Thurs	155	173	96	71	276	(53)	164	114
							95	110

You may have increased your TDD or have an incorrect basal/bolus balance that creates this problem. Try to determine whether it is highs or lows which are the original problem, and review solutions that address the predominant pattern.

One reason a high reading drops quickly to a low one can be a correction bolus that is taken following a meal. The bolus is taken at a time when less insulin is needed to correct a high because much of the recent carb bolus is still working. When a premeal target blood sugar is used for correcting a postmeal high, too much insulin will be given. For example, if 100 mg/dl (5.6 mmol) is used as the target for a postmeal blood sugar, rather than a more realistic postmeal target of 150 mg/dl or 180 mg/dl (8.3 or 10 mmol), the correction bolus would be larger than needed and cause a low. Be sure you have an appropriate postmeal target when you correct postmeal highs.

Another cause for plummeting occurs when two or more carb or correction boluses are taken within four hours of each other without taking into account the unused bolus insulin that is still active from previous boluses. Always take into account unused bolus insulin to avoid giving a bolus that is too large. Review Chapter 14 on the unused bolus rule to ensure lows are not caused by overlapping boluses.

Impatience and frustration can contribute to this problem. If you feel frustrated or uncomfortable when you are high and use extra Humalog or Novolog to lower the reading quickly, try practicing some self-restraint. Waiting a little longer to bring your blood sugar down can stop unnecessary lows. Turn your focus toward preventing the highs in the first place, rather than overdosing to lower high readings too quickly.

Lows After Exercise

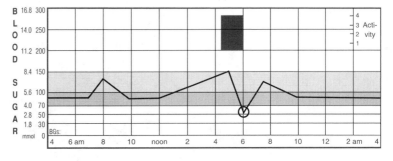

When you are involved in extra physical activity, lows may occur during, immediately after, or several hours following the exercise or activity. The longer and more intense an activity, the more likely that immediate or delayed lows will occur. *Smart Charts* allow exercise to be recorded and matched in time with the low or high blood sugar readings that follow.

What To Do

As will be discussed late in Chapters 23 and 24, the effect that extra activity has on your blood sugar depends on how strenuous it is and how long it lasts, as well as how much insulin you have in your blood at the time. Mild to moderate activity that lasts less than 30 to 45 minutes will not require as much of an increase in carb intake or as much reduction in insulin doses as longer and more intense forms of exercise. Table 24.5 provides guidance for carb and insulin adjustments to make for activity.

First check that your basal and bolus insulin doses are balanced. If they are, the carb bolus taken before the activity can be reduced and/or extra carbs can be eaten before the exercise. How many carbs your exercise will consume can be estimated using Table 24.2. This provides a good idea for how many replacement carbs are needed for your particular activity.

"Take your life in your hands and what happens?
A terrible thing: no one to blame."

Erica Jong

"A blank page is God's way of showing you how hard it is to be God."
Anon.

Patterns
— Correct High Blood Sugars Next

Once frequent and severe lows are reduced or eliminated, look for patterns that involve high readings. If your readings are almost always higher than normal, the best solution is to raise your TDD, basal doses, and/or carb boluses. An exception to this is someone whose highs are largely created by overtreating lows, where a reduction in insulin doses makes more sense.

This chapter presents:

- Causes for morning highs
- Causes for highs after meals
- How to identify common patterns of highs
- Ways to fix unwanted patterns of highs

Morning Highs

Fifty to seventy percent of people with Type 1 diabetes need some extra insulin beginning between 2 a.m. and 3 a.m. to control a Dawn Phenomenon.[51,65] A rise in the blood sugar in the early morning hours is caused by a normal increase in growth hormone and cortisol production at this time of day which reduces insulin's effectiveness. Between 20 and 30 percent of these people need a significant increase in their basal insulin in the early morning hours to keep the blood sugar from rising.

In Type 2 diabetes, high morning readings are common but for a different reason. In a person with insulin resistance, more fat is released from the abdomen into the blood during the night after eating has ended for the day. This fat release includes free fatty acids, which creates additional insulin resistance. Extra resistance to insulin makes the liver think that insulin and glucose levels are low, so the liver increases glucose production, even though the blood sugar is already high. Due to these crossed signals, the person to wake up with a high reading.

Frequent Highs

The blood sugar readings on James' chart on the top of the next page show the consistent highs he has encountered in the past few weeks. This pattern suggests strongly that additional insulin is needed. A person experiencing this pattern will have an A1c level that is well above 7%.

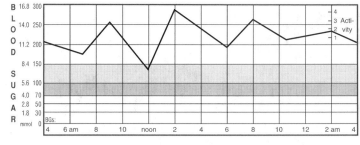

What To Do

If you have this pattern, raise your TDD gradually over time with a series of small increases in your basal and bolus doses. Keep your basal and bolus doses balanced with 50 to 60% of your TDD in your basal doses. If your readings are usually between 120 mg/dl and 200 mg/dl range (6.7 to 11.1 mmol), a 3 to 5% increase in your TDD will help. A 5% to 10% increase should be considered if your readings are often above 200 mg/dl (11.1 mmol). Review your diet, exercise, and whether you need to reduce your weight as other areas that need improvement to reduce these highs. Identify whether it is your lifestyle or insulin doses or both that need to be changed. Always consider whether infection, pain, stress, bad insulin, a steroid medication, or other new medication might be causing the high readings. In some situations, you may need to raise your TDD by much more than 10%, but once the cause is identified and corrected, your insulin doses will again need to be reduced.

Case Study

James' blood sugar is consistently high as shown in the log book. Although he needs to lose weight, he knows his busy

Sugar	Breakfast		Lunch		Dinner		Night	
	Before	After	Before	After	Before	After	Bed	2 a.m.
Sun	163	256	144	292	189	267	212	238
Mon	241	346	212	248	171	283	164	187
Tues	208	219	132	176	143	258	181	206
Wed	233	341	264	217	168	211	145	178
Thurs	204	243	197	236	156	184	173	184
					75		260	467

schedule as a department store manager during the holiday season will not allow this. After discussing the situation with his doctor, he decided to raise his doses as shown in the table. Because his readings were consistently high through the day, he added one unit to each bolus and basal dose. This raised his TDD from 76 units to 81. This total increase of 6.6% brought his readings down until he could focus on losing weight after the holidays. Losing weight takes time, but James realizes it will provide him with far better health in the long run.

James' Dose Change To Stop Frequent Highs

	Brkfst	Lunch	Dinner	Bed	TDD	% Basal
Original dose	12H/20L	12H	12H/20L		76 u	53%
Changed dose	13H/21L	13H	13H/21L		81 u	52%

Highs Before Breakfast

The first blood sugar of the day is often the hardest to bring into the normal range. The chart on the right shows overnight readings starting at 10 p.m. through 8 a.m. the next morning with the three common patterns that cause a high blood sugar at breakfast. When your breakfast readings are high, determine first when your blood sugar begins its rise. Before this rise begins is when you need more insulin. Another cause for morning highs is overtreating a low during the night. More information on dealing with this is covered on page 192.

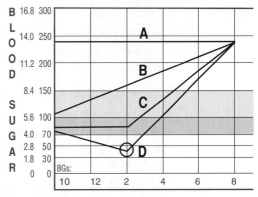

A - already high at bedtime   B - overnight basal too small

C - Dawn Phenomenon   D - overtreated insulin reaction

Already High At Bedtime

Pattern A in the chart above is easy to identify because the blood sugar is already high at bedtime and stays high through the night.

What To Do

If your blood sugar rises after dinner and is often high at bedtime, a larger carb bolus is needed for dinner or the daytime basal dose may need

Sugar	Breakfast		Lunch		Dinner		Night	
	Before	After	Before	After	Before	After	Bed	2 a.m.
Sun	185	212	127	153	76	289	212	207
Mon	204	249	174	156	123	341	238	243
Tues	219	231	84	136	98	207	179	163
Wed	172	187	104	171	143	342	256	268
Thurs	247	233	138	149	107	261	182	196
							260	467

to be raised. After dinner snacks often cause this rise. If snacking is a problem, reduce the size of the snack or fully cover the extra carbs eaten in the evening hours with separate carb boluses. When you find your blood sugar is high at bedtime, take enough correction bolus to bring the high reading down without causing a nighttime low. If taking a correction bolus at bedtime corrects the morning blood sugar, your overnight basal dose is fine.

Jasmine's Dose Change For Highs At Bedtime						
	Brkfst	**Lunch**	**Dinner**	**Bed**	**TDD**	**% Basal**
Original dose	12H/20N	12H	12H/20N		76 u	53%
Changed dose	12H/20N	12H	14H/20N		78 u	51%

If you keep your bedtime reading high because you are afraid you may have a low during the night, discuss this with your physician. You want to recheck your night basal dose to ensure that it does keep your blood sugar flat overnight. You should always be able to go to sleep with a relatively normal bedtime reading.

Case Study

Because Jasmine's blood sugar rises after dinner as shown in her logbook on the previous page, she decided to increase her carb bolus for dinner as shown in her dose change table.

Overnight Basal Insulin Too Low

Pattern B in the chart on the previous page and in the logbook below shows the blood sugar rising steadily during the night. This results from an overnight basal insulin dose that is too low. In Julie's logbook, her Sunday night bedtime blood sugar of 96 mg/dl (5.3 mmol) rises to 151 mg/dl (8.4 mmol) at 2 a.m. and goes higher to 204 mg/dl (11.3 mmol) by breakfast. The rise in the blood sugar through the

Sugar	Breakfast Before	After	Lunch Before	After	Dinner Before	After	Night Bed	2 a.m.
Sun	185	341	188	162	76	142	96	151
Mon	204	289	204	187	123	163	132	187
Tues	219	323	225	156	98	138	105	146
Wed	172	291	198	182	143	189	116	163
Thurs	247	284	233	142	107	154	93	127
							122	167

night hours indicates that the night basal dose is set too low to keep her blood sugar from rising. Remember that a blood sugar test at 1 or 2 a.m. or in the middle of sleep is needed to verify this pattern.

What To Do

Raise the bedtime or dinner basal dose to provide more overnight coverage. Another alternative is to split the evening dose between dinner and bedtime. Review Chapter 11 on how to

Julie's Dose Changes For Low Night Basal Dose						
	Brkfst	Lunch	Dinner	Bed	TDD	% Basal
Original dose	12H/20N	12H	12H/20N		76 u	53%
1st Option	12H/20N	12H	11H/24N		79 u	56%
2nd Option	12H/20N	12H	11H/14N	12N	81 u	57%

set the basals and test the new dose. When you first raise your evening basal dose, test your blood sugar more often and test at 2 a.m. for a few nights to ensure that no drop in your blood sugar occurs in the middle of the night.

Case Study

Julie was feeling frustrated because her blood sugar always rose during the night, even though she ate no bedtime snack. Tuesday night is another example, where her bedtime reading of 105 mg/dl rose to 146 mg/dl at 2 a.m. and then to 172 mg/dl on Wednesday morning. She finally called her physician who suggested she raise her dinner NPH from 20 units to 24 units. Her physician also suggested that if she starts to have any lows during the night after raising her dinner NPH, or if this increase is not enough to keep her morning reading down, that she split her dose and give 14 NPH at dinner and add another injection of 12 NPH at bedtime.

High Protein Or High Fat Dinners

Although this pattern is identical to having too little basal insulin (see pattern B in the chart on page 199), the cause is different. This pattern occurs only after extra protein is eaten for dinner or as a snack in the evening. When protein is consumed, 40 to 50 percent of it changes slowly to glucose over a period of several hours. Most meals contain too little protein to affect the blood sugar, but when larger amounts are consumed, the blood sugar will rise overnight. Examples of heavy protein intake include an 8 to 12-ounce steak, a Mexican dinner with refried beans, or several ounces of nuts.

Higher fat meals can cause a similar overnight rise in the blood sugar. In this situation, a temporary increase in insulin resistance is created by certain fats in certain foods. A dual fat/protein effect may also be at work in some foods.

What To Do

- The wisest thing to do is to eat less of the offending food.
- If you are sure these occasional morning highs are the result of high protein or fat dinners and snacks, try raising your basal dose on evenings when you eat the offending food to offset the increased glucose production or insulin resistance that follows. Correct any high bedtime reading with a correction bolus. Protein that is eaten at dinner will raise the blood sugar for 8 or 10 hours, so an increase in a dose of bedtime NPH or Lente makes sense. Remember, though, that an increase in a 24 hour basal insulin, like Lantus or Detemir, is not a good way to match this particular need that only occurs on certain evenings.
- If you are unsure of a meal's effect, wake up halfway through the night and check your blood sugar. Use a correction bolus at that time if you are high.

A Dawn Phenomenon

This pattern, shown as C in the graph on page 199 and in the logbook below, shows the blood sugar staying level until about 2 a.m. when it begins to rise. In this situation, if the blood sugar is high before breakfast, it often rises even higher afterward and is difficult to bring down until the afternoon. This pattern requires more basal insulin during the predawn hours. For those who sleep typical nighttime hours, an increase in the insulin level is needed around 2 a.m. or 3 a.m. to prevent the subsequent early morning rise.

What To Do

If you use Lantus insulin and take it at bedtime, try taking it at dinner instead. The flat action of this insulin before 2 a.m.

Sugar	Breakfast		Lunch		Dinner		Night	
	Before	After	Before	After	Before	After	Bed	2 a.m.
Sun	185	341	188	162	76	142	96	112
Mon	204	289	204	187	123	163	132	127
Tues	219	323	225	156	98	138	105	121
Wed	172	291	198	182	143	189	116	132
Thurs	247	284	233	142	107	154	93	111
							122	117

may head off the morning rise so that it never occurs. If you use NPH or Lente at dinner, take it at bedtime instead or split the evening dose into one injection at dinner and one at bedtime. Increase the bedtime basal dose by one unit every three or fours days until the morning reading comes down or you begin to have night lows. Monitor at 2 a.m. for a few nights to catch any lows that may start to occur as a result of the increase in the basal insulin dose. You might also try a combination of dinner Lantus with bedtime NPH or Lente.

Highs After Meals

One common and annoying pattern is to have a normal blood sugar before a meal but then lose control after eating. How high your blood sugar will go after a meal depends on which bolus insulin is used, your sensitivity to insulin, how much carbohydrate you eat, your activity level after the meal, and the food's glycemic index. Common reasons for post meal highs are discussed below.

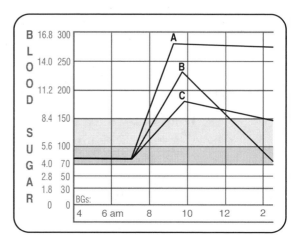

Carb Bolus Is Missed

Line A in the chart shows a typical pattern when a carb bolus is not taken before a meal. Forgetting to take a bolus is hopefully rare, but it can be a real problem when it happens.

If you forget a bolus often, try changing your pattern of injecting boluses, perhaps taking it while the food is being prepared rather than in the bustle of sitting down to eat. Using an insulin pen, like Novo-Nordisk's InDuo, which has a built-in clock to show the time of the last bolus may help. There are also a variety of wrist watches which have up to 12 alarms per day you can preset, and these can assist in remembering doses.

A Late Carb Bolus With A High GI Food

Line B above shows a spiking blood sugar which returns to normal as the insulin finally catches up 4 hours later. After meal spikes that rise above 150 mg/dl (8.3 mmol) should be eliminated whenever possible.

When insulin is injected just before eating a high glycemic index food, the blood sugar spikes because even a rapid insulin cannot open cell doors to glucose that quickly. Learn the glycemic index of the foods you eat, and take your carb bolus earlier than usual for those that have a high glycemic index, when possible.

If you eat 70 grams of carb for a breakfast of old-fashioned oatmeal, your blood sugar will not rise as dramatically as it will after eating most cold cereals. Many common breakfast foods, such as cold cereals, instant oatmeal, yogurt with fruit syrup, or a toasted cheese sandwich are high glycemic index foods and cause mid-morning readings to spike.

A sharp rise in the blood sugar after a meal was common when Regular insulin was used to cover carbs, but this problem can be encountered also with Novolog or Humalog when a bolus is taken too close to eating, especially eating foods that have a high glycemic index. Regular insulin is notorious for this problem because it takes 20 to 30 minutes to have any effect and 2 1/2 to 3 hours to peak in its activity, long after most carbohydrates have already created a marked rise in the blood sugar. Because the high blood sugar would usually return to normal as the dose of Regular finally had its full effect, a correction dose was not needed. Boluses of Regular insulin have to be taken at least 30 or 40 minutes before eating, especially when taken for carbs that have a high glycemic index. When the premeal blood sugar is normal, a carb bolus of Novolog or Humalog works best when taken 15 to 20 minutes before the first bite of food.

Carb Bolus Too Small

Line C shows a pattern when the carb bolus is taken before a meal but the dose is too small for the carbohydrate eaten. Carb boluses frequently can be underestimated if you do not count carbs or you count them incorrectly. Even if you count carbs accurately, you may misjudge carb boluses for a meal when you eat out or for one you do not eat often.

What To Do

Learn how to do carb counting thoroughly and accurately. The time spent doing this will benefit you day after day. If you already practice carb counting, you may want to review carb counting again. The effort it takes to learn how to quantify the effect foods have on your blood sugar becomes invaluable over time.

You may want to retest your carb factor to ensure that the size of your carb bolus is correctly matched to your meals. When a large amount of carbs is eaten, a high blood sugar may result even though the same carb factor is able to control meals which have fewer carbs. Larger quantities of carb may uncover an inadequate carb factor that smaller quantities do not reveal.

Review Chapter 8 on carb counting to be sure you have a good understanding of this excellent tool. At many restaurants, nutritional information is available to guide your doses. Pay particular attention to meals that consistently cause high readings so you can make better decisions when you return and order the same meal. You may want to create a personal list of restaurant meals with their accompanying doses to make postmeal readings more reliable. This can go a long way toward making eating out enjoyable.

"Trust that still, small voice that says, 'This might work and I'll try it.'"
Diane Mariechild

18.1 Start With The Breakfast Blood Sugar

For most people, the breakfast blood sugar is the most important readings to control for the day. When you wake up with a normal reading, your liver is happy and not making the excess glucose that necessitates larger than normal insulin doses through the morning hours.

In someone who does not have diabetes, a low insulin level means the blood sugar is also low. The liver responds to the low insulin level by releasing sugar into the blood. The liver responds in the same way to a low insulin level when someone has diabetes, but here the blood sugar is high rather than low. Unfortunately the liver does not know this. Once the liver starts producing glucose, it is difficult to stop and extra sugar continues to be released through the morning hours. Larger correction boluses than normal are required to lower high breakfast readings compared to similar readings later in the day. When the breakfast reading is high, extra care has to be taken to avoid afternoon lows as correction boluses begin to overlap.

An inappropriate outpouring of glucose from the liver during the night can be prevented by having enough insulin in the blood during the night.

Tips For Preventing Highs After Meals

- If using Regular, switch to Humalog or Novolog for meals. Take carb boluses 20 minutes before eating when possible, while being careful not to delay eating.
- If you plan to eat high glycemic index foods (white bread, white rice, etc.), be sure to take your carb bolus 20 minutes before the meal. Keep glucose tabs handy if your food is not served as expected.
- Eat fewer carbs at the meal and save the rest to have as a snack a couple of hours later. Again, do not forget or delay eating.
- Add extra fiber like psyllium (sugar-free Metamucil) or guar gum to the meal to reduce its glycemic index. A tablespoon or two of psyllium added to cold cereals can dramatically lower postmeal readings.
- Get 30 to 45 minutes of exercise after the meal.
- Discuss with your doctor use of a prescription medication like Precose (acarbose) or Glyset (miglitol) to slow the digestion of carbohydrates.
- Check the glycemic index of any suspect foods on pages 94 and 95 and replace with foods that have a lower glycemic index. For breakfast, try old-fashioned oatmeal, a high-fiber cereal topped with strawberries, or plain yogurt with fresh fruit sliced into it.

If you have between-meal spikes, check the balance between your basal and bolus insulins. If the basal insulin is less than 50% of your TDD, raise your basal insulin during the day while slightly lowering your carb boluses. Having a higher basal insulin level in the blood prior to eating can often help reduce post meal spikes, with the same or even lower carb boluses.

Highs After Breakfast Caused By Unrecognized Night Lows

The pattern to the right shows a typical response during the morning hours following unrecognized nighttime hypoglycemia. Note that the blood sugar often starts near normal before breakfast as shown in the graph but rises above normal after breakfast because of stress hormones that were released earlier in the night as a result of hypoglycemia. Stress hormones often raise the blood sugar for 8 to 10 hours following a major low blood sugar. This can cause the blood sugar

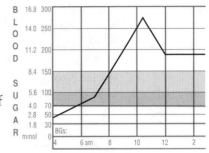

to spike after breakfast even though the breakfast carbohydrate has been correctly covered with a carb bolus. The blood sugar may remain higher than usual at lunch and into the afternoon hours.

If you have unusual spikes in your readings after breakfast, consider whether you may be having unrecognized nighttime lows. See Chapter 20 for signs of unrecognized nighttime lows. For information on setting and testing overnight basal doses, see Chapter 11.

What To Do

This pattern appears similar to taking a carb bolus that is too small for the breakfast carbs, but it is created by an entirely different problem. Learn to recognize the symptoms that may occur the morning after nighttime hypoglycemia on page 222. Set an alarm for 2 a.m. to check whether your blood sugar is dropping in the middle of the night. Reduce the evening basal dose if necessary. It is wise to test the blood sugar at 2 a.m. every week or so, even when you don't seem to be having any problems.

Use of a continuous blood glucose monitor or a Sleep Sentry provides an easy way to identify the problem. Set the alarm feature, and it will warn you every time your blood sugar drops below the limit you set. A download of the data into a PC lets you see the entire night's readings and can open your eyes to a problem you never knew existed.

Fine Tuning

Eventually, you will have made enough adjustments in your doses, or have changed the timing or type of your insulins so that lows and highs are no longer your main concern. Keeping your readings within your target range then becomes your main priority.

Pay attention to matching your meal doses precisely to grams of carbs and their glycemic index, and make additional adjustments for changes in activity. Although the results from fine-tuning may not be as dramatic, making these subtle adjustments every day keeps you involved in your control and lets you see ever better readings and A1c results.

Celebrate small victories. Never feel guilty or blame yourself for a blood sugar reading that is out of your target range. Always recognize that if you don't test because you dread seeing the result, it still affects your body. Only testing allows you to attain really optimal control. When you encounter an unwanted reading or series of readings, stay focused on figuring out what happened and how you can adapt for better control. Aim to get your next reading back into your target range. Allow your mastery over your blood sugar to continue to evolve and improve.

Some people think there is no pattern to their records. Readings may vary anywhere between 30 and 400 mg/dl (1.7 to 22.2 mmol) at different times of the day. Causes for this apparent lack of consistency usually can be identified, however. The next chapter deals with variable blood sugars and can help in attaining optimal control.

"Man is the only animal that laughs and has a state legislature."
Samuel Butler

Why Blood Sugars Vary

CHAPTER

19

When blood sugar readings are often high or low at one time of day, a solution is usually easy to track down. Truly variable blood sugars, on the other hand, seem to have little or no pattern. Readings may stray inconsistently out of your target range at various times of the day.

A little detective work often can find the reason this is happening. Your first step is to discover what causes your blood sugar to vary.

Things that cause the blood sugar to vary:

- Frequent lows caused by too much insulin
- Overeating due to an excessive fear of lows
- Skipping insulin doses
- Erratic or incorrect timing for injections
- Variable absorption of insulin
- An insulin regimen that is too rigid for your lifestyle or a lifestyle too erratic for your insulin
- Poor matching of carb intake with carb boluses or problems with carb counting
- Consuming types or amounts of foods that create control problems
- Stress or pain

Frequent Lows And Problems With Insulin Doses

Frequent lows can be a major source of variability due to excessive stress hormone release or overtreatment. How to prevent frequent lows is reviewed on page 186 in Chapter 17. Focus on stopping lows first whenever your blood sugar is going up and down. Additional information about hypoglycemia can be found in Chapter 20.

Even though insulin doses may be exactly measured, the impact of the dose given may vary from day to day. Table 19.1 shows some of the things that have been shown to cause variability in insulin absorption. Discuss any of these that you suspect may be causing changes in your readings with your health care provider.

207

Variable Lifestyle

If your work or school schedule is erratic and you eat or exercise irregularly, the source for ups and downs in your charts should not be hard to find. You may have started a new job, added exercise to an already jumbled schedule, or changed your meal or sleep times. Lifestyle variability can challenge your skills at giving correct insulin doses.

A consistent lifestyle makes it easier to set appropriate insulin doses. If you have an irregular lifestyle and variable readings, try to create a period where your lifestyle is as stable as possible. Once your insulin doses are sorted out, you can more easily reintroduce flexibility into your life. You'll find you can handle the changes you want more easily from a baseline of consistent readings. Remember that a flexible lifestyle requires frequent testing, consistent recording of these variables, and daily insulin dose adjustments.

> **19.1 Causes For Variable Insulin Absorption**
>
> - Insulin dose
> - Site of injection
> - Depth of injection (IM vs SC)
> - Exercise
> - Local heat/massage
> - Mixing insulins
> - Poor resuspension of NPH, L, or UL
> - Smoking
>
> IM - intramuscular, SC - subcutaneous

What To Do

- Monitor before and after meals. Record your blood sugar results, carb intake, insulin doses, and the timing for each. Make notes on your charts or logbooks about stress, exercise, pain, sleep, and work hours that may affect your readings.
- If possible, eat meals with the same amount of carbohydrate at the same time of day for a while.
- Exercise at regular times. Note whether the type, amount, or timing of your exercise affects your blood sugar.
- Working an overnight shift is usually not a great problem if the weekend schedule does not vary greatly from the weekday schedule. If your weekend schedule varies, discuss with your doctor how to change your workday and weekend doses to match this shift in schedule.
- If you work a rotating shift, see if you can work one shift until your insulin doses are correctly set. If you work a rotating shift and have poor control, seek help from your physician to sort out a workable management plan that uses a flat basal insulin or an insulin pump.

Carb Problems

Varied foods in varied amounts at varied times makes stability hard to achieve, especially if your carb factor has never been accurately determined and your carb measurements are not precise.

Half your TDD is used to cover carbs. Mismatches between carbs and carb boluses are a frequent cause for variable readings. Correct matching of carb intake with carb boluses becomes one of the most critical elements for control. Three areas create problems in matching meals with boluses.

Measurement Errors

Optimal blood sugar control is difficult when carbs are not accurately measured. It is impossible to give an accurate carb bolus unless the amount of carbohydrate in a meal is known. Inexperience in measurement, frequent eating out, or not measuring at all can create problems. If testing shows

> ### 19.2 Questions To Ask When You Have No Pattern
>
> When you're on a rollercoaster and frustrated with the lack of control, calm down, put on your thinking cap, and circle your answer to each question below.
>
> Are you:
>
> | | | |
> |---|---|---|
> | • having frequent or severe low blood sugars? | yes | no |
> | • not counting or measuring carbs accurately? | yes | no |
> | • eating irregularly, different carbs at different times? | yes | no |
> | • skipping meals? | yes | no |
> | • changing insulin doses a lot from day to day? | yes | no |
> | • exercising at different times, intensities, or durations? | yes | no |
> | • not exercising at all? | yes | no |
> | • sleeping at irregular hours? | yes | no |
> | • experiencing stress? | yes | no |
> | • experiencing pain? | yes | no |
>
> If you answer "yes" to several questions or emphatically to one, your control can be improved by dealing with these areas of your life. As you regulate habits, avoid lows and lessen stress for a few days, more consistent patterns will appear on your charts. Consistent patterns enable you to make meaningful changes in your insulin doses.

your basal doses are good but your blood sugar becomes erratic after you eat, the cause will likely be a mismatch between carbs and carb boluses. On your charts, look for high or low blood sugars related to particular meals, especially meals that are eaten out.

When a blood sugar goes high after a meal, may people think "I shouldn't have eaten so much." A proactive approach to this is to think, "Next time I'll take enough insulin to cover those carbs!" When your blood sugar rises and falls in relation to meals, look through your charts and consider whether your carb boluses need to vary more to match the carb content in your meals.

What To Do

• Review how to measure carbs with your dietician or physician. Use food labels, books, measuring cups and spoons, and a gram scale, as needed, to improve your accuracy.

- Measure your carbs carefully for awhile and eat meals with the same amount of carb at the same time each day.

- Carry a PDA, calculator, or other tool to help you measure your carbs accurately. Divide the total carbs in each meal by your carb factor to obtain accurate bolus doses.

- If you eat out often, try eating a favorite meal at the same restaurant several times until you can accurately cover it. Test before, two hours and four hours after the meal. After a few tries it will be obvious how many units are needed for that meal. The carb bolus that is required helps determine how many grams of carb are actually in the meal.

- *The Guide To Healthy Restaurant Eating* and *Eat Out, Eat Right* listed on page 87 are very handy books to have for eating out. They list foods available in different fast food and chain restaurants and how many grams of carbohydrate they contain.

Differences In Glycemic Index

> ### 19.3 Restaurant Tip
>
> Take your gram scale and the carb percentages in Appendix A with you to the restaurant. Weigh your food and calculate the grams of carbohydrate in it. Don't worry. People do strange things in restaurants. Pretend you are a government inspector or food critic. Your self-consciousness will be more than offset by your improved control and the extra service you receive from the waiter.

As noted in Chapter 8 on carb counting, 50 grams of carbohydrate from ice cream can have a totally different effect on your blood sugar than 50 grams from a bowl of cold cereal. Although the amount of carbohydrate is the same, your blood sugar is likely to rise higher and faster after you eat the cereal with its higher glycemic index.

When dieticians realized that different carbohydrates affected blood sugars differently, they attempted to quantify these differences by developing a glycemic index. Fast-acting carbs with a high glycemic index number are more likely to cause postmeal blood sugar readings to spike compared to low glycemic index foods.

If you start with a blood sugar of 82 mg/dl (4.6 mmol), shoot up to 317 mg/dl (17.7 mmol) two hours later, and return to 103 mg/dl (5.8 mmol) before the next meal without taking a correction bolus for the high reading, the carb bolus used to cover the carbohydrate was correct. However, the excessive spiking results from not taking your bolus early enough before the meal or from eating a food which has a high glycemic index.

What To Do

- Check the foods you are eating against those listed in the Glycemic Index on pages 94 and 95. If the foods you eat have a high rating, try foods with a lower rating. Try to keep most of your food choices below 60 on the GI scale.

- If you want to eat a high glycemic index food, take your meal bolus earlier than usual to offset the fast acting carbohydrate.

• Try different types or brands of foods. Instead of a wheat or corn-based cereal, try one made from oats or rice, such as old-fashioned oatmeal, or one that has more fiber, such as All Bran® or Shredded Wheat and Bran®.

> ### 19.4 A Three Day Diet Diary
>
> At your next dietician appointment, bring along a three-day diet diary with brand names, portion sizes, and your estimate of the carb content of meals you typically eat. This not only helps to improve your carb counting, but will allow your dietician to make helpful suggestions to improve your diet.

Instead of a ripe banana, try strawberries. Instead of white rice, try brown or wild rice. The book **The New Glucose Revolution** shows how to shift a diet toward lower glycemic index foods. See page 93 for where to order this book.

Unusual Food Effects

Some foods have unexpected effects on the blood sugar. Candies or foods sweetened with sorbitol may send the blood sugar higher than expected, while foods sweetened with Nutrisweet or saccharine do not. Chips and pretzels often raise blood sugar readings more than expected. Chinese foods and meat pizza are renowned for their tendency to raise the blood sugar. Research has shown that pizza raises the sugar higher than the carb content suggests it should,[50] confirming the experience many people have had with it. Some have noted that pizza which is lower in fat, such as a vegetarian pizza or a particular brand of pizza, does not raise the blood sugar as much. Look for any unusual rise in your blood sugar when you eat a particular food, and adjust your carb boluses or food choices appropriately.

What To Do

• Write down all the foods you eat on your charts, not just the carbohydrates. Record the brand names and quantities of all foods to see if there are any differences in how a particular food affects you.

• If you suspect a particular food has an unusual effect on your blood sugar, compare these readings to other meals with similar amounts of carbohydrate to see if there is a difference.

• If you suspect a particular food, even cheese or meat, is affecting your blood sugar, experiment by omitting it or eating less to see if your readings improve.

• Make an appointment with your dietician or physician to sort this out, and bring with you a three-day food record.

Stress

Stress may have a dramatic effect on blood sugar control. You may experience extra stress during an extended illness, following the death of a family member or friend, or as a result of problems at work or in a relationship. Chronic or low-key stress may be hard to recognize.

Stressful events often make it difficult to continue normal patterns of living. Eating, sleeping and exercise may all be altered. Sleep may be lost, exercise and other calming activities may be put aside, and comfort foods high in sugar and fat may be eaten more often. Controlling the blood sugar during stress becomes difficult because the customary order in daily life has been disrupted.

Fight-or-flight hormones help us remain alert and active during stress. Unfortunately, they also interfere with insulin and cause extra glucose to be produced and released into the blood. This causes higher readings and the need for additional insulin at irregular periods that are determined by the level of stress.

During emotional periods, the blood sugar rises. A high blood sugar, in turn, causes more stress hormones to be released and magnifies emotional reactions. Elevated blood sugars may cause depression and irritability that further impair the ability to deal with the stress at hand.

The challenge of caring for your diabetes may itself cause chronic stress and frustration. During your first attempts at blood sugar control, you may become frustrated when improvements are slow in coming.

If you feel like a totally different person when you are on vacation and your blood sugar becomes easier to control, this provides a good measure for how much stress you are under. Family and friends often see a person's stress before he or she does. Pay attention to their comments. This can be an excellent barometer of your stress and alert you to the need to make changes or seek treatment.

What To Do

- Practice good eating habits all the time. If you avoid candy bars when life is going well, you are less likely to pick up a candy bar when stress hits.
- Keep testing. When you are under stress, testing and exercise are often the first things that are dropped. Testing allows you to have correction boluses for a faster improvement in your readings. Better blood sugar control improves brain function and lowers stress hormone levels. Whatever the source, stress can be handled better when your blood sugar is better controlled.
- Take the time to exercise if at all possible. Moving the feet does wonders for the mind. Exercise releases helpful endorphins so that you feel better. It also reduces insulin resistance so insulin is more effective in controlling your blood sugar.
- The demands of blood glucose monitoring, counting carbs, and blood glucose regulation can be overwhelming at times. Take a break if you really need one. Determine how much time off you need to clear your mind. Take the time needed and come back to your monitoring with new vigor.
- If you feel frustrated by your blood sugar readings or cannot make sense out of your charts, seek help from others. Talk with your physician or ask for a referral to someone who specializes in blood sugar control.
- Stress management classes are offered by many community colleges and employers. Yoga, stretching, meditation, listening to calming tapes, or a good massage help to reduce stress.

19.5 Hypophilia And Hypophobia

One group, though small in number, that is cursed with poor control includes individuals who have hypophobia. These individuals avoid bringing their blood sugars down to normal because they have an inordinate fear of lows. People with hypophobia tend to have very few lows and can usually relate a particular episode where they became so frightened because of a low that they now spend considerable effort avoiding any readings near the normal range. Despite blood sugars that are quite high, when any increase in insulin dose is recommended by a physician, great resistance is encountered.

At the other end of the spectrum are hypophiliacs or individuals who have frequent and severe low blood sugars. Despite repeated efforts over time by health care personnel, serious low blood sugars continue to occur in these individuals.

One gentleman suffered from hypophilia more than two decades, as a result of an encounter on his first visit to a "diabetes specialist" shortly after he began to get serious about improving his control. On entering the physician's waiting room, he found himself in the midst of several amputees. Rather than leave and find a physician who knew how to prevent this from happening, he instead swore that he would never let his blood sugar go high. His zealous efforts led to repeated episodes of hypoglycemia and eventual loss of employment.

Elements of obsessive-compulsive behavior are often present in individuals who are fixated on avoiding low or high blood sugars. Counseling and treatment with an antidepressant medication can be helpful as part of an overall control program. A firm and steady approach by a diabetes specialist or psychologist can gradually improve blood sugar control without exacerbating underlying fears.

© 2003 Diabetes Services, Inc.

- How you respond to stress is largely a learned process. If you note frequent high blood sugars following job pressure, arguments, or bad news, seek the advice of a specialist in how to better handle your responses.
- Some antidepressants help reduce types of stress that originate from an excessive focus on problems.
- Talk. Stress is always worse when carried alone. Share your feelings, worries, guilt and pain with others. No burden is too great to share with others.

Pain

Physical pain is often not recognized as a major player in blood sugar control. Whether caused by an accident or arthritis, when the body hurts, inflammatory particles are released. Inflammatory particles, such as tumor necrosis factor and cytokines, not only cause pain but they also cause the body to become resistant to insulin. Larger insulin doses are always required in the presence of pain. The more you hurt, the higher your insulin doses need to be for good control. Luckily, pain can usually be eliminated or greatly reduced. Talk with your physician about what steps you need to take to do this.

19.6 Why Portal Insulin Delivery Is Better

Location is everything in real estate and in insulin delivery. The pancreas and liver have ideal locations in the body to perform their jobs. When a person who does not have diabetes glances at a plate of ravioli, the brain senses the pending carb intake and signals the pancreas to begin releasing insulin. Even the aroma of food can cause a release of stored insulin.

The pancreas releases insulin into the portal vein which goes directly to the liver. After a carb-rich meal, the liver may see its insulin level rise by 20-fold in a matter of minutes. Alerted by a rise in insulin level, the liver is able to convert about half the incoming glucose which arrives by the same route into glycogen which it stores. This quick removal of glucose keeps after-meal blood sugars from rising above 140 mg/dl (7.8 mmol) even after the largest of meals.

In diabetes, insulin injected under the skin has no direct path to the liver as does insulin released by the pancreas into the portal vein. Because portal insulin levels do not rise following an injection, the liver does not store as much glucose after a meal. Even with rapid insulins, after-meal blood sugars may rise above 140 mg/dl (7.8 mmol).

If insulin could be taken in pill form and quickly absorbed from the stomach, it would go directly into the portal vein along with glucose from food. Two companies are working on modified forms of insulin that can be swallowed and absorbed. This method of insulin delivery would help blood sugar control but would not completely replace premeal injections because oral insulin cannot be given in precise doses.

As another alternative, portal insulin delivery can be created by surgically placing a port on the outer abdominal wall to deliver insulin directly into the peritoneal cavity. About half of this infused insulin is absorbed quickly into the portal vein. Like oral insulin, this approach reduces the ups and downs in post-meal readings and helps avoid low blood sugars.

Despite its less-than-perfect delivery under the skin, injected insulin works amazingly well. The speed of today's rapid insulins helps to lower after meal blood sugars. Their shorter action time helps prevent after meal lows and provides more consistent insulin activity from day to day.

"One who never gets carried away should be."
Malcolm Forbes

Hypoglycemia

People on insulin are often concerned that excess insulin may drive their blood sugar too low. Mild lows can be annoying or embarrassing, while severe lows can be dangerous.

A low blood sugar may cause you to shake, sweat, and feel disoriented, or impair your mental awareness and reaction times. Thinking becomes impaired because glucose supplies, which the brain relies on to function, are unavailable and, unlike other organs, the brain cannot switch to alternate fuels to operate. Loss of coordination, confusion, release of stress hormones, and irritability usually begin when the blood sugar goes below 60 mg/dl (3.3 mmol).

You may misjudge your condition and begin to argue with others who notice the distinct change in your personality and performance. Confusion and irritability during hypoglycemia often cause a person to deny they are having a problem, and may severely challenge the efforts of others who are trying to help.

This chapter discusses the following aspects of hypoglycemia:

- Causes
- Symptoms
- Treatment
- Prevention

Causes

Low blood sugars are most likely:

1. When too much insulin has been given
2. When a carb bolus is given, but eating is delayed, interrupted or skipped
3. When an excessive carb bolus is given because the carb content of a meal has been overestimated
4. When an insulin bolus is given while residual insulin is still active from recent carb or correction boluses
5. After drinking alcohol, which adds to mental impairment and blocks glucose release from the liver

6. During and following increased activity

7. On vacations or long weekends, when stress may be reduced, activity increased, and mealtimes more erratic

Be alert for changes in your routine that cause low blood sugars. Watch for increased activity, travel, a vacation, or loss of weight. Activities, such as a long hike, mall shopping, cleaning the house, fixing dinner for company, a canoe trip, digging the garden in spring, or shoveling snow after a storm, are especially likely to cause lows during or shortly after the activity. A low may occur several hours later as muscles draw extra glucose from the blood to replenish their depleted glycogen stores.

Frequent or severe low blood sugars mean that too much insulin is being given for a person's current weight, activity level, and carb intake. This is especially true if lows occur within one to three hours after a carb bolus or when more than 20 grams of glucose are required to bring the blood sugar back to normal. At the first sign that lows are becoming frequent, call your physician/health care team to discuss lowering your basal and bolus doses by 5% to 10%.

Those who exercise strenuously or for prolonged periods will benefit from reducing their insulin doses to match the increase in activity. When people are more active, they need less insulin. When they are less active, they will need more insulin.

Be sure to consult with your physician or health care team if you are uncertain what to do to stop low blood sugars, or you are gaining unwanted weight because carb intake is the only tool you use to remedy hypoglycemia. Remember or write down the solutions they suggest so you can be on top of things when this or a similar situation reappears. With experience, you will be able to make your own insulin dose adjustments.

Symptoms

Hypoglycemia symptoms vary greatly. Lows may occur with no symptoms, minor symptoms, or full-blown symptoms. They will vary from person to person and from one low to the next in the same person. A single symptom may make you aware that your blood sugar has become low, or you may suddenly become aware of several symptoms at once.

> ### 20.1 "I Feel Bad When I'm Normal"
>
> Some individuals will not feel well when their readings go near the normal range. Reasons for this physical discomfort include having become accustomed to high readings over several months or years and needing to take longer to readapt to normal, or having taken the reading while still in the normal range but the body senses the blood sugar is dropping quickly due to an excess of insulin.

Symptoms are created both by the effect of the low blood sugar on the brain and other organs (weakness, difficulty concentrating, slurred speech, giddiness, confusion, poor judgment, vision problems, sleepiness, yawning), and by the effects of adrenaline and glucagon (sweating, fast heart rate, trembling, irritation, and hunger) which are released in large quantities to raise the blood sugar.

A low blood sugar may first be recognized by the person having it or by others nearby. Check your blood sugar as soon as you suspect you may be low or someone around you suggests this. If someone approaches with a glass of orange juice or asks you to check your blood sugar, do so immediately and cooperatively. You may have to train yourself ahead of time to accept this help without question. Denial and resisting help from others is one of the better indicators of a low blood sugar.

If you live alone or do not have another person around who quickly recognizes lows, you want to focus on prevention. Do this by setting your blood sugar targets higher and insulin doses lower.

Once multiple insulin doses have been closely matched to need, the blood sugar will begin to go low more slowly. Fortunately, a slower blood sugar drop provides more time to respond. Unfortunately, symptoms also appear more gradually and may be harder to recognize. Learn to recognize and pay attention to these more subtle symptoms. Make a list of your personal symptoms and share these with your friends and family or whoever is likely to help you.

> ### 20.2 Signs That You Are Low
>
> - Sweating
> - Shaking
> - Irritability
> - Poor concentration
> - Blurred vision
> - Fast heart rate
> - Hunger
> - Headache
> - Sudden tiredness
> - Dizziness and confusion
> - Numbness or tingling of the lips
> - Nausea or vomiting
> - Frequent sighing
> - Headache
> - Silliness
> - Yawning
> - Resisting help from others

The faster you recognize hypoglycemia, the faster you can respond and bring the blood sugar back to normal. An early response reduces stress hormone release and lessens the chance that your blood sugar will spike afterward. Early testing can alert you when symptoms are minimal and shorten the time when you are out of control.

When you test a blood sugar, consider whether your blood sugar may be moving downward because you still have unused bolus insulin in your system. If your current blood sugar is 120 mg/dl (6.7 mmol) you may smile with satisfaction. Alternatively, you may realize it has been only an hour or two since you took a large bolus and you need to eat to avoid an approaching low blood sugar.

One advantage to using a continuous monitor is that it can track blood sugar trends and warn of lows before they occur. Trends that show a dropping blood sugar signal a pending low before it becomes a real one. To make this happen, select a blood sugar threshold on the device that gives you sufficient warning to take action.

Treatment

Treat Lows Quickly

Not even the most conscientious person can prevent every low blood sugar. Acknowledging that lows will occur should motivate you to keep treatments readily at hand.

Unless you are eating a meal right away, the best treatment for lows is a combination of simple and complex carbohydrates plus some protein. Fifteen to 20 grams of quick carbohydrates, such as glucose, Sweet Tarts™ or honey should raise the blood sugar be-

---

20.3 Treatment Plan For Hypoglycemia

1. Eat 15 to 20 grams of fast-acting carbohydrates immediately.
2. Consider how much unused bolus insulin may still be active. Decide whether complex carbohydrates and/or protein are needed to keep you stable until you eat your next meal. Cheese and crackers, bread with peanut butter, half an apple with cheese, a cup of milk, or another carb/protein combination may be needed after eating the quick carbs.
3. Test your blood sugar 30 minutes later to make sure it has risen. Repeat Step 1 if necessary.
4. After a moderate or severe low blood sugar, wait 30 to 45 minutes before driving or operating machinery. A return to normal coordination and thinking is slower than the return to a normal blood sugar.

When You May Need To Eat More Than 20 Grams For A Low

- When you took a carb bolus for a meal but never ate it.
- When it has been only an hour or two since your last injection of rapid insulin.
- When you have been more physically active.

---

tween 45 and 80 mg/dl (1.7 to 4.4 mmol) depending upon your weight. After treating with quick carbs, eating some additional complex carbs and protein can help keep the blood sugar from dropping later.

Correcting a low blood sugar quickly shuts off the release of stress hormones. You feel better when your body is quickly resupplied with the fuel it needs. Your brain, muscles and other cells will thank you for not prolonging their misery. Remember that many candy bars and cookies do not act quickly, and when consumed in large amounts, cause a high blood sugar to follow.

Glucose is the "sugar" in blood sugar and may also be referred to as dextrose on labels. It comes in tablets, such as Dex4 or BD Glucose tablets, and in certain candies like Sweet Tarts. Glucose breaks down quickly and reaches the blood as 100 percent glucose, which makes it the best choice for raising the blood sugar quickly.

Table sugar consists of one glucose molecule and one fructose molecule, so when it breaks down in the stomach, only half is immediately available as glucose.

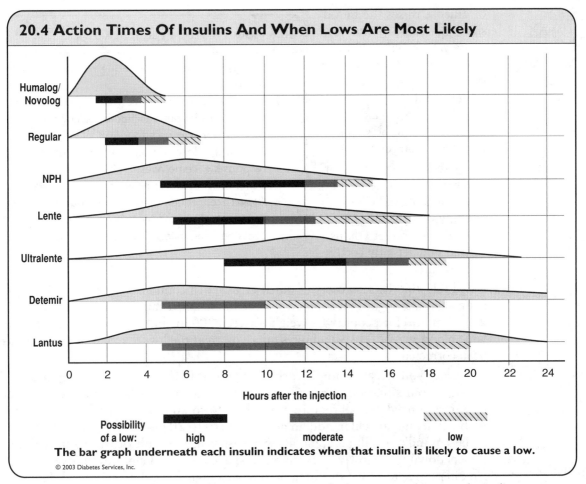

20.4 Action Times Of Insulins And When Lows Are Most Likely

Hours after the injection

Possibility of a low: high moderate low

The bar graph underneath each insulin indicates when that insulin is likely to cause a low.

© 2003 Diabetes Services, Inc.

Fruit juices, like orange juice, contain mostly fructose and are a relatively poor choice for quick treatment of serious hypoglycemia because they take so long to raise the blood sugar. For mild lows, these differences may not be vital, but if a low is serious, you want to choose the fastest carb available to get you back on your feet quickly. Choose a high glycemic food for a quick rise of the blood sugar. See the glycemic index on pages 94 and 95 for more guidance to the highest glycemic index foods to speed up the rise in your blood sugar.

How much glucose do you need to correct a low blood sugar? A good rule of thumb is that 1 gram

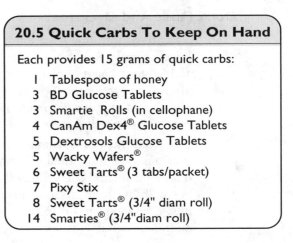

20.5 Quick Carbs To Keep On Hand

Each provides 15 grams of quick carbs:

1	Tablespoon of honey
3	BD Glucose Tablets
3	Smartie Rolls (in cellophane)
4	CanAm Dex4® Glucose Tablets
5	Dextrosols Glucose Tablets
5	Wacky Wafers®
6	Sweet Tarts® (3 tabs/packet)
7	Pixy Stix
8	Sweet Tarts® (3/4" diam roll)
14	Smarties® (3/4"diam roll)

of glucose raises the blood sugar 3, 4, or 5 points for those who weigh 200 lb., 150 lb., and 100 lb. respectively. A 5-gram glucose tablet should raise your blood sugar between 15 and 25 points, with the smaller rise seen in larger people.

Use 15 to 20 grams of quick carbohydrate for all low blood sugars. Check to see how many grams are in each glucose tablet you use so that you actually get 15 to 20 grams.

> ### 20.6 How To Stop Frequent Lows
>
> 1. Identify the time of day during which the most severe lows occur.
> 2. Identify which insulins are working at this time of day. Check your basal/bolus balance to make sure each makes up about 50% of your TDD.
> 3. Reduce the dose of insulin that is most likely responsible, remembering that an excess of either basal or bolus doses can cause lows.
> 4. If lows are frequent and severe, your TDD will need to be lowered by 10% or more. If lows are occasional and mild, a 5% reduction may be perfect.

Table 20.5 lists a variety of quick carbs. Each contains 15 grams of glucose or an equivalent fast sugar that should raise the blood sugar rapidly between 45 and 75 mg/dl (4.2 mmol) for people who weigh between 200 lb. and 100 lb., respectively. Test your blood sugar 20 to 30 minutes after you treat the low to make sure that it has been corrected.

Once you've eaten simple carbs and your thinking is no longer impaired, consider your situation. A recent injection of Humalog or Novolog, extra exercise, or a missed meal will all require more than 15 to 20 grams of carbs for treatment. At bedtime, in particular, add an additional 10 to 20 grams of carbohydrate, such as a glass of milk or half an apple. Raw cornstarch, a complex carbohydrate that breaks down very slowly, is available in special bars to help prevent overnight lows. An alternative to raw cornstarch is to have a high fat and protein food, like cheese or peanut butter, or part of an athletic bar. Protein and complex carbohydrates help keep the blood sugar from dropping for several hours.

Don't Panic And Overtreat

Stress hormone release during a low can cause panic. If you overdose on orange juice, chocolates, candy, or the entire contents of your refrigerator, your goal of a stable blood sugar becomes difficult to achieve. If your blood sugar often goes high after a low, you know you are eating too much for a low blood sugar. If you find yourself gaining weight from overtreating lows, this is another reason to avoid this type of panic.

Keep track of how many carbs you eat for each low. Use glucose tablets whenever possible. Individual tabs have 4 to 5 grams of glucose, which is enough to raise the blood sugar 12 to 25 mg/dl (.7-1.4 mmol) for adults. Three or four tabs are normally sufficient to return the blood sugar to normal. If you do overeat after a low, take a carb bolus to cover most or all of the extra carbs. The wiser and safer method, of course, is not to overtreat lows.

Prepare for the panic by having a preset amount of quick carbohydrate handy at your bedside, in your pocket or purse, at your desk, and in the glove compartment of your car. Memorize that it takes only a little carb to counteract most lows. A low does not mean unlimited treat time! Keep glucose tabs or another quick carb handy and use them

20.7 How Much Does 1 Gram of Carbs Raise Your BG?	
If your weight is:	**1 gram will raise you about:**
50 lbs (23 kg)	8 mg/dl (0.44 mmol)
75 lbs (34 kg)	7 mg/dl (0.39 mmol)
90 lbs (41 kg)	6 mg/dl (0.33 mmol)
120 lbs (55 kg)	5 mg/dl (0.28 mmol)
160 lbs (73 kg)	4 mg/dl (0.22 mmol)
200 lbs (91 kg)	3 mg/dl (0.17 mmol)

© 2003 Diabetes Services, Inc.

automatically. Allow time for them to correct your blood sugar before eating food. Your intense hunger will disappear as you recover, and you will be glad later that you did not overindulge.

If you are fearful because you are having frequent lows, chances are good that your TDD is too high. A simple reduction in your insulin doses can do wonders for sanity. Make the insulin dose change right away before overeating and highs add to your blood sugar management woes.

Lows And Rapid Insulin

With rapid insulins like Humalog and Novolog, it is important to use quick carbs to treat lows. Quick carbs like glucose tablets, Sweet Tarts, jelly beans, or Gatorade work well to reverse a rapid drop in glucose that can be encountered.

Lows with Humalog or Novolog happen within three to four hours of an injection. When a low occurs three or four hours after the last carb or correction bolus, less carbohydrate will be required to treat the low because most of the last insulin activity from the last injection is gone. Ten to 15 total grams of carbohydrate will usually remedy this situation.

A low blood sugar near bedtime becomes easier to treat when a rapid insulin is used to cover the carbs at dinner. When bedtime rolls around three or four hours after the dinner bolus of Humalog or Novolog, most of the bolus activity is gone. A small amount of quick carb should be all that is needed to ensure a sound sleep, provided the night basal has been correctly set.

However, when a low blood sugar happens only two hours after a bolus, much of the insulin has yet to work. Quick carbs will be required to raise the blood sugar quickly along with additional carbs to keep the blood sugar from dropping again.

Remember that thinking and coordination may continue to be impaired for 30 minutes after the blood sugar has been brought back to normal. After a moderately low blood sugar, wait at least 30 to 45 minutes after the blood sugar has returned to normal before driving a car or operating machinery.

Nighttime Hypoglycemia

Waking up in the middle of the night shaking and sweating is not a pleasant experience. When middle-of-the-night lows in blood sugar are experienced, at least one insulin dose needs to be lowered.

Most people do not awaken when they go low in the night and simply sleep through it. If you awaken one night sweating and shaking, there likely have been other nights when you had a low that went unnoticed.

Night lows are a special concern because over half of all severe hypoglycemia occurs during the night. During sleep, mild symptoms of a low blood sugar are unlikely to be recognized, and even serious symptoms may not awaken those who sleep soundly. If you awaken during the night with any of the symptoms below, check your blood sugar immediately or eat quick carbohydrate and then check your blood sugar.

Symptoms Of A Low During The Night :

- Nightmares
- Waking up very alert or with a fast heart rate
- Damp night clothes, sheets, or pillow
- Restlessness and inability to go back to sleep
- Waking up with a vague but persistent feeling that something isn't right

After an unrecognized nighttime low, the following symptoms may occur when you awaken the next morning. If you have any of these, test your blood sugar at 2 a.m. for a few nights to determine whether night lows are occurring.

Symptoms The Morning After An Unrecognized Night Low:

- Waking up with a headache or feeling "foggy-headed"
- Having an unusually high blood sugar after breakfast or before lunch
- A temporary loss of memory for words or names

Use Glucagon For Severe Low Blood Sugars

For a severe low blood sugar, injected glucagon is the best treatment. Glucagon, a hormone made by the alpha cells in the pancreas, rapidly raises the blood sugar by triggering a release of glucose from glycogen stores in the liver. Injected glucagon is the fastest way to raise a low blood sugar, but it requires that an injection be given by someone who has been trained to mix and inject it at the time it is needed.

When someone with diabetes resists treatment, becomes unconscious, or has seizures due to hypoglycemia, glucagon can be injected by another person to rapidly raise the blood sugar. It is also handy for self-injection when someone with diabetes is ill or nauseated and cannot eat to correct a low blood sugar.

20.8 How To Prevent Night Lows

The lowest blood sugar of the day usually occurs around 2 a.m. In an early study of people with Type 1 diabetes using Regular and NPH, researchers found they averaged one low blood sugar every four nights. Fortunately, today's new analog insulins have reduced the frequency of lows, especially at night.

Lows occur in the middle of the night because the body is most sensitive to insulin between midnight and 3 a.m. Around 3 a.m., the liver starts to increase glucose production, causing the blood sugar to rise toward breakfast.

If you suspect you may be having night lows, test at 2 a.m. for a few nights. If your reading is low at that time, lower your evening basal dose and test until you are sure your blood sugar drops no more than 30 mg/dl (1.7 mmol) at any point during the night.

You might also consider another approach if your morning basal dose is much larger than your evening dose. For instance, if you take 40 units of Lente before breakfast, but only 4 units at bedtime, the morning dose is likely the one that needs to come down. Try reducing the morning to 36 units first and later increase the bedtime dose to 6 units if the morning reading becomes high.

If you are still using Regular insulin, switch to Humalog or Novolog to help avoid lows. If you use Lente, NPH, or Ultralente, consider switching to Lantus insulin. Recent unpublished research in a large group of people with Type 1 diabetes by Dr. Satish Garg at the University of Colorado shows Lantus helps to lower the risk of hypoglycemia.

Prolonged exercise or activity can cause the blood sugar to fall for 24 to 36 hours afterward. After a day of increased exercise or activity, it is wise to reduce the carb bolus for dinner and the evening basal dose as well. Extra free carbs at bedtime that you do not balance with a bolus are also wise.

Covering high bedtime blood sugars with too large a correction bolus is another common trigger for night lows. Try bringing down bed time highs with half your normal correction dose.

Glucagon kits are available by prescription and should be kept at home by everyone who uses insulin. The kit can be stored at room temperature or in the refrigerator and is stable for several years after purchase. Dating should be checked periodically to ensure potency. Instructions on how to prepare and inject glucagon should be provided to the person who has diabetes and to the person who is likely to be giving the injection. A diabetes educator, trained nurse, or pharmacist can show how to inject glucagon.

The typical dose in a glucagon kit is 1 milligram, which is sufficient to dose a 200 lb. person. A full dose may cause nausea in a child or small adult and is often more than is needed for those who weigh less than 150 lbs. One half a dose may be all that's required, or you can calculate 10 percent of a full dose for each 20 pounds of weight. If the blood sugar hasn't risen in ten to fifteen minutes after the injection, the other half dose can always be given. Call for emergency services if the person hasn't shown noticeable improvement within 15 minutes.

> ### 20.9 Prevent Follow-up Low Blood Sugars
>
> One low blood sugar increases the risk for another. Researchers in Virginia found that the chance for having a second low after one initial reaction increased by 46 percent over the next 24 hours, 24 percent on the second day, and 12 percent on the third day after the original hypoglycemic event.[35] An enhanced sensitivity to insulin following the first low blood sugar contributes to this increased risk.
>
> Not only is the risk of a second low greater, but symptoms during the second one are milder and harder to recognize. After stress hormones are released during the first low blood sugar, the body's stores are reduced for the next two to three days, causing a reduction in warning symptoms.
>
> Do not take chances. Take steps to keep your blood sugar higher for the next 24 hours after a low by eating free (uncovered) carbs or lowering your carb boluses.

If you are ever unable to handle a low blood sugar by yourself, lose consciousness, or suffer convulsions, notify your physician as soon as possible afterward. Events like this usually indicate that a major reduction in insulin doses is needed. Discuss the situation openly with your physician to prevent a reoccurrence.

Hypoglycemia And Driving

Driving a car can be hypnotic or trancelike. With your attention on the road and other cars, you may not notice that your reflexes, coordination, and ability to think, make decisions and interact with others have all changed. If your blood sugar drops slowly during a drive, a low blood sugar becomes especially hard to recognize, while the risk of injury or death to yourself and others rises. If you drive and become involved in an auto accident due to a low blood sugar, many states automatically suspend your license.

Always check your blood sugar before driving. Do not drive if your blood sugar is below 80 mg/dl (4.4 mmol) before starting the car or if it is likely to drop below 80 mg/dl (4.4 mmol) at any time during the drive. If your blood sugar is between 80 and 100 mg/dl (4.4 and 5.6 mmol) before a short drive, eat 10 to 20 grams of fast glucose. Increase your carb intake for longer drives. Consider when your last bolus was taken and eat extra carbs as needed.

Keep glucose tablets or other quick carbohydrate easily accessible in your vehicle and always be willing to eat them. This applies even if you can't test. It is better to go high temporarily, rather than have a low while driving.

While driving is not a good time to deny that you have a low blood sugar. Be especially willing to treat lows, if someone else in the vehicle suggests this. Some people always eat a small amount of carbohydrate prior to driving, just to be safe. Once on the road, pull over and test your blood sugar if you have any doubts. On long drives, stop, get out of the car, stretch and test your blood sugar every two hours. Do not become a statistic!

20.10 When A Low Occurs Before An Injection, Do You Reduce The Dose?

When a low blood sugar occurs near the time an injection will be given, should you reduce the dose? After eating fast carbs to treat the low, it may be wise to reduce the rapid insulin given as a carb bolus to lower the risk of another low.

However, basal doses are very different from rapid insulins in their timing. Compared to the rapid action of Humalog and Novolog, basal insulin has no immediate effect.

Humalog and Novolog begin to lower the blood sugar about 20 minutes after an injection, but insulins like Lente, NPH, Ultralente, and Lantus have no effect on the blood sugar for at least 90 to 120 minutes.[67] But if a basal dose is reduced, the reduced insulin activity continues to affect the blood sugar over the following 14 to 24 hours. This means that lowering a basal dose for a low blood sugar makes little sense. However, a reduction in the basal dose may make a lot of sense as a way to eliminate a particular pattern of lows over the following days.

Treatment Tips For The Person With Diabetes

Avoid low blood sugars through careful management of insulin doses and carbohydrate intake. This is always the best strategy and is particularly important for people on insulin who live alone. However, even with the best of efforts, hypoglycemia does happen. When a low blood sugar occurs, the following tips can help in treating it quickly and effectively:

• Practice recognizing early symptoms so that a low blood sugar does not become severe. After a low, look back at what might have warned you earlier.

• Never delay treatment. Treat a low as soon as you recognize it.

• Always carry quick carbs like glucose tablets or simple sugar candies to eat when a low occurs or when you have any reason to suspect a low.

• Let family and friends know when you may be more vulnerable to lows because you are changing your insulin doses or lifestyle. Share what is happening with your blood sugar control so that others can help.

• Assume the primary responsibility for handling and treating your own low blood sugars, but always be willing to accept help from others. Be sure family and friends know about your diabetes and what they can do to help, while you stay in charge of your day-to-day management.

• Never resist when someone suggests that you test your blood sugar. Check as soon as the suggestion is given.

• Test more often when you change your insulin doses or food choices, when stress decreases, and when activity increases.

• Unusual upper body activity or exercise often leads to a low blood sugar. Eat extra carbs before digging, raking, moving boxes, washing your car, or playing tennis, and other such activities you do not routinely do. Test often during and after this activity.

Jeremy

Jeremy takes 10 units of Lente before breakfast and another 10 units before dinner, but he has started to have occasional night lows. After discussing the problem with his physician, they decided to lower his dose of Lente at dinner to 9 units and balance this reduction with a rise to 11 units in his breakfast Lente dose

His physician also suggested other options he could try. One was to move the dinner injection of Lente to bedtime. Another was to use a single dose of Lantus at bedtime that was slightly less than his combined two doses of Lente. With no peak and a lesser variable action, Lantus sometimes maintains better blood sugar levels during the night

When NPH or Lente are given at bedtime so that they peak after 3 a.m., they are less likely to cause lows in the middle of the night. Because these insulins may be inconsistent in their activity, this does not always avoid the problem, however.

	Breakfast	Lunch	Dinner	Bed
Lows during the night	6H/10L	6H	6H/10L	
1st option	6H/11L	5H	7H/9L	
2nd option	6H/12L	5H	7H	8L
3rd option	7H/19 Lantus	5H	8H	
4th option	7H	5H	8H	18 Lantus

- Agree with your family on a plan of action before a problem situation occurs.

- Keep glucagon available at home for severe lows. Be sure that a family member or a friend has been well trained in how and when to inject it. Check the expiration date periodically to ensure it is current.

- Although most follow-up lows occur within 24 hours, be especially careful for 48 hours after a low since this is when the risk of another low is greatest.

- Frequent lows are a major cause of hypoglycemia unawareness. Reduce your insulin doses by 5% to 10% as soon as frequent lows begin to occur. You want to retrain yourself to recognize milder symptoms that will warn you to eat, stop driving, or take other action.

Treatment Tips For Helpers

Whenever someone on insulin is acting abnormally, consider a low blood sugar first. The person may appear drunk, on drugs, needy, obnoxious or mentally impaired, but the real cause is an overdose of insulin. Sugar is needed to bring the blood sugar back to normal. Sugar, a soda, glucose or candy can correct abnormal behavior in 10 to 20 minutes.

Being helpful becomes more difficult when the person with the low blood sugar becomes irrational, confused, or angry as a result of the low. Here are some things that may help:

• Control your emotions first. If the person you are attempting to help is stubborn, acts silly, or becomes angry, do not take it personally. Prepare your mind ahead of time to deal with the variety of hypoglycemia-induced attitudes you may encounter.

• Take charge of the situation, using a gentle but firm tone. A non-confrontational stance, such as sitting or standing beside the person, may help.

• Avoid direct questions like "Are you low?", "Do you need to test?", "Do you need to eat?" or "What do you want to eat?" The person who is unable to think clearly is incapable of making rational decisions and will respond with a "NO" as the most convenient answer.

• Instead say, "Here, have this piece of candy." or "I'm going to drink a coke (take a drink yourself); here, have a sip." or "Drink this. It's good and will make you feel better." Get sugar into them in any way possible.

• Do not let the person drive a car, run machinery, or become involved in other dangerous activities that require coordination.

• Ask for help from others when needed. Keep embarrassment to a minimum and the person's cooperation as high as possible.

"Opportunity is missed by most people because it is dressed in overalls and looks like work."

Thomas Edison

Arachnoleptic fit(n.): The frantic dance performed just after you've accidentally walked through a spider web.

Washington Post's Style Invitational

Hypoglycemia Unawareness

One of the more distressing problems in diabetes is hypoglycemia unawareness. Normally, a person who retains physical responses to hypoglycemia will feel warning symptoms when the blood sugar goes low, especially the shaking and sweating caused by release of stress hormones. However, those with hypoglycemia unawareness have reduced warning signals and do not recognize they are low. If they happen to do a blood sugar test and find they are low, they may not realize what they need to do to treat the low.

Luckily, stress hormone release is sufficient to allow the liver to raise the glucose level, although this may take several hours to work. Fortunately, research and clinical experience has shown that this condition can be reversed.

This chapter presents:

- Causes of hypoglycemia unawareness
- How to reverse hypoglycemia unawareness

That hypoglycemia unawareness could occur during sleep is not surprising since people wake up for less than half of the lows that occur at night, but it happens with equal frequency when people are awake.[68] Unless recognized and treated by someone else, serious problems, such as grand mal seizures, can occur. If you have witnessed seizure activity or bizarre behavior, you have some idea of the seriousness of this problem and the danger involved.

What Causes Hypoglycemia Unawareness?

Hypoglycemia unawareness is not rare. It occurs in 17 percent of those with Type 1 diabetes. Symptoms of a low become less obvious after having diabetes for several years because repeated lows impair the body's release of stress hormones. The major counter-regulatory hormone that causes glucose to be released by the liver to raise the blood sugar is glucagon. Glucagon secretion is reduced in most people who have Type 1 diabetes within the first two to ten years after onset.

Women are more prone to this problem because they have reduced counter-regulatory responses and reduced symptoms.[69] Drinking alcohol increases the risk of an unacknowledged low because the mind becomes less capable of recognizing what's happening, the liver is blocked from creating glucose needed to raise the blood sugar, and free fatty acid (the backup to glucose for fuel) release is also blocked.[70] These factors make symptoms milder and harder to recognize.

Severe hypoglycemia occurred in 40 percent of people with Type 1 diabetes in one Danish study. Of those who experienced it, it occurred about once every 9 months with coma occurring once every two and a half years.[71] In studies like this, it is important to realize that the frequency and severity of hypoglycemia depends on how well the individual is using insulin. The 60% who had no severe hypoglycemia likely differ from the first group in how well they adapt their insulin doses to short-term and long-term changes in insulin requirement.

The lower a person's average blood sugar, the higher the risk for hypoglycemia unawareness. Hypoglycemia unawareness was three times as common in the intensively controlled group compared to the conventionally controlled group in the Diabetes Control and Complications Trial, with 55 percent of the episodes in this study occurring during sleep.

The risk of hypoglycemia unawareness is far lower in people who have Type 2 diabetes because hypoglycemia occurs far less often. A study using tight control in Type 2 diabetes done by the Veterans Administration showed that severe lows occurred only four percent as often in Type 2 compared to Type 1.[72] Hypoglycemia occurs in Type 2 diabetes only if the person is using insulin, a sulfonylurea, or Prandin™.

Hypoglycemia unawareness may be triggered by:

- Frequent low blood sugars
- A rapid drop in the blood sugar
- Having diabetes for many years
- Stress or depression
- Situations where self-care is a low priority
- Alcohol consumption in the last 12 hours
- A previous low blood sugar in the last 24 to 48 hours
- Use of certain medications like beta blockers

Frequent low blood sugars appear to be the major culprit in hypoglycemia unawareness. Dr. Thiemo Veneman and other researchers had 10 people who did not have diabetes spend a day at the hospital on two occasions.[73] While they slept, the researchers used insulin to lower their blood sugar below 45 mg/dl (2.5 mmol) for two hours in the middle of the night.

No, they didn't wake up! People do not wake up during most nighttime lows. Five people went through a nighttime low on the first visit and the other five on the second visit. On waking in the morning, all were given insulin to lower their blood sugar to see when they would recognize the symptoms of a low blood sugar.

Dr. Veneman found that after sleeping through hypoglycemia at night, people had far more trouble recognizing a low blood sugar the following day. Their warning symptoms became less obvious because counter-regulatory hormones, like epinephrine, norepinephrine, and glucagon are released more slowly and in smaller concentrations following the occurrence of a low blood sugar within the previous 24 hours. Because a recent low blood sugar depletes a person of the stress hormones needed to alert him, it is more likely the person will fail to recognize a second low. Since this unawareness occurred in people without diabetes, it's even more likely that a recent low would cause hypoglycemia unawareness in someone who has diabetes.

How To Reverse Hypoglycemia Unawareness

Research has shown that people who have hypoglycemia unawareness can become aware again of low blood sugars by avoiding frequent lows.[74] Preventing all lows for two weeks resulted in increased symptoms of a low blood sugar and a return to nearly normal symptoms after 3 months.

A study in Rome by Dr. Carmine Fanelli and other researchers reduced the frequency of hypoglycemia in people who had had diabetes for seven years or less but who suffered from hypoglycemia unawareness. They raised the target for premeal blood sugars to 140 mg/dl (7.8 mmol) and found that the frequency of hypoglycemia dropped from once every other day to once every 22 days. As the higher premeal blood sugar target led to less hypoglycemia, people once again regained their low blood sugar symptoms. The counter-regulatory hormone response that alerts people to the presence of a low blood sugar returned to nearly normal after a few weeks of less frequent lows.

21.1 Reversing Hypoglycemia Unawareness

- Reduce the frequency of your lows
- Be especially careful to avoid another low for at least two days following a reaction
- Test blood sugars often to note dropping numbers and treat them before they become lows
- Set your target blood sugars slightly higher so that you will experience no more than one or two insulin reactions per week
- Always match your insulin doses to changes in your lifestyle

© 2003 Diabetes Services, Inc.

Avoidance of lows enables people with diabetes to regain their symptoms when they become low. To reverse hypoglycemia unawareness, set your blood sugar targets higher, carefully adjust insulin doses to closely match your diet and exercise, and stay more alert to physical warnings for 48 hours following a first low blood sugar. Consider any blood sugar below 60 mg/dl (3.3 mmol) as serious and practice ways to avoid them. Use your records to predict when lows are likely to occur.

You might also consider using a prescription medication like Precose (acarbose) or Glyset (miglitol), which delay the absorption of carbohydrates. This has been shown to reduce the risk of low blood sugars. Use of Precose or Glyset can be combined with a modest reduction in carb boluses to reduce insulin activity and lengthen the time over which carbs are digested.

Be quick to correct problems that arise from stress, depression, or other self-care causes. Avoid drinking alcohol or limit consumption to no more than one or two drinks per day to avoid shutting off the liver's response. For people with a physically active lifestyle, insulin reductions will be needed during and for several hours after increased activity. An occasional 2 a.m. blood test can do wonders in preventing unrecognized nighttime lows. Using a continuous monitor or Sleep Sentry can alert you and your health care team to occurrences of unrecognized hypoglycemia. Once these devices warn of nighttime lows, insulin doses can be changed rapidly to stop the lows.

As continuous monitoring devices become available, they should prevent most episodes of hypoglycemia entirely. Even short-term use of one of these devices may be able to break the cycle of lows with more appropriate insulin doses.

Call your doctor immediately if you require assistance from others to recover from a severe low, whether it occurs during the day or at night. You want guidance because it is very likely to happen again. Discuss how to make immediate insulin reductions.

"Inside every fat book is a thin book trying to get out."

Anon.

Severe Highs and Ketoacidosis

CHAPTER
22

A severe high blood sugar, ketosis (the presence of ketones prior to acidification of the blood), and ketoacidosis (DKA) are serious medical problems. These life-threatening conditions are seen in people with either Type 1 diabetes or long-term Type 2 diabetes when too little insulin is present, or when marginal insulin production is overwhelmed by infection or stress.

This chapter discusses severe highs, ketosis, and DKA:

- Causes
- Symptoms and testing
- How to prevent

Causes

Ketoacidosis is often present when someone is first diagnosed with Type 1 diabetes. After starting insulin treatment, Type 1s may encounter ketoacidosis again with a severe infection or other serious illness, with use of certain medications like prednisone, or if they forget or neglect to take insulin. In children and adolescents, ketoacidosis can be triggered by normal growth spurts that increase the body's need for insulin if recent control was already poor.

Severe highs and ketoacidosis in people with Type 2 diabetes is usually seen under the stress of a severe illness like pneumonia or a heart attack. A person with Type 2 whose insulin production is really low is more likely to encounter ketoacidosis than someone whose production remains high.

When insulin levels in the blood become very low, the body is forced to use fat for fuel even though lots of glucose is present in the blood. Burning fat sounds good if you are trying to lose weight, but excessive fat utilization produces ketones which cause the blood to become acidic. This leads to nausea and vomiting. Vomiting combined with a high blood sugar leads to rapid dehydration. In this situation, immediate hospitalization is necessary as death is the likely outcome without treatment.

In Type 1 diabetes, hospitalization for ketoacidosis occurs about once for every 30 years of insulin use. The prevalence of ketoacidosis in Type 2 diabetes is much lower, but because there are many more people with it, the number of cases of ketoacidosis is actually higher in Type 2 diabetes. The death rate from ketoacidosis is also higher in people with Type 2 diabetes because of older age and because the ketoacidosis is more likely to be triggered by a severe medical problem, such as a heart attack or pneumonia.

Symptoms And Detection

Early symptoms of ketoacidosis include tiredness, great thirst, frequent urination, dry skin, a fruity odor to the breath, abdominal pain, and nausea. Advanced symptoms include vomiting, shortness of breath, rapid breathing, and unconsciousness. Early symptoms are flu-like, but are due to ketone poisoning and should never be ignored. As soon as a person begins to vomit or has difficulty breathing, immediate treatment in an emergency room is required to prevent coma or death.

Everyone with diabetes should know how to recognize and treat ketoacidosis. Ketones travel from the blood into the urine and can be detected in the urine with ketone test strips available at any pharmacy. Always keep ketone strips on hand, but store them in a dry area and replace them as soon as they are outdated. Most people will need to use ketone test strips very rarely, but having them available and knowing how to use them is essential.

22.1 Symptoms Of Ketoacidosis
Early:
• nausea
• increased thirst and dry mouth
• excessive urination
• increased hunger
• excessive tiredness and weakness
• confusion
• an acetone or fruity odor of the breath
• any abdominal pain
Later:
• rapid breathing
• shortness of breath
• unconsciousness
If late symptoms occur or moderate or large amounts of ketones are found, immediate treatment is required.

The Precision Xtra™ meter is able to measure not only blood sugar but also blood ketone levels. This meter measures blood ketones with a special type of strip, so these strips, individually wrapped in foil for freshness, must be kept available.

This ability to measure blood ketones offers a tremendous advantage for people who have a tendency to develop ketoacidosis. For instance, if someone finds his blood sugar unexpectedly high, such as above 300 mg/dl (16.7 mmol), the blood ketone level can be measured immediately on a Precision Xtra™ meter. If ketones are normal, an injection of rapid insulin should correct the problem without any further treatment. But if ketones are present, larger correction boluses and extra attention to increased fluid intake will be necessary.

Measuring ketones in the blood allows them to be detected two to four hours earlier than with urine testing and allows small changes in ketone levels to be monitored rapidly to determine the effectiveness of therapy. The need for insulin and hydration can be evaluated much faster than waiting for ketone levels to rise or drop in the urine where the response is much slower. Anyone who has had more than one episode of ketoacidosis should test ketones in the blood. Ketoacidosis can be debilitating,

> ### 22.2 What To Do When You Are Ill
>
> Illness is often a precursor to ketoacidosis. The following tips for treatment during illness can help you prevent ketoacidosis.
>
> * Monitor your blood sugar every 2 hours
> * Monitor your urine for ketones every 2 to 4 hours when your blood sugar is above 300 mg/dl (16.7 mmol) or use Precision Xtra™ meter for blood ketone testing
> * Increase all basal insulin doses if an infection or pain are keeping your numbers high all the time
> * Never skip a basal insulin injection even if you are not eating
> * Respond to any high blood sugar promptly and realize you may need to use higher than normal correction boluses
> * Drink extra water or noncaloric fluids when your blood sugar is above 200 mg/dl (11.1 mmol)
> * If your blood sugar falls below 90 mg/dl (5 mmol), drink regular soda, fruit juice, or a sport drink in 4 to 6 ounce servings, or eat soup, ice cream, milk shake, pudding, or crackers
> * Call your doctor as soon as vomiting starts or if it lasts more than 4 hours with ketones present

expensive, and frightening. It should always be avoided or treated quickly.

Prevention

When ill, many people fail to identify the seriousness of their situation because they stop testing the blood sugar. A person with a high blood sugar or ketosis may be tempted to go to bed without testing due to extreme tiredness. A rapid change in health from an infection or heart attack requires an equally rapid increase in insulin doses. Frequent monitoring of blood sugar and ketone levels is critical when someone is ill. Otherwise, unrecognized ketoacidosis can complicate an already serious situation.

Some episodes of ketoacidosis occur after several weeks or months of inattention. Insulin doses may have gradually become inadequate due to growth, weight gain, or stress. When monitoring is not done or high blood sugar readings are accepted for weeks, a missed insulin dose or the start of an infection can cascade quickly into ketoacidosis.

To Treat Ketosis And Prevent Ketoacidosis

* Monitor the blood sugar at least 4 times a day at all times.
* Monitor every 2 hours whenever readings are above 250 mg/dl (13.9 mmol).
* Take correction boluses at least every three hours. If available, use a new bottle of Humalog or Novolog insulin to ensure that your insulin is at full strength.

- Check for ketones for any blood sugar above 300 mg/dl (16.7 mmol) and for all unexplained high blood sugar readings

- Correction boluses will need to be much larger than normal when ketones are present. Basal and bolus doses, often two or three times greater than normal doses, may be needed until the situation is resolved.

- Drink as much fluid as possible to correct dehydration. Dehydration is caused by a high blood sugar and excess urination. This worsens rapidly if vomiting begins. Drink plenty of fluids, especially water and noncaloric or low caloric beverages. Continue to drink 8 to 12 oz. every 30 minutes even if you do not feel thirsty. Diluted Gatorade, water with Nu-Salt™, and similar fluids are good because they help restore potassium levels.

- If nausea lasts four hours or more, call your physician.

- If vomiting begins or you cannot drink fluids, call your physician and go to an emergency room immediately. Vomiting means you can no longer hydrate yourself and medical treatment is required.

When an infection or illness is causing the problem, a high blood sugar will be difficult to bring down until the underlying problem is dealt with. If a medication, such as prednisone or cortisone, is causing the high blood sugar, talk with your doctor as quickly as you can about how much to increase your insulin doses. If nausea or vomiting keep you from drinking fluids, call your physician and immediately go to an emergency room for treatment.

> ### 22.3 What To Do When Ketosis Occurs
>
> - Check urine for ketones whenever blood sugars go over 300 mg/dl (16.7 mmol).
> - Drink a large amount of non-caloric or low caloric fluids immediately, followed by another 8 to 12 oz. every 30 minutes. Gatorade and similar fluids are good because they help restore potassium levels.
> - Take larger-than-normal correction boluses every 3 hours until the blood sugar is below 200 mg/dl (11 mmol) and ketones are negative.
> - If vomiting begins or you are unable to drink fluids, call your physician and go to an emergency room immediately.

Any very high blood sugar or ketosis should raise a red flag. The absence of a clear reason, such as illness or infection, may indicate that insulin is bad, insulin doses are incorrect, the basics of blood sugar control are not understood, depression is present or personal care is being neglected. Be sure to discuss any problems you have regarding high blood sugars or ketoacidosis with your physician so they can be resolved quickly and avoided in the future.

During even mild episodes of ketosis, staying hydrated is VITAL. Drink lots of fluids first, then take insulin to start bringing the blood sugar down.

Meters lose accuracy above 360 mg/dl (20 mmol). Readings above this may be much higher or much lower than the reading your meter shows.

Exercise

Exercise sharpens the mind, tones the body, and strengthens the heart and lungs. It increases endurance and resistance to stress and fatigue. It combats depression and creates a sense of well-being. Exercise helps lower body fat and cholesterol levels. Not exercising is as much a risk factor for heart disease as smoking a pack of cigarettes a day!

This chapter explains exercise's

- Benefits
- Risks
- Effects on blood sugar and insulin
- Propensity to cause insulin reactions
- How to better avoid lows caused by exercise

Benefits

In a study of Harvard alumni, researchers found that lifespan increases steadily as exercise levels rise from burning 500 calories a week (couch potato) to 3,500 calories per week (physically fit).[75] The exercise needed to burn 3,500 calories is equivalent to walking at three miles an hour for seven hours a week, bicycling 10 miles an hour for five hours a week, or running nine miles an hour for 2.7 hours a week. One study in men with diabetes found that faster walking is associated with less heart disease and longer lifespan.[76]

It appears that even moderate levels of exercise done regularly protect the heart. If you think burning 3,500 calories a week is too much, try moderate exercise done regularly instead. Getting off the couch can be a major step to cardiovascular protection.

The Harvard alumni study showed that brisk walking or bicycling for 30 minutes five days a week helps prevent heart disease and increases lifespan. Exercise that uses 1,000 calories a week appears to have major benefits for the heart and may be more appealing for those who do not enjoy running marathons. Of special interest to those with diabetes are the benefits of exercise to the heart and blood vessels. Because of the higher risk for heart disease with diabetes, the protection offered by exercise becomes especially important.

In addition to lifestyle benefits, exercise increases insulin sensitivity. Those who exercise regularly find their insulin need is lowered as they become more sensitive to insulin. Once

23.1 Let Your Goal Determine How You Exercise			
Your Goal	**Frequency**	**Intensity**	**Duration**
Reduce Risk of Heart Disease and Illness	2-3 times a week	40% max. heart rate	15-30 min.
Get Physically Fit	4 times a week	70-90% max. heart rate	15-30 min.
Lose Weight	5 times a week	45-60% max. heart rate	45-60 min.
Use this formula to determine your maximum heart rate: 220 - your age = your maximum heart rate			© 2003 Diabetes Services, Inc.

insulin doses have been adjusted downward for the heightened insulin sensitivity, blood sugars are usually easier to control. In one research study, 30 people with Type 1 diabetes on frequent injections who exercised regularly were compared to 23 others on frequent injections who were sedentary. A1c levels were 0.7% lower (7.0% versus 7.9%) in those that exercised.[77]

Research conducted at the University of Wisconsin Medical School also shows a marked lessening of eye damage in those who exercise.[78] This study ranked groups of people with Type 1 diabetes according to how much they exercised, then followed them over four years. When the researchers looked at the amount of eye damage in different groups, they found that proliferative diabetic retinopathy occurred in 36 percent of sedentary women, but in only 16 percent of those who were very physically active. In men, severe eye damage was 48 percent in sedentary men but only 16 percent in those who were very physically active. Beginning an exercise program will not worsen any existing damage to the retina provided it does not involve lifting heavy weights or doing shoulder stands.[79]

Risks

Despite its numerous benefits, exercise also has some risks, especially for those who have had diabetes a long time and those who have existing nerve damage, eye changes, kidney disease, or a history of heart or blood vessel problems. Blood flow and blood pressure increase during exercise to enable more oxygen and fuel to reach muscles. Blood flow in involved muscles may increase 15 to 20 times above resting levels during strenuous exercise and cardiac output may increase fivefold. Increased blood flow and increased pressure place extra strain on the heart and could harm organs and blood vessels weakened by previous high blood sugars.

These risks have to be considered before beginning an exercise program, especially an intense one like heavy weight lifting or scuba diving, which can cause a significant rise in blood pressure. A more gradual increase in training level may be required if blood vessel damage is a concern. Be sure to discuss exercise plans with your physician before you start.

With Nerve Damage

For anyone with existing nerve damage, exercise can present special challenges. The type and level of exercise has to be chosen carefully to protect the feet because insensitivity to pain increases the risk of injury. Swimming or biking, which are non-weight-bearing activities, may be better choices than jogging. Proper footwear is essential for avoiding blisters or calluses that exacerbate the already high risk of foot problems.

Autonomic neuropathy involves damage to the nerves that control processes like digestion, heart rate, and blood vessel tone. It can create an artificially low heart rate and reduce blood flow to exercising muscle. With autonomic neuropathy, a heart rate monitor may not be an accurate way to measure exercise intensity. Autonomic neuropathy creates a higher risk of heart disease. A more gradual training program under supervision is strongly advised when autonomic neuropathy is present.

Autonomic neuropathy can be detected by changes that appear in an EKG or by measuring the change in blood pressure from a reclining to a standing position. If you suspect you have this disorder because of having had diabetes for a long time or a history of poor control, discuss how to diagnose it with your physician.

Blood Sugar And Insulin Levels Affect Performance

When blood sugars are normal, the muscles and heart are able to use glucose and fat for maximum performance (See Table 23.2). With diabetes, performance is affected as the blood sugar goes higher or lower than normal. For optimum performance, an athlete has to know how to replace the carbs burned during exercise and how to adjust insulin doses to enable an ideal flow of fuels. Doing this reduces the number of high and low blood sugars encountered with exercise.

The insulin level in the blood determines how much carbohydrate and fat you use as fuel and where this fuel will come from. It is important to remember that both excess or insufficient insulin creates fuel delivery problems.

Even the amount of oxygen we breathe depends on how well the blood sugar is controlled. Research from Austria reveals that air flow to the lungs is reduced as much as 15 percent when the blood sugar runs high.[80] An oxygen deficit of this magnitude impairs athletic performance.

The person without diabetes can rapidly adjust the amount of insulin in the blood to match activity levels. If someone starts strenuous exercise, like running a marathon, the blood insulin level drops to half of its pre-exercise level over the first 15 to 30 minutes.[81] With moderate exercise, about an hour passes before the same drop in the blood insulin level is seen.

Table 23.2 How Your Blood Sugar Affects Performance		
Blood Sugar	**How Sugar And Insulin Affect Metabolism**	**Impact on Performance**
< 65 mg/dl	Too much insulin and not enough glucose available to cells	Tiredness, poor performance
65 to 180	**Efficient fuel flow**	**Maximum performance**
> 180 mg/dl	Glucose less able to enter muscle cells if insulin level is low, but will come down if insulin ok	Performance may be reduced
> 250 mg/dl	If insulin level is OK, blood sugars come down	Performance is lower, exercise OK to do
> 250 mg/dl	If insulin level is TOO LOW, blood sugars will rise higher	Tiredness and poor performance Check for ketones, take insulin before exercise

© 2003 Diabetes Services, Inc.

This natural drop in the insulin level as exercise begins allows

- glucose to be released from glycogen stores in the muscle and liver
- fat to be released and used as fuel, and
- new glucose to be created by the liver.

A reduction in the insulin level when an activity lasts several hours allows cells to gradually switch from glucose to fat as their primary fuel. This allows the body to access fat for fuel instead of having to rely on its much smaller stores of glucose and glycogen. Glucose levels in the blood are less likely to fall when the insulin level is reduced to allow muscles to access internal glycogen and fat stores.

With diabetes, insulin doses must always be matched to the intensity and duration of exercise. When insulin levels are too high, more sugar enters exercising muscles from the blood, less sugar is released from glycogen stores, and less fat is used to replace glucose. In this situation, the blood sugar will drop rapidly unless extra carbs are eaten during the exercise.

On the other hand, when insulin levels drop too low, more glucose and free fatty acids are released into the blood, and less glucose is able to enter exercising muscles. This causes blood sugars to rise. Ketones are also present in the blood. Table 23.3 shows some of the effects the insulin level has on blood sugar levels, stress hormone levels, and fuel metabolism.

Table 23.3 How Your Insulin Affects Performance

Insulin Level	Effect on Stress Hormones	Effect on Glucose and Fat	Effect on Performance
Low	Increased	Less glucose enters muscles, more glucose and fat are released into blood	Blood sugar usually high, poor performance, possible ketosis
Ideal	**Normal**	**Glucose enters muscles, glucose and fat are released as fuel normally**	**Normal blood sugar and optimal performance**
High	Decreased, until hypoglycemia begins	Increased glucose entry into muscles, reduced release of glucose and fat from internal stores	Blood sugar usually low, poor performance

© 2003 Diabetes Services, Inc.

Estimating Fuel Need

When travelling by car, it is easy to determine how much gasoline will be needed for a trip. If you know how long a trip will take (duration), the car's speed (effort or intensity), and the miles per gallon the car gets at that speed, you can closely calculate how many gallons of gasoline (energy) will be needed. If your gas tank hold this much fuel, you won't run out of gas.

Estimating the fuel needed for exercise is similar. If someone weighs 150 pounds and runs 30 minutes (duration) at seven miles per hour (effort or intensity), he or she can determine the amount of energy needed for the run. In this particular case, it would be 320 calories.

If these calories came only from glucose, calculating how many carbs are needed would be simple. However, the human body is similar to a hybrid car engine in that it uses two fuels. Internally stored glucose and fat, and any carbs that are eaten, can be used as fuel. Both the insulin level in the blood and the intake of carbohydrate have to be considered to keep the blood sugar normal with exercise.

The simplest way for someone with diabetes to balance exercise is to eat extra carbohydrate. If you know how many carbohydrates are consumed in an activity or exercise, you can eat foods containing an identical number of carbs to maintain control. But when an activity lasts longer than 30 or 45 minutes, a reduction in insulin doses will be required as well.

The first fuel source tapped when you start moderate or strenuous exercise is the glucose already present in the blood. As this limited supply is consumed, it is generally restored by the release of glycogen from muscle and liver cells. Although glucose and glycogen are easily accessible and rapidly released, the body's total supply is limited.

For instance, during strenuous exercise, a normal glucose level in the blood can be depleted in about four minutes, compared to 30 minutes at rest.[82] The liver plays a critical role in supplying glucose for exercise by breaking down stored glycogen and releasing it as glucose into the blood. The liver's stores can be largely depleted within the first 20 to 30 minutes of very strenuous exercise, although training for an exercise helps enlarge these stores.

Body fat acts as a large fuel reserve. Fat stores are about 2,000 times as large as stores of glucose and are nearly impossible to deplete even in a thin person, but a fall in the insulin level is required to gain full access to them.

ExCarbs, or Exercise Carbs, is a system that quantifies how exercise will impact the blood sugar and allows more accurate estimates of what is needed to maintain control. ExCarbs allow carb intake to be increased or insulin doses to be reduced to balance various types of exercise. If carbs are eaten to replace the glucose consumed during activity, no insulin is needed to cover them. ExCarbs also can be used to calculate a reduction in insulin doses for longer periods of activity. How to use ExCarbs is covered in the next chapter.

> ### 23.4 Simple Tips For Exercise
>
> **For casual or light exercise**
> (i.e. casual walking, biking, softball)
>
> - No adjustment to insulin
> - Keep fast carbs and your meter and test strips with you.
>
> **For heavy or aerobic exercise**
> (i.e. tennis, baseball, football, jogging, swimming vigourously)
>
> - Test your blood sugar before the exercise and every 30 minutes after you start
> - If less than 120 mg/dl (6.7 mmol), eat 30 grams of carb before exercise.
> - If between 120 and 200 mg/dl (6.7 to 11.1 mmol) eat 15 grams of carb.
> - If over 200 mg/dl (11.1 mmol), don't eat anything but retest in 30 minutes.
> - Test every 30 minutes and follow these tips each time you test.

What Impact Do Intensity And Duration Have On The Blood Sugar?

Intensity

At rest, free fatty acids supply most of our fuel. During mild exercise like walking, energy is still largely obtained from fat rather than glucose, so the blood sugar is less likely to fall than with moderate or strenuous exercise where the percentage of fuel coming from carbs rises.

Whether you walk or run a mile makes no difference in the amount of energy you use. Both will use the same number of calories. However, where these calories come from differs.

In a one-mile walk, only about 20 percent of the calories used come from glucose while 80 percent come from fat. When running the same mile at a strenuous pace, as much as 80 percent of the calories come from glucose. As intensity increases, so does the amount of glucose that is needed as fuel. Because a higher percentage of glucose is used during strenuous exercise, the blood sugar is more likely to drop. Strenuous exercise requires more carbohydrate intake or a larger reduction in insulin doses than mild exercise even though the same number of calories are used.

Duration

How long an exercise lasts also influences how many carbs it will consume. Activities that last longer are more likely to drop the blood sugar. For instance, a leisurely 30-minute walk may have little effect on the blood sugar, but walking for 60 minutes may require extra carbs or a small reduction in an insulin dose.

As moderate or strenuous exercise extends beyond 40 to 60 minutes, the body gradually switches from using its limited stores of glucose and glycogen to using more fat as fuel. For instance, at the start of a six hour period of strenuous exercise or activity, a person normally uses glucose to provide about 80 percent of the fuel they need. After three hours, about equal amounts of energy come from glucose and fat. After six hours, fuel use will have switched, with almost 80 percent of energy being derived from fat.

Remember, though, this person has a normal pancreas which can automatically lower the insulin level. If someone with diabetes does not reduce insulin doses appropriately, body fat will not be as available as fuel, and carbs will have to be eaten to supply the needed energy.

A 150-pound person uses 3,350 calories of total energy in six hours of strenuous exercise. Normally, half these calories would come from carbs that are eaten and from internal glucose stores, with the other half coming from fat stores. With diabetes, more carb intake is required when insulin levels are too high during exercise. If the insulin level is lowered before a long period of exercise, internal glycogen stores can release enough stored glucose to cover much of the exercise.

When insulin levels are high, however, internal glucose and fatty acid stores cannot be accessed as easily. Eating carbs becomes the only way to supply the fuel

Table 23.5 Easy Way To Measure Heart Rate/Pulse

Feel your pulse at the wrist and count your pulse for 10 seconds, then use this table to find beats per minute.

10 second Pulse Count	Beats Per Minute
10	60
11	66
12	72
13	78
14	84
15	90
16	96
17	102
18	108
19	114
20	120
21	126
22	132
23	138
24	144
25	150
26	156
27	162
28	168
29	174
30	180

that is needed. For the six hours of strenuous exercise, most of the 3,350 calories would have to be eaten as carbohydrate to keep the blood sugar from falling. This is equivalent to eating almost two pounds of pure sugar, or drinking twenty 12-ounce cans of regular soda.

Obviously, lowering insulin levels during long periods of exercise can prevent both low blood sugars and stomach aches. Experience helps in estimating how the length and intensity of activities can be balanced with extra carbohydrate or less insulin. ExCarbs, covered in the next chapter, provide a way to make better estimates for carb replacement and insulin reductions.

The longer and more intense an exercise, the less trained you are, and the higher your insulin level, the more likely your blood sugar is to fall!

Advantages Of Physical Training

Someone who is in shape uses 25 percent less glucose than someone who is not trained. Physical training builds glycogen stores, and these stores in liver and muscle cells act as a reserve account to be drawn upon whenever needed to help keep your glucose funds from running low. The physically fit individual has large glycogen stores to draw upon in muscle and can use these as a shock absorber to reduce fluctuations in the blood sugar. If the blood sugar is dropping, more glucose can be released to limit the fall. When the blood sugar is rising, such as after a meal, more of it can be shifted into glycogen.

> ### 23.6 Are You Fit, Trained And In Shape?
>
> The American College of Sports Medicine says you are trained when you exercise:
>
> 1. Three to five days a week
> 2. For an accumulated total of 20 to 60 minutes per day with at least 10 minutes at a time
> 3. At 60 to 90% of your maximum heart rate (or 50 to 85% of VO2 max)*
> 4. Using any large muscle mass
>
> *Do NOT rely on your heart rate if you have autonomic neuropathy

When you exercise regularly, not only do you tone up and slim down, but blood sugar fluctuations can be reduced. Once basal and bolus insulin doses have been reduced, the fit person needs less carbohydrate to prevent insulin reactions. Blood sugar control during and after exercise becomes easier.

Exercise is an important ingredient in anyone's health program and more vital for someone who has diabetes. With planning, monitoring, and balancing of carbs and insulin, you can exercise with a renewed spirit and confidence, knowing that you are strengthening your body and improving your ability to manage your diabetes.

A normal blood sugar during and after exercise is the best indicator that you have an ideal balance between insulin doses and carb intake.

Why The Blood Sugar Goes High After Exercise

When the blood sugar rises after exercise, there are four likely causes.

Lack Of Insulin

A lack of insulin is the most common reason for the blood sugar to rise after exercise. A commonly encountered situation is when exercise starts first thing in the morning with the blood sugar elevated at 140 mg/dl (7.8 mmol) or above. In this situation, the reading that follows the exercise is likely to be higher than 140 because the liver is producing extra glucose. This extra glucose is a result of the relative lack of insulin, indicated by the elevated fasting reading. If the same exercise is done another morning when the blood sugar is 100 mg/dl (5.5 mmol), the blood sugar is likely to fall.

Anaerobic Exercise

During intense, anaerobic exercise a person may gasp for breath. In anaerobic exercise, like running the 100-yard dash or power weight-lifting, glucose becomes almost the only fuel used. A very rapid release of glucose into the blood from glycogen stores is driven by rising catecholamine levels. The hormone shift seen during intense exercise causes glucose production to rise seven or eight times normal levels, while uptake of glucose into the cells rises only three to four fold.[83] In contrast to the reduced need for insulin in less strenuous exercise, a rapid doubling of the insulin level in the blood is required to accommodate the rapid mobilization of glucose seen with intense, anaerobic exercise.[84]

Unfortunately, the speed of the change in blood insulin level in a person without diabetes is so fast that there is no way to mimic it in a person with diabetes with injected insulin. The increased production relative to uptake may cause the blood sugar to rapidly rise. Those who participate in intense or anaerobic sports may need to adjust their insulin doses so they have a higher insulin level at the start of the event. Even so, this may not keep the blood sugar from rising. When a rising blood sugar is seen after intense exercise, the best way to accommodate may be to test frequently before and after the event and use correction boluses to correct high readings as they occur.

Competition

A rise in catecholamines and other stress hormones may be encountered at the start of competitive events and will often cause the blood sugar to rise.

As stress hormone levels rise, the person without diabetes releases extra insulin quickly into the blood. This does not happen with diabetes. At the start of a competitive event, someone with diabetes may see the blood sugar rapidly rise even after beginning the event with a normal blood sugar. Competitive and intense exercise both make insulin adjustments difficult because of the rapid speed at which a change in the blood sugar occurs, as well as uncertainty about how large the stress hormone release will be.

Personal experience is often your best guide, and good record keeping facilitates this process. For activities and events where stress hormone release occurs, a small injection of Humalog or Novolog prior to the event may be needed to prevent the blood sugar from rising. Discuss this with your physician or health care team, and use insulin before your exercise only after testing has demonstrated that the extra insulin is really needed. For short, strenuous events, it may be just as easy, and possibly safer, to correct a high blood sugar after the event is completed.

Dehydration

If your meter displays a high blood sugar after certain exercise, this can be difficult to interpret. The apparent "high" blood sugar may actually be caused or exacerbated by dehydration. In very hot, dry weather, a lack of fluids can concentrate the blood and make the percentage of glucose in the blood appear higher than it really is. Even if the blood sugar is high, combining that with dehydration makes it appear even higher. If you suspect this may be the problem, drink ample fluids and recheck your blood sugar in 30 minutes or so before giving a correction bolus.

Dehydration is a concern for any athlete. Staying hydrated is essential for turning glucose and fat into energy. When blood sugars are high, the risk of dehydration rises, especially during hot weather. Frequent intake of fluid before, during, and after exercise is essential to prevent dehydration and loss of energy. Dehydration also creates confusion and can make recognition of low blood sugars more difficult. Drink fluids regularly during exercise regardless of your thirst, as thirst occurs when you are already 1-2% dehydrated.

How High Is Too High To Exercise?

If the blood sugar is 250 mg/dl (13.9 mmol) or above, exercise often is not recommended because the insulin level may be dangerously low. If the insulin level is low, exercise would only cause the blood sugar to go higher. Although your insulin level cannot be tested directly, in certain situations you can accurately guess it is low. For instance, if your blood sugar was normal at bedtime but your reading the next morning when you awaken is 250 mg/dl (13.9 mmol) or higher, you know your insulin level is low because it was unable to keep your blood sugar from rising. Exercising under these circumstances may cause your blood sugar to rise higher unless you take an correction bolus.

Contrast this situation to one where the blood sugar is raised to 250 mg/dl (13.9 mmol) in preparation for a four hour athletic event. Extra carbs covered by a reduced carb bolus before the event starts created this high blood sugar, but the person can start the event confidently because the blood sugar will begin to drop shortly after the exercise starts. Even though the blood sugar is high, enough insulin is available to move glucose from the blood into exercising muscles.

An alternative to raising the blood sugar this high is to reduce both basal and bolus doses prior to the event so that fewer carbs have to be eaten to exercise safely. With a lower insulin level and less carbohydrate needed at the start of the event, the starting blood sugar can remain in a relatively normal range. Additional carbohydrate will be needed during the event, but less than if the insulin levels had not been lowered.

Ways To Prevent Insulin Reactions

A low blood sugar that occurs during or just after exercise is often more difficult to recognize because symptoms like tiredness and sweating may be caused by either exercise or a low blood sugar. Water sports can be especially difficult because they mask sweating and shaking. Warning signs may also go unnoticed due to a focus on the activity or sport at hand. The blood sugar needs to be checked often during exercise to avoid a low.

Have quick-acting, high-carb snacks on hand during exercise to prevent and treat insulin reactions. Be especially careful during and after exercise that is intense and for which you are not trained. Canoe trips, backpacking, skiing, horseback riding, spring cleaning, snow shovelling, home remodeling, heavy work in the garden, or even washing the car can create an unusually fast drop in the blood sugar when they are not done regularly. Activities which are done only occasionally that use the arm and shoulder muscles are especially likely to cause lows.

Someone who has not trained for strenuous activities like these will need more carb intake or a larger insulin dose reduction to avoid low blood sugars than someone who does them regularly. Use good record keeping and past experience to guide your adjustments for activities you seldom participate in.

Test frequently after any longer-than-normal period of strenuous activity to avoid a delayed insulin reaction that is likely to occur. Lows can occur up to 36 hours later and often happen during the night following the activity. Delayed lows occur as the muscles and liver gradually remove sugar from the blood to replenish glycogen stores depleted during the activity. To prevent delayed reactions, test often, reduce your basal dose that evening, and add extra carbs at dinner and bedtime not covered by bolus insulin.

A drop in the blood sugar becomes more likely when an activity involves a muscle group not normally worked so hard. For example, someone who runs regularly and then begins to bike will experience a larger drop in blood sugar after biking than after running, even if the energy they use for each exercise is the same. This extra drop is caused by the formation of new glycogen stores in the relatively untrained leg muscles that are used when riding a bike.

"The only thing that saves us from bureaucracy is its inefficiency."
Eugene McCarthy

"We have been taught to believe that negative equals realistic
and positive equals unrealistic."

Anon.

Adjustments For Exercise

People with diabetes want to exercise because it is fun, makes them feel better, improves their health, and increases their lifespan. When managed well, exercise will also improve their blood sugar control. But often a long walk, some rollerblading, or painting the house causes the blood sugar to drop. Then a hastily eaten candy bar sends the blood sugar soaring.

Or after exercising for a half hour in the morning, the blood sugar rises rather than falls and it takes most of the day to regain control. A night low that follows a day of exercise also can be frightening.

Can exercise be managed so that it doesn't lead to a loss of control? One way to lessen this risk is to use ExCarbs, a guide to help you make rational adjustments in your carbohydrate intake and insulin doses for exercise or any other increased activity.

This chapter discusses

- What ExCarbs are
- How to use ExCarbs to control your blood sugar during exercise
- How to lower basal and bolus doses with ExCarbs

What Are ExCarbs?

Although exact exercise rules are not possible, ExCarbs provide a good yardstick to measure how a particular exercise will affect your blood sugar. Exercise physiologists have long known how many calories are consumed in different activities and also what percentage of these calories typically comes from carbohydrate as the intensity of the exercise increases. Created with this in mind, Table 24.2 provides a guide for how many carbs will be consumed by these activities. Once you know how many carbs your exercise is using, you can more accurately balance them with carb intake or a reduction in your insulin doses.

ExCarbs allow you to balance exercise

1. By eating more carbs to maintain your current weight
2. By lowering insulin doses to help with weight loss
3. By combining the techniques to allow more flexibility in your response

Eat More Carbohydrate

The easy way to maintain blood sugar control while exercising is to eat the amount of carbohydrate you burn during the exercise. To do this, simply look up your planned exercise in Table 24.2 and determine how many carbohydrates you need for your exercise. Once you know how many carbs will be used, you can eat an equivalent number of carbs before, during or after the exercise to maintain control.

The table is set up for body weights of 100 lbs., 150 lbs., and 200 lbs., as well as for different intensity levels of exercise. For instance, if you weigh 150 pounds

> ### 24.1 Control During Exercise Can Be Affected By:
>
> - A recent history of poor control
> - The length and intensity of the exercise
> - Whether it is aerobic or anaerobic
> - Your training level
> - Timing of the exercise relative to recent meals and injections

and walk 3 miles an hour, you can see from the table that you will use 22 grams of carbs in your walk. This is equal to an average-sized apple or a cup of milk plus a graham cracker. If you walk at the same pace for two hours rather than one, you will need 44 grams of carbohydrate, but if you walk only 30 minutes, only 11 grams will be required.

If instead of walking you run the same 3 miles at a speed of 8 m.p.h., you will need 53 grams of carbohydrate (145 grams times 22 min. ÷ 60 min.), even though it takes only 22 minutes to complete the run. This is more than twice the amount needed for the leisurely one-hour walk over the same ground! Though walking or running 3 miles requires the same total calories, a higher percentage of these calories will need to come from carbohydrates because running is a more intense exercise.

The numbers that are listed in the table provide the maximum amount of carbs needed per hour to prevent a low blood sugar. For an activity which consumes 50 grams or less, replacement carbs can be eaten during or within a couple of hours of ending the activity. For instance, someone who weighs 150 lbs. and rides a bicycle at 10 m.p.h. for an hour will need to replace about 48 grams of carbs. This person could eat or drink 24 grams of carbs before and during the ride, and an equal number of grams within a couple of hours after the ride. Glucose that is derived from muscle glycogen during a ride like this does not need to be immediately re-placed, unless, of course, the insulin level is so high that glucose stored in glycogen is unable to be released.

Immediate replacement of all the carbs used in exercise is not necessary. Depending on the duration and intensity of the activity, and your level of training, extra carb intake or a reduction in insulin doses may be required for up to 24 to 48 hours. A full carb replacement may be needed during an exercise only if excess amounts of insulin are present in the blood to block access to internal fuel stores. In this situation, eating becomes the only way to deliver fuel to exercising muscle.

Table 24.2 suggests the maximum number of carbs required for each type of exercise. Often less than these maximum amounts will be needed for those who are trained for the activity and have already reduced their insulin doses appropriately.

In most situations, all the carbs that are required do not need to be eaten right away. During the first 30 minutes of moderately strenuous exercise, like running at 6 m.p.h., most of the carbs required will come directly from internal glycogen stores in the leg muscles. Only about 10 percent are directly and immediately derived from the blood as glucose, and only this blood glucose has to be replaced by eating carbs or by production and release of glucose from the liver. Even when insulin levels are high during a 30-minute run, only about 16 percent of

Table 24.2 Grams Of Carb Per Hour Of Activity

Activity		Weight		
		100 lbs.	150 lbs.	200 lbs.
baseball		25	38	50
basketball	moderate	35	48	61
	vigorous	59	88	117
bicycling	6 mph	20	27	34
	10 mph	35	48	61
	14 mph	60	83	105
	18 mph	95	130	165
	20 mph	122	168	214
dancing	moderate	17	25	33
	vigorous	28	43	57
digging		45	65	83
eating		6	8	10
golf (pullcart)		23	35	46
handball		59	88	117
jump rope 80/min		73	109	145
mopping		16	23	30
mountain climbing		60	90	120
outside painting		21	31	42
raking leaves		19	28	38
running	5mph	45	68	90
	8 mph	96	145	190
	10 mph	126	189	252
shoveling		31	45	57
skating	moderate	25	34	43
	vigorous	67	92	117
skiing	crosscountry 5mph	76	105	133
	downhill	52	72	92
	water	42	58	74
soccer		45	67	89
swimming	slow crawl	41	56	71
	fast crawl	69	95	121
tennis	moderate	23	34	45
	vigorous	59	88	117
volleyball	moderate	23	34	45
	vigorous	59	88	117
walking	3mph	15	22	29
	4.5 mph	30	45	59

© 2003 Diabetes Services, Inc.

the calories come directly from the blood as glucose. This means that the glucose removed from glycogen stores can, in most instances, be replaced after the exercise is finished, unless, of course, your experience tells you otherwise.

In the first 30 minutes of exercise, local muscle glycogen contributes about five times as much glucose as that contributed by the blood. But as running continues beyond 30 minutes, more and more glucose begins to be drawn through the blood from other sources besides local glycogen stores. The amount of glucose coming from the blood climbs gradually during the first couple of hours of exercise to a maximum of about 40 percent. As time passes, it becomes more and more necessary to eat or drink carbs and the blood sugar becomes more likely to drop as exercise continues.

The longer and more intense an exercise, the more important it becomes to lower insulin doses. It also takes longer to rebuild muscle glycogen stores. Following a few hours of intense exercise, the blood sugar may drop for 36 hours or more as glucose is gradually removed from the bloodstream and used to rebuild glycogen stores. The carbs used to balance activity lasting an hour or more do not need to be eaten immediately but are often better consumed in the hours that follow. Most athletes with diabetes make sure to add uncovered carbs to their bedtime snack to prevent a nighttime drop if they have exercised that day.

Take Less Insulin

To balance easygoing exercise that lasts 30 or 45 minutes in a simple and straightforward way, eat extra carbs. As exercise becomes longer and more intense, a reduction in insulin doses becomes more and more necessary. A lower insulin level will enable fuel to be released from glycogen and fat stores rather than having to eat as many carbs to provide fuel. This helps those who want to lose weight and those who want to participate in long periods of activity without having to consume the large portions of carbohydrate that would otherwise be required.

Long, intense periods of exercise require that bolus and basal doses be reduced beforehand and stay low for up to 24 to 48 hours afterward. Whether bolus or basal doses are reduced depends on the duration of the activity, its timing in relation to meals, and whether the exercise was planned. Keep in mind that following any reduction in insulin doses there will be a time lag before the insulin in the blood actually begins to drop. Take a look at Table 24.3 for more information.

A reduction in Humalog or Novolog meal boluses is ideal when exercise is moderate or strenuous, lasts less than 90 minutes, and begins within 90 minutes of a meal. For exercise that starts after breakfast, the breakfast bolus can be reduced to reduce the insulin level during exercise.

When strenuous exercise lasts 60 minutes or longer or moderate exercise lasts for 90 minutes or longer, a reduction in the basal dose should be considered as well. Remember that basal insulin must be lowered two to four hours before the insulin level in the blood can actually begin to drop. Therefore, basal reductions typically have to be started several hours before exercise begins and more planning is required.

24.3 How Long Before Exercise Do I Lower My Insulin Doses?

Below are suggestions for how long before an exercise to lower various insulin in order to reduce insulin levels at the start of exercise. Included also is how many hours the reduction will last.

Insulin	Starts	Lasts
Humalog or Novolog	15 to 20 min	3.5 to 4.5 hrs
Regular	30 to 40 min	5 to 6 hrs
NPH or Lente	2 to 4 hrs	14 to 18 hrs
UL	3 to 4 hrs	16 to 22 hrs
Detemir	1 to 4 hrs	18 to 20 hrs
Lantus	2 to 4 hrs	18 to 26 hrs

For instance, a bedtime basal dose must be lowered the night before to cover a long period of exercise or activity that begins the next morning. Table 24.3 provides a timetable to show how long before exercise you should reduce each type of insulin so that your blood insulin level will be lower at the start of an exercise.

Your level of fitness and your training for a specific exercise can make a large difference in your fuel need. When you rarely engage in a particular exercise, you will need larger basal and bolus reductions than for an equivalent amount of exercise that is routine. Before beginning a training program, some reduction in boluses and basal doses likely will be needed. People who exercise regularly and have their current insulin doses correctly adjusted will require only small reductions in their insulin doses before doing their regular exercise routine.

Using Your Carb Factor To Help Reduce Insulin For Exercise

ExCarbs can be used to guide not only an increase in carb intake but also a reduction in insulin doses. You only need to know your carb factor or insulin-to-carb ratio to convert the carbs required for exercise into an equivalent insulin dose reduction.

Let's use the 500 Rule to determine the carb factor for someone who wants to lower a bolus dose for exercise after a meal. This person weighs 150 pounds and uses 38 units of insulin a day to stay in good control using multiple daily injections with about half of the total insulin coming from basal doses. As shown in Table 24.4, the TDD of 38 units is divided into 500 to determine that one unit of Humalog or Novolog will cover about 13 grams of carbohydrate.

Now look at Table 24.2. For someone who weighs 150-pounds, a 30-minute run at 8 m.p.h. translates into about 72 grams of ExCarbs (145 grams per hour times a half hour). By knowing how many carbs are required for the run, we can divide these carbs by the person's carb factor to find out how much insulin the exercise is equal to. Dividing 72 grams of carb by 13 grams per unit of insulin tells us that the run is equal to about five units of Humalog or Novolog insulin (72 grams/13 carbs per unit = 5.5 units).

Having determined both the carb and insulin equivalents of the run, our runner can choose to eat extra carbohydrates, lower a meal bolus, or both. (A basal reduction will not be needed because the run lasts only a half hour.) Using only carbs to replace the glucose burned in the run, our runner could consume 24 grams of carb before the run, another 24 after the run, and the rest as needed later in the day. This runner would eat as many as 72 extra grams of carbohydrate that, of course, would not be covered with insulin.

If our runner chose to only reduce carb boluses to balance the run, one or two meal boluses that are close in timing to the exercise can be reduced. For a run at an hour after breakfast, four fewer units could be taken for the carbs at breakfast and one or two units could be taken out of the lunch bolus that follows.

Add Carbs As Well As Reduce Insulin

A combination of increased carbs and reduced carb boluses would be the preferred choice for most runners. For example, our 30-minute runner could reduce the breakfast bolus by 2 units and the lunch bolus by 1 unit. Three units times 13 grams per unit = 39 grams. Subtracting the 39 grams covered by insulin reduction, the other 33 grams of carb (72 – 39 = 33)) can be eaten as needed.

Suggestions for carb and basal/bolus adjustments that are based on the duration and intensity of exercise are also given in Table 24.5. Both intensity and duration of an exercise affects how it is balanced with extra carbs or reduced doses. Basically, the longer and more strenuous an exercise, the greater the adjustment that will be required, and the more likely that insulin doses will need to be lowered.

Length of exercise is easy to determine with a watch or clock, but intensity is highly specific to the individual. Two people may be running side by side, but one may be running at maximum intensity, while the same exercise might be mild for the other.

In Table 24.5, mild exercise is any physical activity that is relatively easy for you to do, such as casual walking. Moderate exercise involves something that makes you breathe harder but which you could do for some time, such as brisk walking or jogging. Intense exercise involves anything that causes deep breathing but usually allows you to carry on a conversation. Examples are race walking or a steady, fast bike ride.

24.4 The 500 Rule*

If Your TDD is:	Your Carb Factor is:
15 units	33 grams
20	25
25	20
30	17
35	14
40	13
45	11
50	10
55	9
60	8
70	7
80	6
90	5
100	5

*500 ÷ TDD = # of grams of carb covered by 1 unit

Table 24.5 Carb And Insulin Adjustments To Balance Exercise Per 100 lbs. Weight									
	Exercise Intensity								
Exercise Duration	**Mild**			**Moderate**			**Intense**		
	Carbs*	Bolus	Basal	Carbs*	Bolus	Basal	Carbs*	Bolus	Basal
15 min	+ 0 g	normal	normal	+ 0 g	normal	normal	+ 20 g	- 10%	normal
30 min	+ 10 g	normal	normal	+ 20 g	- 10%	normal	+ 40 g	- 20%	normal
45 min	+ 18 g	- 10%	normal	+ 30 g	- 20%	normal	+ 50 g	- 30%	normal
60 min	+ 25 g	- 15%	normal	+ 40 g	- 30%	normal	+ 60 g	- 40%	- 10%
90 min	+ 38 g	- 20%	normal	+ 55 g	- 45%	- 20%	+ 90 g	- 50%	- 20%
120 min	+ 50 g	- 30%	normal	+ 70 g	- 60%	- 20%	+ 110 g	- 70%	- 30%
240 min	+ 80 g	- 50%	- 10%	+ 120 g	- 60%	- 20%	+ 200 g	- 70%	- 40 %

These are only estimates and must be individually adjusted through testing.
*Important: The carb values above are for a person who weighs 100 lbs. If you weigh 200 lbs, you will need twice these amounts. If you have not trained for an activity, you may need slightly more than these amounts. Once you are trained, you may need substantially less.   © 2003 Diabetes Services, Inc.

How To Lower High Blood Sugars With Exercise

Exercise can be used to lower a high blood sugar. Exercise will usually lower a high reading and reduce or eliminate the need for a correction bolus.

For example, Jeremy weighs 200 pounds and uses 50 units of insulin a day with generally good control. Using Table 12.1 on page 141, he will need one unit of Humalog or Novolog for each 10 grams of carbohydrate, and one unit of Humalog for each 36 mg/dl reduction in blood sugar. Let's say Jeremy finds his blood sugar is 172 mg/dl (9.6 mmol) before dinner and he wants to eat 100 grams of carb for the meal. If he were not planning any exercise, he would take 10 units of rapid insulin for dinner plus 2 more units for the high blood sugar (72/36 = 2.0). But let's say he wants to ride his bike at 14 m.p.h. for an hour after dinner.

From Table 24.2, riding at 14 m.p.h. for an hour will use 105 grams of carb.

These 105 grams can be replaced with:

- 105 grams of carbohydrate that is not covered with a bolus
- 10.5 fewer units of insulin (105 grams of carb ÷ 10 grams per unit)
- A blood sugar drop of 378 mg/dl (21 mmol) (36 per unit X 10.5 units)
- Some combination of the above

Jeremy wants to lower his high blood sugar with the exercise. The blood sugar of 172 mg/dl is 72 mg/dl above his dinner target of 100 mg/dl, so he wants to lower it by 72 mg/dl. His blood sugar elevation is equivalent to 2 units of insulin (72 mg/dl desired drop divided by 36 mg/dl drop per unit) and also to 20 grams of carb (2 units X 10 grams per unit = 20 grams).

Two of several options:

1. He can take only his normal bolus of 10 Humalog to cover the 100 grams of carb he plans to eat, but no insulin to lower his high blood sugar. Instead, he can allow the bike ride to lower his blood sugar. The fall in blood sugar of 72 mg/dl is equivalent to 2 units times 10 grams of carb per unit or 20 grams of carbs. The blood sugar is unlikely to go low if the ride occurs within two hours of dinner, but he will pay attention in case his blood sugar does fall as a result of the 10 unit bolus plus exercise. He will check his blood sugar after the ride and start consuming some of the additional 85 grams of carb he is likely to need through the evening to offset the carbs consumed by the ride. (85 grams of carbohydrate equals five average slices of bread.)

2. He can also take only 6 units to cover his dinner carbs rather than 10 and no insulin to lower the blood sugar. This would be 6 fewer units of insulin than normally taken, or 6 times 10 grams of carb per unit or 60 grams of carbs. He would eat his usual 100 grams of carbohydrate for breakfast, but here no more than 45 grams of additional carbs are likely to be needed after the ride (105 grams required for the ride minus the 60 grams that were not covered by insulin).

Contrast this situation to a similar one where the blood sugar is 172 mg/dl before breakfast and the bike ride will occur after breakfast. Here, the liver is actively producing glucose and the blood sugar may not drop as much as it would before dinner when the blood sugar had started in a normal range at lunch. When the liver is activated after several hours of higher readings, the blood sugar will not come down as much as it would if the blood sugar had been high for only a few hours.

When To Reduce Insulin Doses

How long before exercise do you need to lower an insulin dose to have a lower insulin level in the blood when you start? The type of insulin you use determines when it needs to be lowered, but remember that there is always a lag between when insulin is injected and when the level of insulin in the blood actually begins to change.

If a Humalog or Novolog bolus for a meal is lowered prior to exercise following a meal, this reduction will take 30 minutes or more to have an effect. If you want to

---

> ### 24.6 Highs And Lows With Exercise
>
> - The longer and more strenuous an exercise or activity, the more likely the blood sugar will go low and the greater the need to lower your insulin doses.
> - The less trained you are for an activity, the more likely your blood sugar will go low and the greater the need to lower insulin doses.
> - Strenuous or anaerobic exercise may raise the blood sugar if glucose is mobilized faster than it can be moved into cells by the prevailing insulin level.

lower the insulin level in the blood by a reduction in the basal dose, the wait is much longer. It takes two to four hours for the blood insulin level to go down. See Table 24.5. It will stay down until the end of the action time for that insulin, although its peaking action may also change insulin levels. Reducing the basal insulin for longer periods of activity can be very helpful, but you must experiment to make it work.

For example, if a Lantus dose is reduced, less insulin will be available for the next 24 hours. If a bedtime Lantus dose is lowered, the blood sugar may be higher by morning.

> ### 24.7 Fast And Slow Carbs For Exercise
>
> Not all carbs are the same. Different foods are digested and raise the blood sugar at different speeds. Knowing these speed differences can be useful.
>
> Fast carbs are ideal for raising low blood sugars before or during exercise and also for balancing exercise that uses carbs rapidly. Fast carbs include glucose tablets, Sweet Tarts, honey, corn flakes, raisin bran, athletic drinks (Exceed, Body Fuel, Gatorade, Power Ade), raisins, dried or ripe fruits, and regular soft drinks.
>
> Slow carbs help prevent the blood sugar from dropping during long periods of activity. They can be eaten before exercise starts and every 45 minutes thereafter. Slow carbs can also be used to replenish glycogen stores following exercise. These include PowerBars, PurePower bars, oatmeal, Swiss muesli, fruit, Teddy Grahams, Fig Newtons, ginger snaps, pasta al dente, brown rice, and many candy bars.

A correction bolus might be added to the carb bolus for breakfast, but because of the increased activity that day, the total bolus dose would be less than the amount normally taken. You may need a bolus for breakfast that partially covers the carbs and partially brings down a high blood sugar. If your exercise is long and strenuous, is unusual or uses untrained muscles, or if you are starting an exercise program, you may benefit from the lower insulin level after the exercise. You might even want to lower the Lantus dose the following night, too.

How Far Can Insulin Doses Be Reduced For Exercise?

When calculating basal and bolus reductions for exercise, realize there are limits to how far insulin doses can be reduced. Let's say your current insulin dose is correct (i.e., your control is quite good). You start a strenuous running program in preparation for a marathon. With multi-mile runs on your training days, you find your activity is equal to enough ExCarbs that it would seem possible to skip your insulin entirely.

Can your insulin really be eliminated if you exercise long enough? Someone with Type 2 diabetes who retains adequate internal insulin production might be able to do this. With Type 1 diabetes, however, basal and bolus insulin can never be totally eliminated.

Consider what happens with a marathon runner who does not have diabetes. Even during maximum training, a marathoner's blood insulin level will drop no further than to about half of its original level. This tells us that in Type 1 diabetes, total insulin intake should be reduced by no more than 40 to 50 percent from the original dose for even the most intense exercise programs.

So keep in mind that, while carbohydrates can be added as needed, insulin doses can be reduced only so far. Even during something like training for a competitive marathon, your TDD cannot be reduced more than 40 to 50 percent, unless you are also losing weight or your original insulin doses had been set too high.

Insulin can be lowered only so far because:

1. It is needed to cover meal carbohydrates to keep the blood sugar from rising.
2. It is needed as background insulin to allow glucose to enter cells and to keep internal stores of glucose and fat from being released in massive amounts.
3. It is needed to prevent ketoacidosis, which results from the uncontrolled release of internal glucose and fat.

Never take a dose of insulin that seems inappropriate. If you usually take three units of Humalog for your meal prior to the start of your exercise and your blood sugar control has been great, do not take more or less than this amount, even if a different dose is suggested by the ExCarb system, the 500 Rule, or any other rule. Your own blood sugars are always your best guide. Check with your physician before using ExCarbs as a system for controlling blood sugars with exercise.

Wise Exercise

Be sure your insulin doses and carbohydrate intake are matched to your normal daily lifestyle before attempting to make adjustments for exercise. Discuss your exercise program with your physician or health care team. Keep in mind your personal experiences with similar exercise in the past.

Test your blood sugar often during and after exercise, or use a continuous monitoring device. This feedback lets you adjust your insulin doses more accurately the next time you exercise. Carry fast carbs, like glucose tablets, SweetTarts™, or Gatorade,™ at all times for rapid correction of low blood sugars. To stay hydrated, always carry water or a sport fluid.

If you plan to participate in a strenuous activity like a triathalon, marathon, or century bike ride, tap the experience of other athletes with diabetes who have encountered these challenges before you. You can usually get a quick referral to another athlete who participates in your sport through the Diabetes Exercise and Sports Association at www.diabetes-exercise.org or (800) 898-4322. Always discuss your ideas and findings with your physician.

When ExCarbs Don't Work

Sometimes the ExCarb system doesn't seem to work and you may need to consider competing factors that can affect your exercise and insulin needs:

Incorrect Insulin Doses

A key question to ask if the ExCarb system does not seem to be working is, "Are my current basals and boluses set properly?" If someone's insulin doses are set too high, consider what will happen if he already experiences frequent low blood sugars in the afternoon but decides to start exercising at 3 p.m. anyway without eating extra carbs or lowering the morning basal insulin or the lunch bolus. The severe insulin reaction that follows should not be blamed on the exercise. Blame it instead on the underlying problem: in this situation the person already had excess insulin and made matters worse by consuming inadequate carbs for the exercise.

Someone with insulin doses set too low may wake up in the morning with a reading of 180 mg/dl (10 mmol) because the overnight basal insulin is too low. She then goes jogging for 30 minutes and is surprised to find her blood sugar has risen to 240 mg/dl (13.3 mmol) on her return. Again, the exercise is not to blame. The cause is the underlying lack of insulin, which allows excess glucose to be released from glycogen stores in the liver and muscles. The inadequate insulin level also makes it hard for the released glucose to move into muscles to be used as fuel. Her blood sugar control would have been improved by taking a small dose of Humalog before starting to jog, or, even better, by maintaining blood sugar control during the previous night by raising the nighttime basal dose.

Stress Hormones

A less predictable factor affecting exercise is the action of stress hormones. Large amounts of stress hormones can be released at the start of a competitive event, like a swim meet, a 10K run, or a century bike ride. Nervousness at the starting line is a sign that stress hormones are at work. Blood sugars often rise unexpectedly in these circumstances.

The impact that stress hormone release may have on the blood sugar is hard to predict. Extra insulin may be needed for a consistent blood sugar rise during shorter events like a 10K run, but seek the advice of your doctor on this. Extra insulin won't be needed for a century bike ride because the exercise itself will lower the high blood sugar during longer events. Again, your personal experience in similar events can be a great aid, as can frequent testing, if that is possible.

Unusual Circumstances And Unpredictability

Problems can also creep in when exercise conditions change. If you usually walk two miles on flat ground but decide to walk the same distance in hilly country, you will use more fuel climbing the grades. A strong headwind can increase carbohydrate consumption by about one percent for each extra mile per hour of headwind (i.e., for a 10 m.p.h. headwind, increase carbs by 10 percent). Walking in dry sand or soft snow can double the amount of carbohydrate compared to the same walk on firm ground.

Activities that have uneven pacing, like spring cleaning or playing football, can also cause problems. With cleaning, it's hard to predict whether you'll spend the next hour sorting through the closet for throwaways or moving furniture. In football, maybe you'll sit on the bench during the entire game or perhaps you'll be giving your all on the field. Luckily, most activities don't suffer from this much unpredictability.

Be Your Own Guide

Insulin and carb adjustments vary greatly from individual to individual. These variations are complex and not completely understood. Some people may need to lower their boluses and basals only slightly for exercise, while others find that a large insulin reduction is the only way to control their blood sugars for the same exercise. For some, the breakfast bolus does not need to be lowered for morning exercise, but when they do the same exercise later in the day, they have to reduce their lunch or dinner bolus. The only way to determine your own response is to experiment, record your results, and discuss these with your physician. ExCarbs are helpful, but your own experience is your ultimate guide. Experience will help you only if you look back over your records before deciding how to manage a particular situation.

Exercise Tips

• Test blood sugars often before and during exercise, as well as during the 24 to 36 hours that follow. Wear a continuous blood sugar monitor, if possible, and set the low blood sugar warning alarm.

• For weight loss, enhance the availability of internal stores of glucose and fat and lessen the risk of a low blood sugar during long periods of activity by lowering your basal and bolus doses appropriately rather than having to eat lots of extra carbs.

• For performance and safety, keep the blood sugar between 70 and 150 mg/dl (3.9 to 8.3 mmol) during exercise, and try to keep it from dropping below 65 mg/dl (3.6 mmol) afterward. Properly adjusted insulin and carb levels let you do this.

• Normal meal boluses may need to be lowered by 50 percent or more before or during vigorous exercise or heavy work. For example, if you normally take one unit for each 10 grams of carbohydrate, try taking one unit for every 20 grams when you may be working or exercising hard. Some vigorous exercise may require the total elimination of a bolus for the carbohydrate in a meal.

• A bolus taken to bring down high blood sugars will also need to be lowered by 50 percent or more when it is given before or during longer periods of moderate or strenuous exercise.

• For intense activities that last a day or two, such as a weekend backpacking trip, try lowering the basal dose by 20 percent to 40 percent and the meal bolus by 50 percent. Lower the basal insulin the night before the activity. Keep the basal dose somewhat lower than normal for about 24 to 36 hours following the end of the exercise.

• The basal insulin dose rarely needs to be lowered for short, random periods of exercise, although it may need to be reduced before starting a new exercise training program or reduced gradually as your overall fitness improves.

• Never lower your TDD more than 50 percent for even the most strenuous exercise.

• Before making any changes in your insulin doses, discuss the changes with your physician to be sure they are appropriate for you.

"The two hardest things to handle in life are failure and success."
Anon.

Kids And Teens

by Shannon Brow, R.N., B.S., C.D.E.,
Diabetes Nurse Consultant, Houston, TX

Kids and teens benefit from intensive management more than adults as they face frequent small dose adjustments for growth and development. Only an intensive management program with multiple daily injections can provide precisely sized and timed insulin doses needed by little ones. Kids and teens are often very sensitive to insulin, have a strong Dawn Phenomenon, and face maturation issues that require an individual approach. Basal and bolus doses that are carefully matched to carbs and exercise can improve blood sugar control, growth, and school performance.

Why Choose Intensive Therapy

Kids and teens may object to or be lukewarm about intensive management because it requires more planning, thought, attention, injections, and finger sticks. They may see it as just more shots and more sugars. Although lifestyle flexibility increases, they may think the extra planning required means less spontaneity. Training and support are needed to put the program in place so that kids and teens feel better and have better A1c's.

Parents often are willing to do their part in intensive therapy in order to provide better control of their child's diabetes now and better health for their child in the future. However, a child who has not reached the age of reason or a teen with other issues to face can present major challenges to these parents, who already face the extra burdens of diabetes.

Diabetes professionals need to discuss quality of life issues with the kid or teen and family to show them how intensive management can improve life. Is it frustrating to have to eat a snack before P.E. each day? Is it embarrassing to have to be home to eat dinner the same time every night? Do meal times conflict with weekend soccer tournaments and little league games? Are there days when all your carbs are eaten and you still want more? Would you like to do brunch on a weekend instead of breakfast and lunch? Are there times when all you really want to eat is a small salad? Are there days that you just want to sleep in? The flexibility, precision and discipline of intensive management gives positive answers to all these situations that improve the quality of life.

Health professionals also look to intensive management for children and teens to delay or prevent diabetes complications, to prevent repeated hospitalizations, to decrease episodes of severe hypoglycemia, and to help control blood glucose during the Dawn Phenomenon or during growth spurts.

Myths Of Intensive Management

Parents and their child or teen have to be realistic about what intensive therapy can do. Here are some common myths:

Myth: My child or teen will have perfect blood sugar control once on intensive management.

Truth: Blood sugar control will improve as insulin is better matched to need, but no one's control is perfect with any method.

Myth: Intensive management will prevent all complications.

Truth: Better control with intensive management decreases the risk of complications greatly. However, some complications may still occur.

Myth: Intensive management will be easier and take less time.

Truth: Intensive management becomes easier as you do it, but learning the techniques takes time. Many aspects are at first time consuming, but they become easier to do and more habitual with use. Like any learning task, it will be intense at the start before rewards are seen.

Myth: We will know what to do and will understand what we are doing.

Truth: Intensive management is systematic and is based on analysis of patterns and use of formulas for solutions. But formulas cannot make every decision and assist every situation. Mysteries and unexplained blood sugars will always exist, so "feel" or intuition may help in some circumstances.

Myth: More shots mean worse diabetes.

Truth: Frequent, small injections of insulin are more physiologic, contributing to better blood sugar control. The number of injections a day has nothing to do with "better" or "worse" diabetes.

Myth: Intensive management sounds too complicated. Just use a general correction scale.

Truth: Most correction scales are broad generalizations that are retrospective and not customized to the person's needs. A customized correction scale can play a useful role within a completely customized program.

Myth: Adjusting your own insulin doses based on what you eat is just playing Russian roulette with your life.

Truth: Russian roulette is picking a random number and sticking to it. It depends on pure luck. Intensive management uses science, experience and formulas to customize a program to match each individual's needs.

Overview Of Intensive Management

In the Diabetes Center in Houston where I previously worked, we put children and teens on intensive insulin management. To support this, we have a diabetes educator and diabetes dietitian conduct an Intensive Insulin Management Class for parents and their child or teen. We group four families with children of similar age together so that the group process provides support and raises and answers issues common to all. During this time, the child or teen switches from intermediate insulin to multiple injections, with a long-acting insulin to cover the body's basal need, plus with a rapid insulin taken before meals and large snacks to cover carb intake.

The starting TDD and ratios of basal and bolus doses to the TDD are determined, set and reset based on blood sugar patterns as they develop. Then participants begin to use carb factors to test out flexibility in their meal plan, and use a correction factor to calculate doses needed to lower high blood sugars. During this time, the child or teen learns how important it is to count carbohydrates correctly, dose insulin correctly, and record the information needed as a basis for future decisions.

25.1 When Is A Child Ready To Inject?

Children differ in the age at which they can self-inject. By age 10, most children are able to do so with minimal assistance. Encourage self-care at a young age. Start by allowing the child to clean the skin with alcohol and to push the plunger on the syringe.

Relapses in self-injection skills may occur, but the desire to self-inject is often reintroduced by the desire to stay overnight with a friend or to attend diabetes camp.

Proper injection technique should be checked occasionally by the parents and by a health care provider.

Any child or teen going on intensive therapy must have at least one adult around who is also trained in its use. The child or teen's primary caregiver must acquire the skills needed: how to set and test basal doses, calculate and give carb boluses, record data, analyze patterns, and troubleshoot when problems arise.

Whether the diabetes educator or physician trains other caregivers or the parent or child or teen trains them, they all must have appropriate knowledge of the goals and methods of intensive care. Babysitters, school nurses, camp nurses, and coaches need to know the basics: usual doses, appropriate foods, the symptoms and treatment for hypoglycemia and hyperglycemia, and who to call for further help. Diabetes supplies need to be with the school nurses and coaches and carried by the kid or teen in a fanny pack or bag of their choosing.

Setting The TDD, Basals, And Boluses For Kids And Teens

Selecting an initial intensive program for children or teens is very similar to the procedure for adults. However, there are a few differences to consider.

Children and teens often have a more pronounced Dawn Phenomenon than adults. Because of early morning surges of growth hormone and cortisol, growing children and teens often need additional basal insulin during the predawn hours. Some may need a relatively large bedtime basal dose or even a combination of basal insulins, such as Lantus taken before dinner along with NPH taken at bedtime or Lente and Ultralente mixed in one syringe at bedtime, to counteract a strong Dawn Phenomenon. In order to match insulin to need, especially at first, frequent night-time blood sugar monitoring is necessary to determine whether the Dawn Phenomenon is present and its severity. These blood sugar results are used to determine whether and when increased basal doses are needed.

Children and teens often require one or two snacks in addition to their three meals, to provide enough calories for growth and development. Some may want to snack a lot at times and not so much at other times. How to best cover these snacks needs to be considered when setting basal and bolus doses.

Teens have notoriously inconsistent routines and eating patterns, and teens with diabetes are no

25.2 Grams of Carbs For Treating Lows In Children			
Age	**1-6 yrs**	**6-10 yrs**	**10 yrs -Adult**
Grams of Carbs	**5 - 10 grs**	**10 - 15 grs**	**15 - 20 grs**
Lg Glucose Tabs 5 grs each	1 - 2 tabs	2 - 3 tabs	3 - 4 tabs
Med Glucose Tabs 4 grs each	1 - 2 tabs	3 - 4 tabs	4 - 5 tabs
Orange Juice 1/3 cup = 10 grs	1/4 - 1/2 cup	1/2 - 3/4 cup	3/4 - 1 cup
Apple Juice 1/3 cup = 10 grs	1/4 - 1/2 cup	1/2 - 3/4 cup	3/4 - 1 cup
Table Sugar 4 grs per tsp	2 tsps	3 tsps	4 - 5 tsps
Regular Soda 3 grs per oz	2 - 3 ozs	4 - 5 ozs	5 - 6 ozs
Lifesavers 3 grs each	2 - 3	4 - 5	5 - 7
Milk 8 ozs = 12 grs	4 - 5 ozs	6 - 7 ozs	8 - 10 ozs

Adapted from **Understanding Diabetes**, 10 ed., by H. Peter Chase, M.D., 2002

different. While intensive management is the ideal tool for such a lifestyle, as this process starts and doses are being determined, the teen will need to keep a consistent schedule to set insulin doses correctly. We suggest about two weeks. Then when the schedule changes, such as the start of school or vacation, doses may be set again.

The hormones of puberty often challenge any insulin program. Hormonal changes can make this month's insulin program obsolete next month. During "growth spurts," growth hormone and cortisol are higher than usual and require a higher basal rate. It is unlikely that any starting insulin doses, no matter how perfect, will stay perfect for long. Teen hormones and growth bring humility to the best clinicians in diabetes. Expect to adjust insulin doses frequently to keep up with growth.

> ### 25.3 Testing And Kids
>
> When giving an injection or drawing blood for monitoring from young children, remember that their imagination can be vivid and reassurance about their fears may be needed. Let them know that the syringe needle will not affect their heart or puncture a large blood vessel and cause bleeding, and that they easily recreate the small amounts of blood removed for blood tests. Encourage them to ask questions so their fears are allayed.

Setting The Total Daily Dose

See Chapter 11 for a full discussion of setting the TDD. Like adults, a child's TDD always is determined before basals and boluses, which then are calculated as percentages of the TDD.

Certain guidelines suggest that a child or teen decrease his TDD as he switches to more frequent injections. This may not be appropriate for some teens who may need to increase their prior totals, including teens who have not had adequate blood sugar control before switching to intensive management, those who need to increase their food intake for growth, and those who have had wide blood sugar fluctuations with relatively few low blood sugars.

We calculate a starting TDD by looking at their current TDD, their A1c, and units/kg/day. With A1c's less than 7% we may reduce the current TDD to create a starting TDD that won't cause hypoglycemia. If over 9%, no reduction is made.

Setting And Testing Basal Doses

See Chapter 11 for a full discussion of setting and testing basal doses.

Even though they often have a Dawn Phenomenon, we prefer starting children and teens with the simplest approach: a basal dose that provides the same amount of insulin over a 24 hour period. Lantus is good for this because of its flat action, although Lente or NPH can be combined in premeal boluses to provide three or four injections that flatten out the insulin's peaking action. We then gather blood glucose data by testing these first basal doses and make adjustments as needed.

Many guidelines recommend starting youngsters with 40% of their TDD as basal insulin. This may be too low for teens who need more basal insulin. Our experience suggests that many teens need closer to 60% of their TDD as Lantus or other long-acting insulin due to their higher levels of circulating pubertal hormones.

One of the basal dose adjustments we make for a child or teen who often forgets to take a carb bolus for snacks is to use the peaking action of a long-acting insulin to cover snack time. With this, a carb bolus does not have to be remembered. However, the child must remember to snack because the insulin is already in the body. NPH at breakfast works well for covering lunch, while Lente or UL at breakfast can be tried to cover afternoon snacks. Any of the peaking insulins can be taken in addition to Lantus, which has a flatter profile and a more consistent action.

Kids or teens who take one shot of Lantus at night and have lows during the night may need to take Lantus in the morning instead. Lantus may have a slight peak for some users. It is better if this occurs during waking hours so that it can be treated then.

Breast fed and bottle fed infants who feed on a schedule of every few hours which causes minute rises and falls in blood glucose levels may benefit from three daily injections of NPH eight hours apart. This takes the place of diluted doses of rapid insulin given every time the baby feeds.

Setting And Testing Carb Boluses

Chapter 12 has a full discussion of setting and testing boluses and gives a good presentation of using the 500 Rule for Humalog to get the correct carb factor.

We will sometimes use another approach, which is simpler but may not be as exact. We divide the number of carbs in the child's meal plan by the amount of TDD left over after the basal doses are subtracted. For example, if the TDD is 60 units and we use 60% for the basal, that leaves 24 units (60 units times 40%) for boluses.

If the child has a meal plan with a total of 195 grams of carb in the day (breakfast=45, lunch=60, supper=60, and snacks=30), then 24 units must cover 195 grams of carb. We divide 195 by 24 and get 8.1, so 1 unit covers 8 grams of carbohydrate, which means 2 units will cover 15 grams of carb, which we call a carb choice. For some people, this is simpler than counting carbs.

Not all snacks need to be covered with an injection. A small carb snack of 8 to 15 grams might be "free," without the need for an injection if the blood sugar does not rise unacceptably. Bedtime snacks are not covered completely, especially during testing. For instance, for a 32-gram bedtime snack, we let the first 8 to 16 grams of carb be "free" and only cover the 16 to 24 remaining carbs using a carb factor of 8 (rounded from 8.1 for this sample child). So 24 divided by 8 = 3 units, one unit less than normally taken for a 32-gram snack.

A safer method would cover only 16 grams and require a 2 unit bedtime bolus to protect against night lows. This is especially important if the child or teen's exercise or activity level has been sporadic or inconsistent. Large snacks may need to be counted fully for carb bolus amounts, although activity during the day and experience can reduce these bolus amounts.

Be sure the child or teen works out several examples of using carb factors to ensure the child understands how to determine bolus doses for various foods and snacks.

All boluses have to be timed. Usual guidelines suggest that when using Humalog or Novolog insulin, boluses should be given 5 to 15 minutes before the meal. Boluses of Regular insulin are normally given 30 minutes before the meal. There are some instances, however, when the timing of the bolus must be individualized:

Premeal bolus: Give a normal bolus before the meal when you are certain of the food and the time you will eat.

Split bolus: Sometimes it is safer to use a "bolus now, bolus later" approach. This is useful when you don't know how much food you will be eating or the

> ## Jack
>
> Jack is 12 years old and has had diabetes for 4 years. He is very athletic and stars on the school's track team and swim team. He has been on a 2 shot per day program, but he hates having to eat an afternoon snack to avoid going low. Eating dinner late because of sports practice can also make him low. His last A1c was 8.5%. He wants to do intensive management because he wants flexibility with his meals, workouts and practices.
>
> Jack's current insulin program is a TDD of 44 units, a morning shot mixture of 20 units of NPH and 6 units of Humalog, and an evening shot of 10 NPH and 8 Humalog. Jack's weight is 42 kg (93 pounds) and he takes about 1 unit of insulin for each kg (typical for 12 year old boys entering puberty).
>
> Jack's new insulin program starts with about 10% less TDD which is 40 units a day. This reduction works because intensive management, closer to the way the normal pancreas works, uses less insulin. His basal is 20 units of Lantus at bedtime, his carb factor is 1 unit for 12.5 grams of carbohydrate, and his correction factor is 1 unit for every 45 mg/dl above 100 mg/dl. For the first week, Jack agreed to test before each meal, at bedtime, at midnight and at 2 a.m. each night and bring these records to his medical team.
>
> Within 2 months, Jack had become accustomed to his new program. His parents helped him adjust his Lantus so his morning blood sugars were in target. He had flexibility with his meals which made his workouts and training safer. And his A1c was down to 7.6%.

time it will be available or served. This might happen during parties, restaurant dining, or all-you-can-eat buffets. It may also happen during holiday feasts, snacking on chips and salsa, or expecting to eat more than you really can, called the "my eyes are bigger than my stomach" phenomenon. A child should always keep in mind that taking an extra injection when food intake turns out to be more than expected is far better than having a high blood sugar.

After-meal bolus: This approach calls for a meal dose of Humalog or Novolog given immediately after the meal. It is especially useful for small children who may have unpredictable appetites or for anyone during sick days.

Setting And Testing Correction Boluses

See Chapter 13 for a complete discussion of setting and testing correction boluses. Have the child or teen determine how far she drops on a unit of insulin and test this correction factor for accuracy.

Roles And Responsibilities

Intensive management is a great program, but it also carries responsibilities. It is wise to discuss the roles of parent and child or teen with your health care team. In general, the diabetes care team should provide thorough training and complete recommendations for the insulin program. After the program is started, the same team should be available for consultation, especially during the first few days after starting new insulin doses.

Intensive management means planning, thought, and attention must be involved even though teens may complain about a loss of spontaneity. Point out that with this program they have more freedom and flexibility in some ways, like going out to eat with friends after the ballgame.

Any time a child or teen is switched to a different basal/bolus approach or doses are being adjusted, a TDD must first be selected. Basal doses then need to be tested and adjusted, usually over two to three weeks. After this, carb and correction boluses can be fine-tuned. Be sure to have close phone availability and followup during these times. Some diabetes centers use a system of faxed or emailed reports every few days. The most important information to provide in these reports includes basal doses, the carb boluses given and their times, amounts and times for all carbohydrate, and when a correction bolus was used. Some teams also will want to know the total daily dose injected each day and exercise patterns.

If you are new to reviewing blood glucose log books, here is a simple system. Use three different highlighter pens to see patterns quite readily. First choose the target range for blood sugars and then highlight in different colors the blood sugars within range and the ones outside.

For example, if the target range is 80-150 mg/dl,

- Highlight all blood glucose levels below 80 mg/dl with blue.
- Highlight values between 80 and 150 mg/dl, or in the target range, with yellow.
- And highlight values over 150 mg/dl with a pink highlighter.

For another method of recording, use the *Smart Charts* discussed in Chapter 6 . They provide a handy, convenient record of everything that affects your blood sugar on one day on the same page. They also have a place for you to graph readings, which is an excellent way to visualize blood sugar problems, such as when values are regularly too high or too low.

Evaluating Outcomes

How well intensive therapy is working will depend on evaluating the reasons that the child or teen chose this therapy. For example, if the goal was for fewer hospital admissions, then clearly the measure of success is the number of hospitalizations.

Other measures of therapy success are based on a range of goals. Are the child or teen and the parents happy with the program? How often do they report complaints or problems with injections and blood sugar tests? Has the child or teen explained the program to friends and relatives? Has the child or teen benefitted medically or emotionally?

Samantha

Samantha is an 8 year old who has had diabetes for about 5 months. She is a good student and is in the second grade. Her blood sugars during the day are within target and above 100 mg/dl (5.5 mmol) at bedtime. Recently Samantha has been waking up with headaches. Her parents started checking her blood sugar at 2 a.m. and found she is having low blood sugars during the night.

Samantha has been taking 2 shots a day, NPH and Novolog for breakfast and again at dinner. Her last A1c was 7.2%. This suggests she's in good control except overnight. Samantha doesn't mind taking more shots but she doesn't want to take a shot at school.

With these concerns in mind, her diabetes team started her on a program of NPH and Novolog for breakfast, Novolog before dinner, and Lantus at bedtime. This program gives her flexibility at breakfast and dinner, and the NPH covers her lunch at school. Lunch is at a scheduled time and contains a set amount of carbs so Samantha does not have to take a noon shot. With Lantus, her bedtime dose is not peaking during the night and she no longer has nightime lows.

Special Child And Teen Issues

There are several areas that a child or teenager may have concerns about. The following guidelines in these areas may help reduce concerns.

Growth Spurts

Growth spurts and the onset of puberty can signal a time of blood sugar upheaval for teens because the hormones responsible for growth also cause glucose to be released. In addition, the pubertal hormones cause a type of insulin resistance that necessitates increasingly higher doses of insulin. These changes are unpredictable which can make the control of blood glucose during adolescence frustrating. However, intensive management allows the teen to make rapid dose adjustments, as the need arises.

Most children require a total of about a half unit of insulin per pound of body weight each day. Teenagers, on the other hand, can require up to one unit for each pound of weight. This increased insulin is not an indication that the teen's diabetes has become "worse." It is simply a physiological need caused by normal growth. As a teen's overall total daily dose increases, his or her basal, carb, and correction boluses also need to be raised to maintain good control. During the growth years, anticipate needing extra insulin every few weeks or months and increase insulin doses as soon as the need is apparent.

Identification Tags

While wearing ID tags has always been a good idea for the child or teen with diabetes, it is even more important for anyone practicing intensive management. Ordinary ID tags may not appeal to many kids and teens, but newer ID tags include colorful sports bands complete with medical insignia. Some jewelry stores are also making more attractive bracelets. An ID card carried in a wallet is not enough. A child needs clear identification that is visible so emergency people will not miss seeing it. It's a good idea to have "diabetes," any allergies, and a phone number on the ID bracelet or pendant. Don't leave home without it!

School

Key school personnel need to know about your diabetes, the procedures you typically follow, and what to do in case of emergencies. Many schools have "zero tolerance" when it comes to medications and syringes, but to receive federal funding schools must also follow a 504 Plan that is developed by parents of qualifying children in cooperation with their child's school. Sample 504 Plans for diabetes are available at www.childrenwithdiabetes.com/504/ for your use. To avoid problems, the child or teen and parent should prepare the school nurse, coach, teachers, and principal by providing them with adequate printed materials, including a 504 Plan. Your diabetes educator or physician can also write a letter introducing diabetes to your school.

Check with your school officials about where they would like you to test your blood glucose and give injections. Because of health regulations or school policies, it may be customary to do all diabetes care in the nurse's office, but again this is open to the 504 Plan that is developed. Use of an insulin pen or lancets may require your physician to write a letter or place a phone call to a principal or appropriate school official. Work out with school officials a health program that enables your child to stay healthy and to have the freedom other children have.

Keep your school kit filled and handy with these necessities:

- insulin (Humalog, Novolog or Regular)
- insulin syringes and/or an insulin pen
- blood testing supplies
- low blood sugar supplies
- ketone test strips or a Precision Xtra™ meter
- fast-acting carbs

Physical Exercise

The exercise in school P.E. classes is often not consistent in intensity. One day you may be playing a vigorous game of soccer and the next day watching a movie. Consequently, you must decide whether to eat an additional snack during vigorous exercise. Request to do this when you need extra carbs during an unplanned exercise event. If you don't have it in your pocket, you may have to be excused from the workout.

If you have a practice session for a sport you participate in every day after school, consider setting your insulin up so insulin levels are low at that time. Also eat carbs that are not covered by a carb bolus.

Ted

Tad is a 3 year old with diabetes for about a year. He is on a program of 3 shots of NPH a day. His parents check his blood sugar several times a day and see wide fluctuations but seldom a pattern. His last A1c was 9.4%. His activity and food intake are much more variable now than when he was a little baby. His parents know how to do carb counting and want to begin an insulin program that gives better control and predictability.

His diabetes team keeps him on 3 shots a day of Ultralente and Humalog at breakfast, Humalog at lunch, and Ultralente and Humalog at dinner. They mix Ultralente and Humalog in the same syringe and give injections after Tad has eaten, basing the dose on how many carbs he ate.

Athletics

Intensive management is ideal for athletes. Adjustments in carbohydrates, basal doses, and carb boluses may be made so that blood sugar control can be maintained. It is vital to get good guidance on fine-tuning your care so that you can become successful rather than discouraged. You may have required lots of carbohydrates to get through afternoon practices while using the peak of NPH or morning Lente before intensive management. Now when you use a peakless insulin, such as Lantus or Detemir, you can get through practice without having to eat so much. Often a temporary decrease in basal doses may be needed for long and intense activities. You have to plan ahead to do this before you give your breakfast doses or even before giving your doses the night before. In addition, lower doses will often be necessary following the exercise to avoid post-exercise hypoglycemia.

If you test your blood sugar immediately after exercise, you may see that your sugar rose due to the action of adrenaline during exercise, especially after a competitive sports event. Do not immediately give a correction bolus for this high blood sugar reading! Drink lots of water and retest in 60 minutes. Within an hour, the blood sugar often comes back down as adrenaline levels drop. If the blood sugar doesn't come down after an hour, give a correction bolus to lower the high reading. Be sure to test in an hour to see whether the correction bolus worked. Continue to test frequently for the next 24 hours, eat extra carbs and lower insulin doses because blood sugars may continue to drop for up to 36 hours after strenuous exercise. When available, a continuous blood sugar monitor is ideal for monitoring blood sugar changes during and after exercise.

You may need to eat extra carbs before, during, and after exercise to prevent hypoglycemia. Sports drinks or glucose gels are handy choices. Extra carbs for exercise may not need to be covered by carb boluses if the amount is not excessive.

See Chapters 23 and 24 on exercise and intensive management for systematic guidelines about adjusting basal and bolus doses and carbohydrate consumption for various durations and intensities of exercise, as well as physical training. Teens who are interested in exercise may want to join the Diabetes Exercise and Sports Association (www.diabetes-exercise.org or 1-800-898-4322), which holds regional conferences and an annual convention with information sharing, workshops, and group activities.

Fast Foods And Restaurants

Fast food guides and restaurant carbohydrate guides are extremely useful when children and teens are eating away from home. Most chain restaurants have nutrition information available in pamphlet form or upon request. In addition, books are available that give specific nutritional values for items on the menu at many family and chain restaurants. See Chapter 8 on carbohydrate counting, as well as Appendix A.

For high fat meals, it may be necessary to use the "bolus now, bolus later" approach. For example, a pizza may require an initial carb bolus to match part of the carbohydrate intake and a later bolus dose to match the digestion of carbohydrate slowed by the fat. Never be afraid to experiment with your doses, but when doing so test a lot and keep dose changes reasonable!

Most condiments, such as ketchup, dipping sauces, and barbecue sauce have carbohydrates that should be considered when counting carb grams. For instance, ketchup may contain from 3 to 5 grams of carbohydrate per teaspoon or packet which can usually be ignored, but barbecue sauce may contribute enough carbs to create problem readings.

Some carbs in non-starchy vegetables are hard to quantify. Here is a guideline for estimating carbs in vegetables such as green beans, asparagus, lettuce, and other nonstarchy vegetables:

1 cup raw or 1/2 cup cooked vegetables = 5 grams of carbohydrate

Use this guideline to count carbs on vegetable plates and at salad bars!

Dating

To tell or not to tell? It is a personal decision. Friends and dates are often inquisitive about diabetes if they see you test, count carbs or inject. This may serve as an "ice breaker" to start talking about your diabetes. On the other hand, you may feel more comfortable concealing your diabetes for awhile. Even if you don't want to reveal your diabetes at first, do not skip testing and taking your injections. Excuse yourself and go to the restroom for these procedures.

Driving

Always test your blood sugar before driving. If this is inconvenient, eat a snack of at least 15 grams of carbohydrate, such as 3 glucose tablets, before driving to ensure no low blood sugar occurs.

Menses

Some young women may experience drastic changes in blood sugar levels a few days prior to the beginning of their menstrual periods and during the first 2 days of their period. Some have highs that require increased basal and bolus injections, others will tend to have lows following their period, and some will notice little difference around their cycle. It is helpful to record both menstrual and blood sugar history to discover the effect of the cycle on blood sugars and to enable better dosing decisions to be made.

Many teens do not have regular, predictable cycles for several months after the onset of puberty. After you have your first period, start recording your periods even though they may be irregular so that you can see any pattern in how they affect your blood sugar. If you have regular cycles, you can anticipate their effect and check where you are in your menstrual cycle as a possible explanation for control problems.

Alcohol

Drinking alcohol can have several adverse effects for teens on intensive therapy. Aside from the moral or legal issues about alcohol, alcohol prevents the liver from releasing sugar during hypoglycemia and may leave you without the regulator that usually kicks in to bring you out of a low. This can be quite dangerous. The symptoms of hypoglycemia can look strikingly similar to those of intoxication. Not knowing the difference may delay the treatment that is needed. Alcohol impairs judgment and makes it difficult for people to recognize their hypoglycemia, as well as impairing the accuracy of carb intake and insulin dosing decisions.

To stay in control and make the best decisions, consider these tips:

- Know the laws in your state about drinking.
- Remember, you have the choice to say, "No thanks!"
- If you plan to drink, be sure to eat carbohydrates first!
- Limit the amount of alcohol by drinking one or two drinks slowly or alternating alcoholic with nonalcoholic beverages.
- Never drink before you drive. Never drive after drinking.
- Wear your diabetes medical ID tags.
- Let your friends know you have diabetes and how hypoglycemia might make you look or act.
- Test your blood sugar before going to sleep. Eat an extra snack after alcohol for safety.

Sleep-Overs

Some parents and children may feel apprehensive about nights or weekends away from home. Having a sleep-over plan can help relieve some of this anxiety. It is difficult to predict which direction the blood glucose will go during a sleep-over. With the excitement and extra snacks, blood glucose levels may be higher than usual. On the other hand, being awake during usual sleep time with extra activity may actually cause lower blood sugar levels. The only way to know for certain is to test and be prepared to eat carbs to raise a low or to take extra insulin if a high occurs!

Sleeping In On The Weekends

When you first begin intensive therapy, your diabetes team is likely to ask you to follow a specific schedule of waking, eating, and sleeping while they are customizing your basal rates. It is important to know that your overnight basal dose will maintain a safe blood sugar through the night and into the morning. To check this systematically, test your basal doses as shown in Chapter 11. Once your basal doses have been set correctly, the blood sugar results you collect should have values that are similar. Only when this is achieved is it safe to hit the snooze button and go back to sleep! You want to know that when you wake up, you'll be able to eat and enjoy the day ahead without struggling to regulate out-of-control blood sugars.

Eating Disorders

With all the focus on food, it is not surprising that some teens with diabetes have eating disorders. Most often these teens are young women who have a distorted image of themselves and who want to lose inappropriate amounts of weight. They may discover a quick weight-loss technique by continuing to eat what they want while decreasing their insulin doses. Soon blood sugar, calories and ketones start to spill into the urine, resulting in weight loss but also in a very risky medical condition.

Parents and diabetes professionals must stay aware of teens who are overly concerned about food and weight. These teens typically have poor glucose control because they do not calculate basal and bolus doses appropriately. For teens with these behaviors, psychological assessment and intervention are imperative.

If you are using any of these techniques or think that you have problems with food and weight, seek professional help. Untreated eating disorders are very dangerous and can be life threatening, especially with diabetes.

Camping

Diabetes camp is a great way to meet other children and teens with diabetes. The American Diabetes Association maintains a listing of camps throughout the U.S., as does Children With Diabetes at www.childrenwithdiabetes.com. These camps are great for helping a child realize they are not alone with their diabetes. Lasting friendships through life can be developed.

Immunization

We don't often think about the effect immunizations may have on blood glucose. In some children and teens, blood glucose can be elevated for a few days following an immunization. Typically, this means insulin doses need to be raised a small amount over a few days.

"What doesn't kill me makes me stronger."
Albert Camus

Considerations For Infants And Toddlers

A cooperative effort between diligent, well-educated parents and their diabetes team is critical for success with a toddler. Extensive education and evaluation should include carbohydrate counting, how to evaluate insulin needs, sick day management, and troubleshooting skills.

Basal and bolus doses used in toddlers are much smaller than those needed by older children. Doses, often in fractions of units, need to be carefully monitored by a team that is experienced in working with small children. Small doses become easier to give when insulin has been diluted with a special diluent solution available from the insulin manufacturer. For instance, when a rapid insulin has been mixed with an equal volume of diluent, a one unit dose in the syringe will now be a half unit of insulin. Of course, a bottle of diluted insulin has to be carefully marked so that a bottle of full strength insulin will not be used instead, as this would double the insulin dose given.

Babysitters And Daycare

Babysitters and daycare providers can be trained to deliver an injection. During training, parents should always directly supervise the injection. Simple worksheets should be created to give instructions to the childcare provider regarding how to test blood sugars and give injections. In toddlers, we recommend giving the carb bolus after the meal in those who may be finicky, picky or unpredictable eaters.

Instructions should also be given in writing as well as verbally on when to immediately contact the parent, for instance if the blood glucose is abnormally high or low, if the child is vomiting, etc. It is not appropriate that the parent expect the babysitter or daycare providers to be as efficient or as competent in managing the child with diabetes as they themselves are. Parents must be accessible at all times. Any delay in response time can cause significant harm to a child as a result of ketoacidosis or severe hypoglycemia. A simple piece of advice to give to all caretakers is that if something is wrong and you cannot test, always start by giving fast-acting carbs.

Expectations

Parents as well as the diabetes care team of the toddler with diabetes should have realistic expectations for age appropriate goals of control. The desire for 'tight control' or for A1c's of less than 7% for the infant or toddler who is unable to perceive and treat hypoglycemia or hyperglycemia can be dangerous. Instead, parents and healthcare providers should rely on safer measures of success: Does the child have fewer episodes of hypoglycemia? Are the fluctuations in blood glucose levels more controlled? Has the child's quality of life improved? Are the parents less fearful and anxious? Is the child growing and developing normally? If the answers to these questions are "Yes," then the child and family are successful intensive management users.

Consider Pump Therapy

Parents and health care providers may want to consider pump therapy as an option for toddlers and children who experience frequent episodes of severe hypoglycemia or for those who experience rapid and wide fluctuations in their blood glucose levels. Intensive injection programs may be frustrating and difficult to manage when toddlers refuse to eat, are napping, or are ill. Pumps can make these situations easier to handle, allow very precise insulin doses, and provide more stable insulin delivery which reduces hypoglycemia compared to injections. However, the risk of ketoacidosis is greater with pump use. Since this is usually caused by accidental detachment of the infusion set, frequent monitoring is a must when a pump is used.

Troubleshooting

Problems with insulin doses for children and teens are not terribly different from those encountered by adults. The real difference is in the individual's problem-solving skills. Developmentally, youngsters may not be ready to analyze problems. Children and teens can be taught the basics, but they still require good supervision from a knowledgeable adult.

Parents need to know how to verify that insulin doses are accurate and that they are being given, how to evaluate the child's blood sugars, and how to discuss issues in ways that produce positive outcomes. Recording carbs, blood sugars, and insulin doses will help you recognize patterns of poor control and their causes. Then analyzing this data is needed to adjust the amount and timing of basal and bolus doses and carbs for the best results.

Summary

For many years, the need for intensive insulin management in the care of diabetes in children and teens was not fully appreciated, but this is no longer the case. Any insulin program must take into consideration the individual abilities and needs of the child or teen with diabetes. We have seen the success and safety from properly used insulin doses in the well-trained and professionally supported child or teen and family. This ideal setting is not always available, but when it is, the well-being of the child makes all the training and care fully worthwhile.

"You can be sincere and still be stupid."

Anon.

Pregnancy

Gestational diabetes or GDM, which is an elevation of the blood sugar during pregnancy, affects 7% of all pregnancies and over 200,000 women a year in the U.S.[85] GDM is a form of Type 2 diabetes that begins during pregnancy, often near the end of the second trimester or during the third trimester.

Diabetes affects another 10,000 pregnancies annually in women who have Type 1 diabetes prior to conceiving. In addition to these, an increasing number of cases are seen of pregnant women with preexisting Type 2 diabetes as more women develop Type 2 at a younger age and the age at which women become pregnant rises. All of these women have a compelling reason for controlling their diabetes – to promote not only their own health but the health and wellbeing of their unborn babies.

This chapter covers

- Why blood sugar control is necessary during pregnancy to avoid complications to the mother and baby
- Why blood sugar control is more difficult during pregnancy
- Preparing for pregnancy
- Pregnancy management in Type 1, Type 2, and GDM
- Gestational diabetes
- How to distribute carbs through the day with the Rule of 18ths
- Insulin adjustments during pregnancy
- Labor, delivery, and followup after delivery

Complications Found In Pregnancy--Type 1, Type 2, GDM

For good health, a person with diabetes needs to keep her blood sugars close to normal all the time. Control becomes even more important during pregnancy because only strictly controlled glucose levels can create the environment needed to produce a healthy baby. High blood sugars before conception and during the first eight weeks of pregnancy are often associated with serious birth defects. High levels in the second and third trimesters may result in fetal complications and problems at or following birth.

First trimester complications include

- Birth defects
- Spontaneous miscarriage

The risk for these complications increases when Type 1 or Type 2 diabetes is present but poorly controlled near the time of conception.

Second and third trimester complications include

- Premature delivery
- Delayed growth and development
- Large birth weight (over 9 pounds), often requiring a C-section

Dangers to the child at birth include

- Injury during delivery
- Severe low blood sugars after delivery
- Seizures
- Respiratory distress syndrome
- Enlarged heart
- Low calcium level and tetany (jitters)
- Jaundice
- High red blood cell count or polycythemia

These complications may occur due to poor control in Type 1, Type 2, or GDM. One complication resulting from high blood sugars during pregnancy is that the baby at birth does not have fully developed lungs even though it is full term and normal weight. Underdeveloped lungs may cause the baby to have respiratory distress or difficulty in breathing after delivery.

A mother's high blood sugar during pregnancy can also cause severe low blood sugar in the newborn baby. In the womb, the fetus will produce large amounts of insulin to compensate for a high blood sugar in the mother. If the mother's control is poor near delivery, the baby will continue to produce excess insulin after delivery, triggering severe low blood sugars.

How Does Control Affect Complications?

Since 1949, blood sugar control has been directly linked to the survival of the infant. In that year, Priscilla White, M.D., reported from the Joslin Clinic in Boston that 18 percent of the babies of mothers with diabetes were stillborn or died shortly after birth. She also noted that "good treatment of diabetes" clearly improved the outcome.[86] In 1965, Jorgen Pedersen, M.D., studying pregnant women in Copenhagen, reported that women who had none of the Bad Signs in Table 26.2 had a 6.9 percent rate of fetal and neonatal deaths.[87, 88] In contrast, in 130 diabetic pregnancies where one of these signs was present, the death rate rose to 31 percent.[89]

Table 26.1 Blood Sugar Goals During Pregnancy

Time	Whole Blood	Plasma
Before meals and at bedtime:	60-90 mg/dl (3.3-5 mmol) (3.3-5 mmol)	65-100 mg/dl (3.6-5.6 mmol)
1 hour after starting to eat:	<120 mg/dl (6.7 mmol)	<135 mg/dl (7.5 mmol)
2 a.m. to 6 a.m.:	60-90 mg/dl (3.3-5 mmol)	65-100 mg/dl (3.6-5.6 mmol)

Note: Keep your A1c at least 20% below the lab's upper limit for normal for nonpregnant women, i.e, in a normal range for pregnancy. You should know whether your meter is reading whole blood or plasma. © 2003 Diabetes Services, Inc.

During the late 1960's and early 1970's it became clear that the higher the average blood sugar level of the mother, the higher the risk that the child would be lost near birth. By the early 1980's, the mother's blood sugar and the child's metabolic environment could be normalized through blood sugar testing at home. This helped reduce complications after the mother became aware she was pregnant. At the same time, birth defects emerged as a major cause of infant deaths in babies born to women with Type 1 diabetes.[90, 91]

In several studies that looked at this problem, birth defects were found to occur in 4% to 11% of infants born to women with Type 1 diabetes, compared to a rate of 1.2% to 2.1% in the general population.[92-93] Researchers and physicians realized that blood sugar levels needed to be normalized before conception occurs. The child's organs

26.2 Dr. Pederson's Bad Signs
Things to avoid in pregnancy

1. Ketoacidosis
2. Preeclampsia toxemia of pregnancy: a combination of high blood pressure, headaches, protein in the urine, and swelling of the legs, usually occurs late in the pregnancy
3. Kidney infection
4. Neglect of prenatal care

form rapidly during the first eight weeks after conception, often before a woman realizes she is pregnant.

Several researchers also noticed that higher A1c values during the first trimester were associated with more spontaneous abortions than were seen in nondiabetic women.[94, 95] Interestingly, one researcher found that women with diabetes who have excellent control throughout pregnancy actually have a lower rate of spontaneous abortion than nondiabetic women.[95] An A1c that is in the normal range or no higher than one percent above the upper limit of the normal range minimizes the risk of both birth defects and spontaneous abortions.

The conclusion from these early studies was that maintaining normal blood sugars throughout pregnancy reduces the risk of complications. Furthermore, women with Type 1 or Type 2 diabetes who plan to conceive should keep their blood sugars at the same lower levels recommended for pregnancy before they conceive so that a tightly controlled environment exists from the day of conception through delivery. The guidelines that follow provide a good way to maintain tight control during pregnancy.

> ### 26.3 Can Insulin Harm The Child?
>
> Some women are concerned that injected insulin will harm the fetus. This cannot happen because the majority of the insulin does not pass through the placenta and the little bit of insulin that does pass is not biologically active. Glucose, on the other hand, passes easily through the placenta. As the child's own pancreas develops and begins producing insulin during the second and third trimester, the baby will try to lower any high blood sugar by producing insulin. Because insulin is a growth hormone, these excess amounts of insulin created by the baby adds excess and unneeded weight. Macrosomia (or "large body") develops and can make delivery difficult or dangerous for both mother and child.

Control Issues In Pregnancy--Type 1, Type 2, GDM

Blood sugar control is more difficult during pregnancy for several reasons. A nondiabetic pregnant woman's blood sugar is normally lower than a woman who is not pregnant. Recent research has shown that blood sugar levels for a woman without diabetes during pregnancy is 55 to 65 mg/dl (3 to 3.6 mmol) in the morning after an overnight fast and always less than 120 mg/dl (6.6 mmol) even one hour after eating a high carbohydrate meal. This means that target blood sugars for the pregnant woman with diabetes are very close to a hypoglycemic range.

For good control and a healthy baby, A1c levels should be kept within a normal range for pregnancy. Here again, A1c levels in pregnancy are 20 percent lower than a lab's normal range for healthy adults. See Table 26.1. Control can also be complicated when the nausea and vomiting caused by morning sickness make eating and insulin coverage difficult. Control is further complicated by the hormone changes and gradual weight gain that cause insulin need to rise during the course of the pregnancy.

Preparing for Pregnancy--Type 1, Type 2

If you have Type 1 or Type 2 diabetes, you should have your blood sugar under control before you try to conceive. If you have Type 2 diabetes and are using an oral medication, this should be discontinued prior to conception to avoid any possible effects on the fetus. A program using diet, exercise, and insulin, if needed, can be worked out with your physician to achieve optimal control before conception.

Until your blood sugar is controlled, use adequate birth control. Low dose birth control pills appear to be both safe and effective. Once your A1c is in the normal range, you are ready for pregnancy, and birth control can be discontinued.

Achieving optimal control before conception is necessary because the fetus begins to develop specialized organs and tissues from the time the egg is fertilized. This development phase, which lasts through the first three months of pregnancy, determines more than anything else whether the baby will be normal. High blood sugars at this time interfere with cell division and can lead to DNA damage and birth defects. There is a 20 percent chance that the infant will develop complications or die if control was poor prior to conceiving the child and optimal control is achieved only by the second trimester.[96]

If you are planning a pregnancy, you can benefit from following a healthy food plan, exercising regularly, and supplementing your diet with a vitamin/mineral capsule designed for use during pregnancy. If you already have diabetic complications prior to pregnancy, such as damage to the eyes, kidneys, or vascular system, there is a greater risk of complications in pregnancy for yourself and the baby.[97] This does not rule out a healthy pregnancy but should be taken into consideration before pregnancy begins.

> ### 26.4 What If My BG Is High Before A Meal?
>
> Take the carb bolus plus enough correction bolus to lower the high reading. Check the blood sugar every 30 minutes until it is below 120 mg/dl (6.7 mmol) before eating. If the blood sugar is still high two hours later, decide whether to take an additional correction bolus, after you have determined how much unused bolus insulin is still active. If you cannot delay eating, eat the fat and protein portions of the meal first and have the carbohydrate as late into the meal as possible to allow time for your blood sugar to drop.

Testing For Prediabetes or Diabetes Prior To Pregnancy

If you have a high risk of GDM (See Table 26.5) and are attempting to conceive, you should have fasting and glucose tolerance tests to determine if you have prediabetes (also known as glucose intolerance) or diabetes before conception. If these tests are positive, follow Preparing For Pregnancy – Type 1, Type 2 on in the section above. If these tests are negative, they should be repeated as soon as pregnancy is confirmed and, if again negative, repeated at 24 to 28 weeks of gestation.

> ### 26.5 High Risk Factors For GDM
>
> - Age over 35
> - Being overweight
> - Previous history of GDM
> - History of multiple miscarriages and stillbirths
> - Previous baby weighing over 9 pounds at birth
> - Elevated blood sugar in the past
> - Family history of Type 2 diabetes

These tests detect prediabetes as shown by a fasting plasma glucose that is equal to or above 110 mg/dl (5.8 mmol) and less than 126 mg/dl (7.0 mmol) or a random plasma glucose equal to or above 140 mg/dl (7.8 mmol) and less than 200 mg/dl (11.1 mmol) at the two hour point during a 75 gram glucose tolerance test.

A diagnosis of diabetes is made if a fasting plasma glucose is equal to or above 126 mg/dl (7 mmol) or a random glucose

> ### 26.6 Low Risk Factors For GDM
>
> - Women who are < 25 years of age
> - Normal body weight
> - No family history of diabetes
> - No history of abnormal glucose metabolism
> - No history of poor obstetric outcome
> - Not a member of an ethnic/racial group with a high prevalence of diabetes (e.g., Hispanic American, Native American, Asian American, African Amercian, Pacific Islander)
> - No family history of Type 2 diabetes

equals 200 mg/dl (11.1 mmol) or above two hours into a 75 gram OGTT. A third diagnostic test involves diabetes symptoms plus a random plasma glucose equal to or above 200 mg/dl (11.1 mmol). A diagnosis of prediabetes or diabetes can be made only after a second test on another day shows the same result on one of these tests. The diagnosis of prediabetes or diabetes occurs at blood sugar levels that are higher than the tight control desired during pregnancy with diabetes.

Gestational Diabetes

The most common form of diabetes during pregnancy is gestational diabetes mellitus (GDM), which is defined as glucose intolerance that is first recognized during pregnancy. It typically develops late in the second trimester or early in the third trimester of an otherwise normal pregnancy due to an increasing demand for insulin production at this time. Gestational diabetes puts both the mother and baby at risk for serious complications during the pregnancy. The mother also faces a greatly increased risk of developing Type 2 diabetes later in life.

Gestational diabetes is most often a form of Type 2 diabetes uncovered by the increased insulin requirement that occurs during pregnancy. Blood sugar elevation during pregnancy can also result from early Type 1.5 diabetes. If a woman with GDM also has GAD65 antibodies, this indicates Type 1.5 diabetes is likely and that insulin therapy is seven times as likely to be needed as in Type 2.[98]

A woman retains the diagnosis of gestational diabetes even if unrecognized glucose intolerance may have preceded the pregnancy or diabetes persists after the pregnancy. In most cases, glucose regulation returns to normal after the delivery, although the underlying problem persists and is important to address through lifestyle changes.

Screening For GDM

An accurate diagnosis of gestational diabetes is important to reduce health risks to the mother and baby, especially to prevent a large baby (macrosomia), which

26.7 Screening And Diagnosis Of Gestational Diabetes (GDM)

When a test is done, a blood sugar above the threshold indicates GDM.

ADA Screen	Fasting	1 hr	2 hr	3 hr
Screen with 50g GCT*	–	>140 mg/dl* (7.8 mmol)	–	–
ADA 1 Step				
Diagnose with 100g OGTT	>95 mg/dl (5.3 mmol)	>180 mg/dl (10 mmol)	>155 mg/dl (8.6 mmol)	>140 mg/dl (7.8 mmol)
ADA 2 Step				
Screen with 50g GCT	–	>140 mg/dl (7.8 mmol)	–	–
Diagnose with 100g OGTT	>95 mg/dl (5.3 mmol)	>180 mg/dl (10 mmol)	>155 mg/dl (8.6 mmol)	>140 mg/dl (7.8 mmol)
Alternative 1 Step				
Diagnose with 75g OGTT	>95 mg/dl (5.3 mmol)	>180 mg/dl (10 mmol)	>155 mg/dl (8.6 mmol)	–

GCT = glucose challenge test; OGTT = oral glucose tolerance test

* Two research studies have used this as a cost-effective diagnostic tool. One study used the 50g GCT screening test at 16 weeks and found values above 135 mg/dl (7.5 mmol) to be a sensitive diagnostic tool.

often necessitates a C-section and problems for the newborn. Pregnant women who are at high risk of GDM should be tested at the first prenatal visit.

If the high risk characteristics don't exist, the current recommendation is that all pregnant women be screened for GDM with a shortened glucose tolerance test. This is routinely done in pregnant women between the 24th and 28th weeks (the sixth month) of pregnancy.

All pregnant women should be screened for GDM because traditional risk factors have a low probability of predicting who will develop GDM, especially for the first pregnancy.[99] It is important to use both fasting and glucose tolerance tests to detect GDM because an elevation of either one may be the only clue that GDM is present.

Fasting hyperglycemia may be particularly important. One research study involving over 145,000 births in Dallas, Texas, found that a fasting plasma glucose of 105 mg/dl or higher was over three times as likely to be associated with fetal malformations than in women without diabetes and those with GDM who had a fasting value below 105 mg/dl. Women who had diabetes prior to pregnancy were at the highest risk of fetal malformations at 6.1%, followed by those with GDM and an elevated fasting plasma value at 4.8%, then women without diabetes at 1.5% and finally those with GDM and a low fasting plasma glucose value of 1.2%.[100]

Be aware that serum and plasma glucose values are 10% to 15% higher than whole blood values. Some home blood sugar meters measure whole blood, while others measure plasma values. See Table 26.1 for the appropriate target blood sugar values for pregnancy using plasma and whole blood values.

The first test done should determine whether diabetes is already present. A fasting plasma glucose with a reading over 126 mg/dl (7 mmol) or any random glucose higher than 200 mg/dl (11.1 mmol) provides half the testing normally required to diagnose diabetes. If one of these tests is positive in the presence of pregnancy, there is no need to do a glucose challenge test because diabetes exists. The second confirmatory test that is normally done at the lab on another day may be replaced by a test in the clinician's office or by home monitoring results to speed treatment and normalize glucose levels.

If the glucose results are not high enough on these tests to warrant a diagnosis of diabetes, evaluation should be done with one of two approaches:

ADA One Step Approach

An oral glucose tolerance test (OGTT) using 100 grams of glucose. Criteria for diagnosis of GDM using the 100 gram OGTT are shown in Table 26.7. If the blood sugar is equal to or higher than two of these values, a diagnosis of GDM is made. This one step approach may be cost-effective in high-risk populations, such as Native Americans.

ADA Two Step Approach

Two steps are used. An initial screening is performed by measuring the plasma glucose one hour after a 50 gram glucose load which is called a glucose challenge test or GCT. A glucose threshold of 140 mg/dl (7.8 mmol) or higher will pick up 80% of women who have GDM, while a value of 130 mg/dl (7.2 mmol) or higher will pick up 90%. The problem with using the lower value, however, is that it gives more false positives than the higher value and many women without GDM are reported as having it. A diagnostic OGTT is then performed on the women who exceed these threshold values on the GCT.

Regardless of which approach is used, a diagnosis is based on the OGTT. This three hour glucose challenge is done in the morning after an 8 to 14 hour fast and after at least three days of unrestricted eating that includes plenty of carbohydrate. On the morning of the test, the woman drinks a solution containing 100 grams of glucose. If two or more of the glucose results exceed the values in Table 26.7, a diagnosis of GDM is made.

Pregnancy Management Program--Type 1, Type 2, GDM

Every effort should be made to keep your blood sugar normal throughout pregnancy. (See Table 26.1 for blood sugar targets during pregnancy.) You need to manage your diabetes in the following ways:

- Frequent blood sugar and A1c tests to determine your exact level of control
- An eye exam for retinopathy
- A 24-hour urine collection for creatinine clearance, total protein, and microalbumin to assess the health of your kidneys, done each trimester
- An evaluation of your cardiovascular system
- A detailed diet program, using the Rule of 18ths (Table 26.9) or a similar plan
- A regular exercise program

Treatment of Diabetes in Pregnancy--Type 1, Type 2, GDM

Blood Sugar Monitoring

In order to adjust insulin to need in Type 1 during pregnancy, you must maintain a very strict regimen of blood glucose monitoring. Check at least eight times a day, before each meal, an hour after each meal, at bedtime, and at 2 a.m., to alert yourself and your health care team quickly to any increased need for insulin. The tests done at one hour after eating should be the highest blood sugar readings of the day with a desired target at this peak of less than 130 mg/dl (7.2 mmol) on a plasma meter or below 120 mg/dl (6.7 mmol) on a whole blood meter. A test result in the lower end of the target range could indicate you should eat more carbs to avoid a low blood sugar. Table 26.10 shows the typical rise in insulin requirements throughout pregnancy for women with Type 1 diabetes.

For women with Type 2 and GDM, daily self-monitoring of blood sugars with four to seven tests a day are required to reduce exposure of the fetus to elevated glucose readings. Readings done while fasting and one hour after each meal are the most important times to test and are often the minimum testing requirement to ensure adequate control of glucose levels. Tests before meals and at bedtime are also very helpful. Blood sugar targets should be set with therapy adjustments based on how well the targets are met.

For all women who have diabetes during pregnancy, the last three months of the pregnancy are an especially critical time to test because it is at this time that the baby can produce its own insulin. The baby will overproduce insulin if the mother's blood sugar is higher than the normal values of pregnancy.

Other Testing

The following tests are essential for all women with diabetes and pregnancy. Monitoring of ketones at home with a urine test first thing in the morning is essential to detect whether there are too few calories or carbohydrates in the diet. Blood pressure should be measured at home and at each clinic visit to avoid hypertension, and a severe disorder called preeclampsia or toxemia of pregnancy. This is a combination of very high blood pressure, swelling, and protein in the urine that starts middle to late in about 5% of pregnancies. A sonogram is done early in the third trimester to assess the size of the fetus and warn of macrosomia.

Medical Nutrition Therapy (MNT) And Carbohydrate Adjustments

Medical nutrition therapy (MNT) should be started by all pregnant women with diabetes after nutritional counseling by a registered dietitian. MNT should be consistent with ADA guidelines and include adequate calories and nutrients for the woman based on weight and height. These should meet the needs of pregnancy as measured by set blood sugar goals.

Eating a balanced diet every day is important for a pregnant woman with diabetes. Because the fetus is continually removing glucose from the mother's blood for growth, eating many meals and snacks throughout the day becomes important.

During pregnancy, a diet comprised of 40 percent carbohydrate, 40 percent fat, and 20 percent protein is generally recommended. Spreading the carbohydrate portion throughout the day makes blood sugar control easier. An easy way to spread these carbohydrates is by using the "Rule of 18ths." With the help of your dietician, estimate your total daily caloric need. Then distribute the carbohydrate portion throughout the day (see Table 26.8) based on the number of 18ths of total carb needed at that time.

26.8 Carb Distribution With the Rule of 18ths		
Meal or Snack	**Portion of The Day's Total Carbohydrate:**	**Percent of Total Daily Carbs**
Breakfast	2/18	11.0%
Midmorning Snack	1/18	5.5%
Lunch	5/18	27.5%
Midafternoon	2/18	11.0%
Dinner	5/18	27.5%
After-Dinner Snack	2/18	11.0%
Bedtime Snack	1/18	5.5%

As an example, if you require 1800 calories per day, eat 180 grams of carbohydrate (1800 calories times 40% of calories as carbs divided by 4 calories per gram of carb). This total of 180 grams divided by 18 (Rule of 18ths) equals 10 grams per 18th. According to Table 26.8, your breakfast would include 20 grams of carbohydrate.

The breakfast carbohydrate is kept low in comparison to the rest of the day because most women with Type 1 diabetes have at least a mild Dawn Phenomenon and therefore are more resistant to insulin at the beginning of the day. Women with Type 2 and gestational diabetes often have insulin resistance, which can also cause high morning readings. Keeping carb intake low until noon helps in dealing with this. Since strict control is of such importance, staying away from high glycemic foods which can spike the blood sugar is a good idea at any time. Consult a list of foods with their glycemic index ranking and primarily choose foods ranking 60 and below.

Your caloric need will rise during pregnancy, usually adding between 500 to 1,000 extra calories per day over the nine months. These calories supply fuel for

26.9 Rule of 18ths: Grams of Carb Per Meal Based On Total Calorie Need

Meal	Carbs as 18ths	Total Calories Per Day							
		1600	1800	2000	2200	2400	2600	2800	3000
Breakfast	2/18 =	19 g	20 g	22 g	24 g	26 g	29 g	30 g	34 g
Morning Snack	1/18 =	9 g	10 g	12 g	14 g	14 g	14 g	16 g	17 g
Lunch	5/18 =	44 g	50 g	55 g	60 g	66 g	72 g	78 g	82 g
Afternoon Snack	2/18 =	18 g	20 g	22 g	24 g	27 g	30 g	31 g	82 g
Dinner	5/18 =	44 g	50 g	55 g	60 g	66 g	72 g	78 g	34 g
Evening Snack	2/18 =	18 g	20 g	22 g	24 g	27 g	29 g	31 g	82 g
Bedtime Snack	1/18 =	9 g	10 g	12 g	14 g	14 g	14 g	16 g	34 g
Total Carbs/Day =		160 g	180 g	200 g	220 g	240 g	260 g	280 g	300 g
40% of Total Cal/Day =		640 cal	720 cal	800 cal	880 cal	960 cal	1040 cal	1120 cal	1200 cal

your higher metabolic rate and your required weight gain. The distribution of carbohydrates changes along with the calorie change. Table 26.9 provides guidance for distributing the carb portion of these calories.[101]

Exercise

Increased exercise is a critical part of blood sugar control during pregnancy. An ideal way to do this is to walk for 15 to 20 minutes after each meal. When this can be done, post meal blood sugars are greatly improved. A total of 45 to 60 minutes of walking a day is ideal during pregnancy. Starting or continuing an exercise program is recommended during pregnancy.

Insulin Therapy

If you have well-controlled Type 1 diabetes when you become pregnant, you can begin adjusting your normal basal doses and boluses through the pregnancy. If you have Type 2 diabetes, you may be controlling your diabetes with diet and medication. When you become pregnant, if you are on a diabetes pill, it will be replaced immediately with insulin, since oral agents may have a negative effect on the fetus. If your diabetes is diet-controlled, your blood sugar should be monitored carefully at home and in the clinic with the goal of staying within the targets in Table 26.1. Insulin will be started whenever the blood sugar rises above the targets required for a healthy pregnancy.

Insulin requirements generally rise steadily throughout pregnancy and will usually double by the last month.[102] The rising need for insulin is caused by several factors, including weight gain, increased caloric intake, creation of new tissue, and an increase in hormones made by the enlarging placenta. The action of placental hormones, especially estrogen, cortisol, and human placental lactogen, conflict with the action of insulin. Each woman's experience varies so an insulin program must be tailored to each individual's need.

However, there are two periods during a pregnancy when a reduction in insulin need may be noted. The first period occurs in Type 1 diabetes during a five week interval between weeks 7 and 12 of gestation. In one clinic's experience, after an initial rise in insulin doses of 18% between weeks 3 and 7, a significant drop in insulin requirement averaging 9% was seen in weeks 7 through 12.[103] The reason for this insulin change is not clear, but may be caused by a rapid

26.10 Typical Rise In Total Daily Insulin Doses By Trimester For Type 1 Diabetes

| If your weight is: | At this trimester: | | | |
	Pre	1st*	2nd	3rd**
100	27 u	32 u	36 u	41 u
120	33 u	38 u	44 u	49 u
130	35 u	41 u	47 u	53 u
140	38 u	45 u	51 u	57 u
160	44 u	51 u	58 u	65 u
180	49 u	57 u	65 u	74 u
200	55 u	64 u	73 u	82 u

In contrast to Type 1 diabetes, the TDD for women with Type 2 diabetes and recently diagnosed gestational diabetes varies greatly.

* From week 7 to 12, the need for insulin may decrease about 9%.
**In the last 4 weeks, the need for insulin may decrease slightly.

Adapted from Jovanovic L, et al. Am J Med. 71: 925-927, 1981

increase in doses to correct past hyperglycemia, followed by improved sensitivity as a result of the better control. It may also be caused by a decline in progesterone secretion. This drop in insulin need appears to have been first noted by physicians in the 1950's who found that unexpected, sudden hypoglycemia in women with Type 1 diabetes was often the first sign of pregnancy.

The second exception to the general rise in insulin requirements as pregnancy progresses occurs in the last four weeks of pregnancy. At this time, the fetus starts to draw more glucose from the mother's blood for its own use causing the mother's insulin need to fall slightly. If a decreased need occurs, the basal dose and boluses are reduced. A reduced overnight basal and a larger bedtime snack may be required to keep the blood sugar from dropping during the night at this time. Reduce your carb boluses as needed if you are unable to eat a substantial meal because of the enlarging uterus.

Caution: If you experience a drop in your need for insulin that does not occur at these times and is not caused by these obvious reasons, contact your obstetrician for consideration of immediate delivery.

With Type 1 diabetes, multiple injections based on matching insulin to need, using a basal and bolus approach, works best for maintaining control in the face of a largely constant rise in the need for insulin, especially in the last four months of pregnancy. With GDM and Type 2 diabetes, where significant insulin production remains, control can often be achieved with two or three injections a day. The usual dose is an injection of Regular plus Lente or NPH before breakfast, and an injection of Regular plus Lente or NPH before dinner.

An alternative for the evening is Regular before dinner with Lente or NPH taken at bedtime. The peaking action of the breakfast Lente or NPH is used to cover lunch. If a larger lunch is desired, an additional injection of Regular can be given before eating lunch. In Type 1 diabetes, during pregnancy the normal percentage of basal insulin at 50 to 60% of the TDD usually stays the same. In GDM and Type 2 diabetes, the presence of insulin resistance may necessitate that 70% of the TDD be used for basal insulin. The remaining 30% is used for meal boluses.

Correction boluses should be used when necessary to bring down a high blood sugar. This should be done quickly so the fetus is not harmed. If the blood sugar continues to rise above your targets, it is time to raise your basal dose and boluses. Increased doses usually are required every 5 to 15 days through most of the pregnancy as determined by charting the blood sugars and the amounts of carbohydrate eaten. See Table 26.10 for the typical rise in TDD. We recommend a graphic charting system, like Sm*art Charts*, during pregnancy to track everything that may affect your control.

Insulin Choices

ADA guidelines say human insulins, such as Regular, should be used when insulin is prescribed and that home glucose testing should guide the dosing. Insulin analogs, such as Humalog, Novolog, and Lantus have not been approved for use in diabetes in pregnancy. The problem with using a new analog insulin arises from its structural differences compared to human insulin. Research has yet to prove that these structural differences will not cause unwanted changes during the rapid cell division and organ development that is seen during pregnancy, especially during the first three months.

Before release by the FDA, all insulins are studied carefully to detect unwanted effects on cell growth. Neither Humalog nor Novolog have shown abnormal effects on cell growth in these tests. In real life testing, one measure of cell change is whether those using an analog insulin have any more retinopathy compared to existing insulins, and again no difference has been detected in studies involving large numbers of users.

Humalog (lispro) has been available since 1997 and has been in use by many women during the time in which they conceived and through the subsequent pregnancy. To this point, research studies have found no detrimental effects on the child with the use of Humalog in Type 1 or Type 2 diabetes.[104-107] Several studies have concluded that use of Humalog in Type 1 pregnancy results in outcomes that are comparable to other large studies of diabetic pregnancy. Though not approved for use in pregnancy, some clinicians prefer to use Humalog in Type 1, Type 2 and GDM for improvements that are seen in postmeal control.

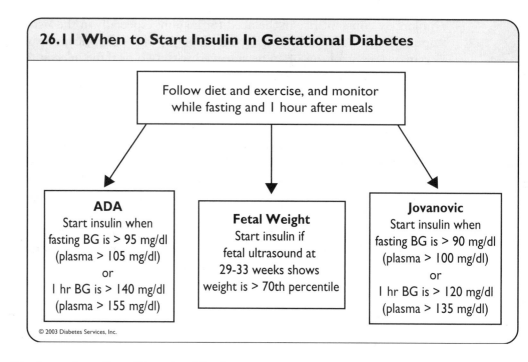

26.11 When to Start Insulin In Gestational Diabetes

Follow diet and exercise, and monitor while fasting and 1 hour after meals

ADA
Start insulin when fasting BG is > 95 mg/dl (plasma > 105 mg/dl)
or
1 hr BG is > 140 mg/dl (plasma > 155 mg/dl)

Fetal Weight
Start insulin if fetal ultrasound at 29-33 weeks shows weight is > 70th percentile

Jovanovic
Start insulin when fasting BG is > 90 mg/dl (plasma > 100 mg/dl)
or
1 hr BG is > 120 mg/dl (plasma > 135 mg/dl)

© 2003 Diabetes Services, Inc.

When To Start Insulin – Type 2, GDM

Ten to fifteen percent of women with gestational diabetes require insulin to control high blood sugars. You need insulin as soon as blood sugars rise above the range in Table 26.1. Insulin doses for GDM and Type 2 must be handled on an individual basis. Starting insulin doses depend on how much insulin the woman is producing, how high the blood sugar is, her current weight, and when during the pregnancy insulin is started.

For women with Type 2 diabetes or GDM, the American Diabetes Association recommends adding insulin therapy to MNT and exercise when fasting home monitoring values are above 95 mg/dl (5.3 mmol) whole blood or above 105 mg/dl (5.8 mmol) plasma, or one hour postprandial values are above 140 mg/dl (7.8 mmol) whole blood or above 155 mg/dl (8.6 mmol) plasma.

These plasma values recommended for starting insulin by the ADA are higher than the plasma glucose values seen during a normal pregnancy. Some pregnancy specialists lower the thresholds and recommend that insulin be started as soon as home blood glucose testing on whole blood shows values greater than 90 mg/dl (5 mmol) while fasting or greater than 120 mg/dl (6.6 mmol) 1 hour after a meal.[100] These values are equivalent to plasma values of 100 mg/dl (5.5 mmol) fasting and 135 mg/dl (7.5 mmol) one hour after eating. Home monitoring values are more indicative of actual control and are easier to obtain and monitor during the pregnancy than tests done in the medical office.

Another reason to begin insulin therapy is when a fetal ultrasound at 29 to 33 weeks shows the fetal weight is greater than the 70th percentile. Insulin is started for this reason regardless of the mother's glucose levels.[108]

When macrosomia is controlled, the need for a C-section becomes less likely. Gestation should last 38 weeks when possible, but not go beyond 38 weeks because longer pregnancies increase the risk of macrosomia and do not decrease the risk of a C-section.

How To Use Insulin When Nausea Occurs – Type 1, Type 2

Nausea and vomiting often occur in the first trimester. This becomes a concern for a pregnant woman with Type 1 diabetes who may think that because she cannot eat when she's nauseated, she does not need any insulin. This is not the case. Since the liver continues to make glucose and release it into the bloodstream, basal insulin is needed to keep the blood sugar from rising even when no food is eaten. This means that a background basal insulin like Lente or NPH will be needed even if nausea prevents eating. No carb bolus is needed if eating can't occur.

Glucagon should be kept available for use anytime the carb bolus has been taken for a meal but you find you are unable to eat due to nausea. An injection of glucagon raises the blood sugar by causing the liver to release some of

26.12 Glucagon: How Much Do You Need?

Each 0.15 mg of glucagon (or 1/6 of the standard 1 mg. dose) raises the blood sugar 30 mg/dl! Avoid taking too much glucagon, as this raises the blood sugar too high and may cause nausea, which is what you are trying to avoid.

its stored glucose. If nausea occurs frequently, as it will in some pregnancies, you may want to take only part of your carb bolus and then attempt to eat. If you find you are able to eat food and keep it down, you can take the rest of the bolus as soon as you are sure of this.

If food or caloric drinks won't stay down but a meal bolus has been taken, you may inject a partial dose of glucagon to quickly raise the blood sugar. Usually, one third to one half of a standard one milligram glucagon kit is all that is needed to prevent a low blood sugar.

Ketoacidosis And Pregnancy--Type 1

In Type 1 diabetes, the greatest threat to the fetus and the mother are high blood sugars leading to diabetic ketoacidosis. If the mother develops severe ketoacidosis, there is a 95 percent probability that the fetus will die. The following precautions help to avoid ketoacidosis:

- Test the blood sugar frequently to ensure that control is constant
- Take a correction bolus to lower any blood sugar over 160 mg/dl (8.9 mmol)
- Check the urine for ketones every morning and when the blood sugar is above the target level

Oral Diabetes Medications

Oral diabetes medications are not FDA approved for use in pregnancy with Type 2 diabetes or GDM and are generally not used. However, one study used glyburide successfully to achieve tight control in a head to head study with insulin involving over 400 women with gestational diabetes who were not able to achieve blood sugar control with MNT. This study took place after conception. No differences were found in control or outcomes between the two groups.[109] However, a full scale clinical trial at various locations will need to be done to confirm this study. Glyburide has not yet been approved for use in pregnancy.

Older sulfonylureas are known to cause fetal damage so they are avoided. Prolonged hypoglycemia lasting four to ten days has been seen after delivery in women receiving a sulfonylurea, so glyburide, if used, should be discontinued at least 2 weeks before delivery.

Metformin is not used during pregnancy. However, women of child bearing age with Type 2 diabetes or PCOS may be treated with metformin, which improves fertility so pregnancy may occur. See page 40 for more information on PCOS. Metformin is generally an excellent diabetes medication. However, one important issue that arises with its use is that it can lower blood levels of folic acid and vitamin B12. Folic acid intake is generally low in the diet and a lack of folic acid is associated with spina bifida and other neural tube defects in the child.

Loss of folic acid and vitamin B12 can also raise homocysteine levels in the blood, a risk factor associated with an increased risk of heart disease. Absorption of vitamin B12 appears to be corrected by taking a calcium supplement. Women of child bearing age, particularly those who use metformin, would be wise to take a calcium supplement along with a prenatal vitamin that contains 400 mg of folic acid and other B vitamins.

Labor And Delivery

During active labor at the hospital, muscle contractions can be similar to strenuous exercise. This activity reduces insulin need dramatically. The goal is to maintain blood glucose levels between 60 and 100 mg/dl (3.3 and 5.6 mmol). If you have Type 1 diabetes, you may attain this by reducing your basal dose quickly and temporarily discontinuing all boluses. An intravenous line will be started to give insulin as needed to lower the blood sugar or glucose to raise it. Test your blood sugar hourly or have someone else test it to ensure that the intravenous line is controlling the blood sugar well. If you have GDM, both basal doses and carb boluses are discontinued when active labor begins.

After Delivery

After the baby has been delivered, the hormones in the placenta that antagonize insulin are no longer at work. Insulin requirements rapidly drop. Most women with GDM who required insulin during their pregnancy no longer need it. Women with GDM may continue to have diabetes and need some type of treatment, but often they return to impaired glucose tolerance, impaired fasting glucose, or to normal blood sugars. Between 20% and 50% of women with gestational diabetes develop Type 2 diabetes, either immediately or at some point within the next 20 years.

The reduced demand for insulin after delivery, together with the prolonged "exercise" of labor, may be so dramatic that even in Type 1 diabetes insulin may not be needed for a day or two. If the woman has had a C-section, her eating will be limited for the next two to three days, which limits her insulin need also. In a few days, the woman with Type 1 will be back to her pre-pregnancy insulin requirements.

Care Following Delivery

In GDM, tests are performed six weeks after birth to determine whether the mother's blood sugar has returned to normal. The criteria for a diagnosis of diabetes at this time are the same as for diagnosing the general population. See Testing For Prediabetes Or Diabetes Before Pregnancy on page 285. Women with a diagnosis of prediabetes or diabetes should be counseled on diet, exercise and medications to treat the condition.

Babies born to women with GDM should be followed closely to prevent the development of obesity or abnormal glucose tolerance.

Breast Feeding--Type 1, Type 2

If you breast-feed (which benefits the baby's immune system), insulin requirements may be lower than before conception because more glucose is needed for breast milk. Adjust your calorie intake to match the child's breast-feeding habits. If the baby consumes most of its calories at bedtime or in the middle of the night, you must do the same. Many Type 1 women with this breast-feeding pattern need only a low basal rate to cover eating in the evening.

"When I was a kid my parents moved a lot
— but I always found them."
Rodney Dangerfield

"Diabetes is a symptom, not a disease, and insulin... does no more than palliate this symptom. The drug throws no light upon the cause, it does not act in the manner described, and, had the cause been found and eradicated as it can be, there would have been no need to use it. "

J.E.R. McDonagh, F.R.C.S.
in The Nature of Disease Journal, Vol. 1, pg.1, 1932

"There are days when it takes all you've got just to keep up with the losers."
Robert Orben

Insulin And Diabetes Medications

Insulin and oral diabetes medication have been combined to treat Type 2 diabetes with measured success since medications became available. With today's new insulins, medications, and treatment options, an unprecedented opportunity to improve blood sugar control and health has arrived. The number of drug and insulin choices and the urgency of treating to blood sugar and A1c targets means that you and your health care provider must stay up-to-date on the latest approaches to treatment.

This chapter covers

- The five classes of oral diabetes medications
- Treating prediabetes with medications
- Why medications fail over time
- New combination treatments for Type 2
- Oral medication and insulin approaches for Type 1
- Weight gain with insulin
- Special concerns in using different medications

The Five Classes Of Oral Diabetes Medications

The oldest class of diabetes medications, the sulfonylureas, has been used in the United States for 50 years. A second class, the biguanide metformin, has been in use in Europe since 1957, although it and a third class, the starch blockers, were introduced into the United States in 1995.

Another class, called glitazones (currently Avandia and Actos), was introduced in 1997. Unfortunately, the first glitazone drug, Rezulin, had to be taken off the market because of serious side effects and several deaths. Actos and Avandia, fortunately, do not share these problems. Another class, the rapid insulin releasers, became available in 1998 and includes Prandin (repaglinide) and Starlix (nateglinide).

Each drug class works by a different mechanism. Sulfonylureas and rapid insulin releasers stimulate the pancreas in several ways to increase insulin production of insulin. The starch blockers (alpha glucosidase inhibitors) work on the digestive system to slow the entry of glucose into the bloodstream after meals. A biguanide decreases glucose production by the liver, while glitazones work at the cell level to overcome insulin resistance and enhance glucose uptake. This wide choice of medications allows treatment to be tailored to individuals with different levels of insulin resistance and insulin production.

Drug combinations have allowed many people with Type 2 diabetes to delay the start of insulin. Some people who previously used insulin and needed it at that time have been able to stop using it or to reduce their dose through judicious use of some of the newer classes of drugs. However, since A1c values for nearly half of those with Type 2 diabetes are over 8.5%, many people would improve their control by adding insulin to their diabetes medications or replacing one or more medications with insulin. Even though insulin is more effective than any medication, it is not used early enough nor aggressively enough in most people with Type 2 diabetes.

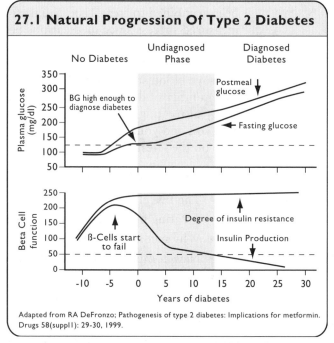

27.1 Natural Progression Of Type 2 Diabetes

Adapted from RA DeFronzo; Pathogenesis of type 2 diabetes: Implications for metformin. Drugs 58(suppl1): 29-30, 1999.

Insulin use would rise dramatically if everyone who could benefit from it were actually using it. Unfortunately, people resist the idea of injections because it is easier to think first of the discomfort rather than the benefits. Physicians who have encountered this reluctance in previous patients may hesitate to suggest insulin until late in the course of the disease, despite its proven benefits.

Some physicians use the threat of insulin as a motivator to encourage a patient to improve their diet or increase their exercise. Unfortunately, this puts negative connotations on insulin use so that it appears to be a punishment imposed because of personal failure.

Because Type 2 diabetes is a progressive disorder, as shown in Graph 27.1, people with Type 2 diabetes often need to adjust their therapy several times through their lives. When a combination of therapies is used to advantage, they will remain in good control over time. By encouraging their medical team to work with them, they can customize a combination of insulins and medications that will match their particular needs.

Sulfonylureas

Sulfonylureas, the oldest drug group introduced into the U.S. in 1955, stimulate the beta cells to produce more insulin. These drugs have kept many Type 2's off injected insulin, but will not work in those with Type 1 diabetes nor in anyone with Type 2 whose beta cells no longer produce insulin. Loss of insulin production, as shown by a low C-peptide level, is universal in Type 1 diabetes, in many who have Type 1.5 diabetes, and in many others who have had Type 2 diabetes for more than 6 or 12 years.

When someone retains insulin production, this production can be increased by stimulating beta cells with a medication. Insulin from the beta cells is released directly to the liver via the portal vein, allowing it to work more effectively.

Sulfonylureas can cause low blood sugars, although they occur much less often than with insulin injections. Severe low blood sugars occur about 500 times more often with insulin than with sulfonylureas. Emergency room visits for low blood sugars occurred only once for every 4,000 person-years of sulfonylurea use during a large 10 year study done in Switzerland between 1975 and 1984.[110] Low blood sugars brought on by sulfonylureas are generally infrequent and mild.

The original "first generation" sulfonylureas include Orinase (tolbutamide), Tolinase (tolazamide), and Diabinese (chlorpropamide). These drugs work well in lowering the blood sugar, but they have a major drawback. Because they bind to proteins in the blood, they can be dislodged by other medications that bind to these same proteins. Once dislodged, their activity can increase rapidly and lead to low blood sugars.

Diabinese lasts longer in the blood and on rare occasions can cause a severe and long-lasting form of hypoglycemia. Its use was phased out as newer, safer sulfonylureas became available. However, chlorpropamide, the generic form of Diabinese, can still be encountered in many nonprescription oriental "herb mixtures" that are imported and used as over-the-counter treatments for diabetes within the U.S. The product label is unlikely to list chlorpropamide, so the wise approach is to avoid use of any herb mixtures for diabetes.

Second generation sulfonylureas include Glucotrol (glipizide), as well as Micronase, Diabeta, and Glynase (all contain glyburide). A third generation called Amaryl (glimepiride) is also available. These drugs have an advantage for those who use other medications since they do not bind to carrier proteins in the blood. Because of this, drug interactions that may cause low blood sugars are less likely.

Sulfonylureas work best when taken at the same time each day. Glyburide and glipizide are shorter-acting versions. Glyburide (Micronase and Diabeta), and glipizide (Glucotrol) are usually taken twice a day, half before breakfast and half before dinner. Sustained-release versions called Glynase or Glucotrol XL are also available. Long-lasting versions can be taken once a day instead of twice a day. These medications can be used once a day before the evening meal when a person has high blood sugars at bedtime or before breakfast if care is taken to monitor the daytime blood sugar until the safety of the dose is assured.

As well as stimulating insulin production, Amaryl (glimepiride) may cause a mild reduction in insulin resistance and may be less likely to cause low blood sugars than other sulfonylureas. It is also safer for people who have advanced kidney disease indicated by an elevated creatinine level. Other sulfonylureas are usually not recommended when the creatinine level is elevated. Glimepiride also does not block the normal relaxation of blood vessels and does not affect coronary arteries. These unwanted side effects may occur infrequently with other sulfonylureas.

When starting a sulfonylurea, the greatest risk of a low blood sugar occurs during the first few days to first four months of use. Be careful during this time and check your blood sugar often when you exercise, increase activity, or skip a meal. Drinking alcohol or taking certain medications like decongestants can also increase

27.2 Sulfonylureas

Target organ: Pancreas
Action: Increase insulin release
Lowers HbA1c by 1% to 2%
Taken: with or without food

	Drug	Acts Over	Dose Range	Rel. Potency	Doses/Day
1st Gen	Orinase (tolbutamide)	6-10 hrs	500-3000 mg	1	2-3
	Tolinase (tolazamide)		100-1000 mg	3	1-2
	Diabinese (chlorpropamide)	24-72 hrs	100-500 mg	6	1-2
2nd Gen	Glucotrol (glipizide)	12hrs	2.5-40 mg	75	1-2
	Glucotrol XL (ext. rel. glipizide)	24 hrs	2.5–20 mg	150	1
	Micronase, Diabeta (glyburide)	18-24 hrs	1.25-2.0 mg	150	1-2
	Glynase (micronized gly.)	24 hrs	3-12 mg	250	1-2
3rd Gen	Amaryl (glimepiride)	24 hrs	1-8 mg	350	1

Side Effects: low blood sugar (bloating, nausea, heartburn, anemia, weight gain metallic or change in taste in 1% to 3%)

Contraindications: Type 1 diabetes, advanced liver or kidney disease, sulfa allergy the risk of a low. Medications, such as steroids, beta blockers, niacin, and Retin-A, may decrease the action of a sulfonylurea and cause the blood sugar to rise.

Rapid Insulin Releasers

Two drugs in this class are now available – Prandin, derived from benzoic acid and approved by the FDA in 1997, and Starlix, derived from D-phenylalanine and approved in 2000. They raise insulin levels rapidly by stimulating the beta cells by mechanisms different from the sulfonylureas. They enhance insulin release from the pancreas over a short period of time only when the glucose level is high. Therefore, the risk of hypoglycemia is reduced. Their activity more closely mimics normal first phase insulin release when food is eaten by a person without diabetes. Peak activity is seen in one hour and the short action time of three hours makes them ideal for matching carbs in meals.

Prandin or Starlix are taken 10 to 15 minutes before meals and do not need to be taken if a meal is skipped. Like sulfonylureas, they do not work in Type 1 diabetes and work in Type 1.5 and Type 2 only as long as the beta cells are capable of producing insulin.

People who eat carbs and then have their blood sugars spike more than 40 or 50 mg/dl above their premeal readings are the most likely to benefit from these drugs. However, most people do not check to see how high their blood sugar is spiking after eating. Testing at one or two hours after a meal is of real value because it can identify those who may benefit from one of these drugs. One minor inconvenience of the drug is the need to remember to take it several times a day before meals.

27.3 Rapid Insulin Releasers

Target organ: Pancreas
Action: Increases first phase insulin release, glucose driven, lowers after–meal glucose
Lowers HbA1c by 0.5%–2.0%
Time to reach maximum effect: 1 hr
Taken: Slarlix is taken right before each meal while Prandin is taken 15–30 minutes before each meal

Drug	Acts Over	Dose Range	Doses/Day
Prandin (repaglinide)	3 hrs	0.5-4 mg before each meal	2-3
Starlix (nateglinide)	3 hrs	60 to 120 mg before each meal	2-3

Side Effects: low blood sugar, nausea, vomiting, diarrhea, muscle aches, upper respiratory infection, cold and flu like symptoms, headache, joint aches, and back pain

Contraindications: Type 1 diabetes, liver disease

In people who retain residual insulin production, one of these medications can be combined with a basal insulin like NPH, Detemir, or Lantus to provide great control. The injected insulin provides basal coverage to keep the fasting blood sugar at a good level, while one of the rapid insulin releasers can enhance internal insulin release to control the blood sugar after meals.

Interactions with other drugs may occur, so be sure your physician knows what else you are taking. Certain drugs may increase the effect of these medications, including large doses of aspirin or Motrin type medications, sulfonamides, chloramphenicol, coumadins, monoamine oxidase inhibitors, and probenecid. Drugs that may decrease their effect include calcium channel blockers, corticosteroids, oral contraceptives, thiazide diuretics, thyroid preparations, estrogens, phenothiazines, phenytoin, rifampin, isoniazid, phenobarbital, and sympathomimetics. One advantage to the medications is that they can be taken safely by people with impaired kidney function or sulfa allergies.

Metformin

Two drugs from the biguanide class, metformin and phenformin, were developed in 1957. Unfortunately, phenformin reached the U.S. market first and resulted in several deaths from lactic acidosis. When this risk surfaced, phenformin was pulled from drugstore shelves worldwide. Metformin was eventually found to be 20 times less likely to cause lactic acidosis, but it was tainted by the history of its cousin. Metformin first became available in France in 1979 and has been widely used in Europe since then, but it was not cleared for use in Type 2 diabetes in the U.S. until 1994.

> ### 27.4 Metformin
>
> Target organ: Liver, secondary effects on muscle and fat.
> Action: Lower glucose production by liver, increase number of insulin receptors on muscle and fat cells
> Lowers HbA1c by 1.5%–2.0%
> Time to reach maximum effect: 2–4 hrs
> Taken: with meal
>
> | Drug | Acts Over | Dose Range | Doses/Day |
> |------|-----------|------------|-----------|
> | Glucophage (metformin) | 8-12 hrs | 500-2550 mg | 2-3 |
> | Glucophage XR (metformin) | 24 hrs | 500–2250 mg | 1 |
> | Glucovance (metformin plus glyburide) | 12-18 hrs | 250/1.25 to 2000/20 mg | 2-3 |
>
> Side Effects: bloating, fullness, nausea, cramping, diarrhea, vit B12 deficiency, headache, metallic taste, agitation, lactic acidosis
>
> Contraindications: DKA, alcoholism, binge drinking, kidney or liver disease, congestive heart failure, pregnancy, use of contrast media, surgery, heart attack, age > 80

Metformin is a chemical kin to the French lilac plant, which was noted in the early 1900's to lower the blood sugar. However, French lilac, like phenformin, turned out to be too toxic for use in humans. Metformin, with a much shorter action time than phenformin, has a much lower risk for severe side effects and is quite safe for use by anyone who is otherwise healthy. In fact, in the major UKPDS study, it was the only drug that reduced diabetes-related death rates, heart attacks, and strokes.[111] It should not be used by those who use more than two ounces or two drinks of alcohol a day, who have congestive heart failure, or who have significant kidney, liver, or lung disease.

Metformin lowers fasting blood glucose levels by an average of 25% (17 to 37%), postprandial blood glucose up to 44.5%, and the A1c by an average of 1.5%

(0.8 to 3.1%). Metformin reduces raised plasma insulin levels in cases of metabolic syndrome by as much as 30% and reduces the need for injected insulin in Type 2s by 15 to 32%.[112]

Metformin is available under the trade name Glucophage, or as an extended-release tablet called Glucophage XR. It works well when combined with sulfony-lureas. A combination of glyburide and metformin is available as Glucovance. Combined therapy leads to a greater reduction in blood sugar than can be attained by either class alone. Generic metformin is available at a reduced cost.

Metformin possesses some distinct advantages in treating diabetes. Excess glucose produced by the liver is the major source of high blood sugars in Type 2 diabetes and is typically the reason for high blood sugars on waking in the morning. Metformin reduces this overproduction of glucose. It helps in lowering the blood sugar, especially after eating, with no risk of hypoglycemia when used alone. Modest improvement in cholesterol levels are also seen.[113] The 10 year UKPDS Study of over 3,000 people with Type 2 diabetes found that those who were placed on metformin had a 36% decrease in overall mortality and a 39% decrease in heart attacks.[111]

Because metformin shuts off the liver's excess production of glucose, it reduces the amount of injected insulin needed to control the blood sugar in both Type 1 and Type 2 diabetes.[114, 115] People with Type 2 diabetes who are on insulin usually are advised to lower their insulin doses prior to starting metformin. The full improvement in glycemic control and cholesterol levels may not be seen until 4 to 6 weeks of use have passed.

Side effects from metformin include a change in taste, loss of appetite, nausea or vomiting, abdominal bloating or gas, diarrhea, or skin rash. These may occur during the first few weeks of taking the medication but are seldom long-lasting. Taking the medication with food and starting out with a low dose help reduce side effects. The dosage can be gradually increased as side effects diminish.

Lactic acidosis, the serious but rare side effect originally seen with phenformin, results when a buildup of lactic acid occurs due to an inability to clear metformin from the system. Lactic acidosis occurs very rarely, only once in every 30,000 person-years of use. It almost always occurs in older people who have another major health problem, especially one that may impair breathing or circulation. Warning signs of lactic acidosis include fast and shallow breathing, diarrhea, severe muscle aches, cramping, unusual weakness or tiredness, or feeling cold. Because lactic acidosis has a mortality rate of about 40%, anyone who has significant lung disease, congestive heart failure, or kidney disease should never take this drug.

Because drinking alcohol while taking metformin may also trigger lactic acidosis when other health risks are present, be sure to ask your doctor about alcohol consumption if you are taking this drug. Be aware that Tagamet, a gastrointestinal medication, may enhance the effects of metformin. Therefore, the dose of metformin may need to be lower if you already take Tagamet.

Although not yet FDA approved, metformin is now in clinical trials for treatment of teens who have developed Type 2 diabetes. Some pediatricians also prescribe it, on occasion, to help control a strong Dawn Phenomenon seen in a growing teen with Type 1 diabetes. This use is also not approved. It also helps lower insulin resistance in women with polycystic ovary disease. One side-effect for these women, sometimes a desired outcome, is a greater likelihood of pregnancy.

Glitazones

Thiazolidinediones or glitazones are the first class of medication designed to reverse the basic problem in Type 2 diabetes of resistance to insulin. Insulin resistance appears to be associated with high blood pressure and the high triglycerides/low HDL cholesterol problem that puts many people with Type 2 diabetes at risk for heart disease.

The drugs currently available in this group, Avandia and Actos, reverse insulin resistance by improving the sensitivity of insulin receptors in muscle, liver, and fat cells. This helps the body use insulin better. They improve sensitivity partly by reducing levels of inflammatory cytokines like tumor necrosis factor alpha, while increasing activity of the PPAR gamma receptor. They also help keep the liver from overproducing glucose. They have been shown to lower blood sugar levels about 15% while at the same time lowering insulin levels by 20%. In Type 2, insulin levels are raised as the body produces more insulin than normal to try to overcome insulin resistance. Lower insulin levels indicate that these drugs are decreasing insulin resistance.

In addition to improving insulin sensitivity, glitazones may decrease cardiac risks. They raise the LDL level slightly, but increase the size of the LDL molecule. This may make LDL less harmful, because small, dense LDL is the type most likely to clog blood vessels. Glitazones also lower alpha tumor necrosis factor, an inflammatory particle that is associated with an increased risk of heart disease. Blood pressure and triglyceride levels are somewhat reduced, while HDL levels are slightly raised. Newer glitazones, which work on other PPAR receptors and are currently in clinical trials, also seem to lower high triglycerides and raise the low levels of protective HDL cholesterol commonly seen with insulin resistance.

27.5 Glitazones

Target organ: muscle, fat, and liver
Action: improve receptivity of insulin receptors, reduce glucose production by liver
Lowers HbA1c by 0.5%–1.5%
Time to reach maximum effect: 6–8 weeks
Taken: with or without food

Drug	Dose Range	Doses/Day
Actos (pioglitazone)	15-45 mg	1
Avandia (rosiglitazone)	2-8 mg	1-2

Side Effects: swelling of the legs, fluid retention, weight gain (upper respiratory tract infections, headaches, muscle aches, tooth aches, sore throat in less than 1%)

Contraindications: kidney or liver disease, enlarged heart, congestive heart failure, edema, pregnancy

Glitazones decrease insulin resistance and improve cholesterol, lipid and glucose levels around the clock. Their greatest effect on the blood glucose occurs after eating. They do not cause hypoglycemia when used alone, but can cause lows if used with a sulfonylurea or insulin.

Less insulin is required to control blood sugars when glitazones are used. This means that doses of other drugs that increase insulin production, like sulfonylureas and Prandin, or insulin itself may need to be reduced when a glitazone is started.

Avandia and Actos may produce side effects, such as water retention and swelling of the ankles, especially in older people. Other possible side effects include weight gain, muscle weakness, and fatigue. Because they lower insulin resistance, they also increase fertility in younger women who have polycystic ovary disease, called PCOS. If pregnancy is not desired, a premenopausal woman using one of these drugs should be careful to use birth control. Although they have been shown to rarely cause liver damage, the FDA requires that liver tests be done before treatment start, every two months for the first year and periodically thereafter. If the liver enzyme ALT shows a value more than three times the upper limit of normal, the drug must be stopped.

The glitazones work well in Type 2 diabetes only when insulin resistance is present. People with Type 1.5 diabetes, caused by a lower production of insulin rather than resistance to insulin, are unlikely to benefit from a glitazone. The presence of excess abdominal weight, a low HDL level, high triglycerides, or high blood pressure, all associated with insulin resistance, are good indicators that glitazones may be worth trying.

Starch Blockers

Alpha-glucosidase inhibitors or starch blockers help control blood sugars by slowing down the digestion of complex carbohydrates. This greatly reduces the spikes that may be seen in blood sugar after meals and, surprisingly, also tends to lower the fasting blood sugar. The two medications in this group, Precose and Glyset, are taken with every meal.

Like metformin, Precose had been used in Europe for several years before it was approved in the U.S. Its action is quite different from other diabetes medications in that it works by inhibiting enzymes in the intestine that break down carbohydrates. This slows the digestion of carbohydrates in the small intestine, which, in turn, slows the rise in the blood sugar after a meal. This slower rise in glucose level matches a person's reduced internal production of insulin to improve blood sugar control.

The way in which starch blockers work is also the source of their side effects. Although they are very safe because they usually enter the bloodstream in negligible amounts, their side effects within the intestine can be annoying. If digestion is greatly inhibited, abdominal bloating, gas, and diarrhea can result.

A very good way to minimize or prevent intestinal side effects is to start these medications at minimal doses and then gradually increase them as tolerance improves in a week or so. Half of the smallest tablet can be started before one meal a day, then gradually the dose can be increased and extended to all meals this way. Side effects tend to decrease over time, allowing doses to be increased. Anyone who has problems with digestion or absorption will need to take extra care with these medications.

If Precose and Glyset are taken with insulin or another diabetes medication that can cause low blood sugars, the lows are best treated with glucose tablets or a glucose gel. Digestion of sugar, fruit, and fruit juice is delayed by starch blockers, so they will not raise a low blood sugar as quickly.

27.6 Starch Blockers

Target organ: Intestine
Action: Slow breakdown of carbs in intestine
Lowers HbA1c by 0.7%–1.0%
Time to reach maximum effect: 1 hr
Taken: before meals with first bite of food

Drug	Acts Over	Dose Range	Doses/Day
Precose (acarbose)	4 hrs	25-300 mg	3
Glyset (miglitol)	4 hrs	25-300 mg	3

Side Effects: bloating, diarrhea, nausea, excess gas, abdominal pain

Contraindications: liver disease, bowel or intestinal disease, intestinal obstruction

Like metformin, these drugs do not cause low blood sugars when used alone, nor do they cause weight gain or raise insulin levels. Because they work in a unique way, they can be added to other oral agents to improve blood sugar results. They can reduce after meal spiking in Type 1, Type 1.5, or Type 2 diabetes.

Treating Prediabetes With Medications

Insulin resistance is relatively easy to identify long before Type 2 diabetes actually begins. A history of diabetes in the family, previous gestational diabetes, PCOS, high triglycerides, low HDL, an apple figure, or the presence of high blood pressure all signify that a person is at risk for Type 2. These are often characteristics of prediabetes, also called impaired glucose tolerance or impaired fasting glucose. Fortunately, there are good options for delaying the onset of diabetes.

Acarbose, metformin, and a glitazone have each been shown to delay diabetes when prediabetes exists. On average, these medications reduce the risk of developing Type 2 by about 30%. The best preventive medicine, however, turns out to be an improved diet and exercise, which have been shown to reduce the risk of diabetes in people with prediabetes by 57%! Because diet and exercise improvements are difficult to maintain, clinicians today are likely to consider combining diet, exercise, and medications to delay the start of Type 2 diabetes. The benefits of retaining normal glucose levels is important in the bigger battle of preventing cardiovascular disease.

Why Medications Fail Over Time

The oral agents used to treat Type 2 diabetes can delay and occasionally overcome the need for injected insulin. However, they have not been found to stop the progressive loss of insulin production. Table 27.1 shows the natural progression of Type 2 diabetes. Insulin resistance, glucose toxicity from high readings, and one or more gene defects cause less and less insulin to be produced over time. Since insulin is a critical hormone for good health, it must be injected when too little is produced internally. Needing to inject insulin does not mean that you have failed to control your diabetes well. Rather, it means it is time to start an excellent therapy that improves quality of life and health. Make this positive choice and learn all you can about how to use insulin to ensure that good blood sugar control can continue in the future.

One or more defects in insulin production is almost always present by the time Type 2 diabetes is finally diagnosed. This defect worsens over time and the use of insulin becomes necessary for most people with this type of defect. Although insulin is currently used in about 36% of people with Type 2 diabetes, well over half of those with Type 2 eventually go on to need it. If insulin were added as soon as the loss of beta cell activity made this necessary, the percentage currently using insulin would likely be closer to 50%.

New Treatment Options For Type 2 Diabetes

Recently, treatment goals in diabetes have been set more stringently for tighter control by WHO, AACE, and other groups to help people avoid complications. Suggested treatment goals in Type 2 diabetes include:

- a fasting plasma glucose of 110 mg/dl (6.1 mmol) or less
- blood sugars 2 hours after eating of 140 mg/dl (7.7 mmol) or less
- an A1c of 6.5% or less

Whenever current therapy is not controlling the blood sugar, medication and insulin doses are increased or supplemented with different types of medications and insulin. Many people are unable to reach these target goals through lifestyle changes alone because they have had diabetes for several years before being diagnosed. The length of this disease means that medication or insulin are required to support the failing beta cells. Blood sugars may be so high at the time of diagnosis that insulin is required immediately to overcome glucose toxicity and bring high blood sugars down to target.

Sometimes an injection of insulin is needed at the first clinic visit to overcome glucose toxicity which has created additional resistance to insulin. In the first few days of diabetes, short term use of an insulin pump or multiple daily injections of insulin to aggressively normalize glucose levels may also be attempted.[32-34] Lifestyle changes may then enable many to maintain normal blood glucose levels for several months without the need for insulin. However, because of the progressive nature of Type 2 diabetes, most people eventually benefit from using both medications and insulin.

A treatment approach used in the past was to start one medication and increase it to a maximum dosage. When this maximum dose no longer controlled the blood sugar, one or more other medications were added or a long-acting insulin was started before dinner or at bedtime.

Today's approach to therapy is different. Doctors now are aware that there are two distinct defects in metabolism in Type 2 diabetes and they have a variety of medication options to treat these defects. People with Type 2 usually have impaired beta cell activity that causes less insulin to be produced and insulin resistance that causes insulin to be poorly utilized. Multiple treatments can be selected so that each defect is treated at the same time.

The new approach is to use small to moderate doses of one, two, three, or four medications that work on different aspects of these defects. Combinations of different medications can succeed where taking large doses of a single agent may fail. In addition, one or two injections of insulin may be added to the medications at a fairly early treatment stage. Continuation of the medications after insulin is started means less insulin will be needed. Combined treatments work to allow both lost insulin production and insulin resistance to be treated.

In Type 2 diabetes, insulin is typically started when two or more diabetes medications can no longer keep the blood sugar under control. The preferred way to start insulin is to add it to the diabetes medications currently in use, while gradually adjusting insulin doses and the number of injections until control is reached. Once control is achieved with insulin, the role of each medication may be reconsidered. In some cases, an oral medication can be reduced or stopped. If control worsens, the medication is helping and can be restarted. Keep in mind that when a particular medication, such as a glitazone, is stopped, it can take six weeks for its full effect to wear off.

Advantages to using insulin and medications together:

1. Lower insulin doses are required to achieve control
2. Weight gain is less likely using some combinations
3. Hypoglycemia is less common because less insulin is used
4. Medication side effects are less likely because smaller doses are used

Each class of diabetes medication works in a different way on a different organ. To take advantage of these different mechanisms, combinations of medications, such as a sulfonylurea plus metformin, a sulfonylurea plus starch blocker, a glitazone with metformin, or a rapid insulin releaser plus glitazone plus metformin are becoming common today.

Drug companies are also creating combo pills that combine two different medications. Although this may increase the cost per tablet, taking fewer pills is attractive to many people and may lower insurance costs when two medications can be obtained for a single copay.

Another advantage of newer medications is they allow health care providers to address specific control problems. For example, if someone with Type 2 has high morning blood sugars but normal postmeal readings, metformin alone might be the perfect solution. If morning blood sugars are normal but postmeal readings are high, taking Prandin or Precose before meals may help. Even with these new medications that target specific problems, insulin remains the most potent and most cost-effective tool for lowering blood sugars.

A good way to measure treatment effectiveness is the A1c test. Although it is difficult to reach for most people, the ideal goal is to keep the A1c less than 6.5% or at most 7% when the lab's upper limit for normal is 6%. Research studies consistently find the average A1c among people with Type 2 diabetes is over 8%, well above the levels considered safe for health. The average A1c for Type 1's is even higher in the 9% range. These elevated blood sugars indicate that control tools like insulin, medications, and testing are underutilized. Because of the excessive cardiovascular risk associated with higher blood sugar levels, the World Health Organization, the International Diabetes Federation, and the American Association of Clinical Endocrinologists recommend that the A1c level be kept at 6.5% or lower.

Keeping the blood sugar normal most of the time is the goal of treating Type 2 diabetes just as it is for Type 1 diabetes. Due to Type 2's slow onset, people with it often feel well even though their blood sugar has been elevated at 150 or 250 mg/dl (8.3 or 13.9 mmol) for several years. Organ damage will progress with these high blood sugars, even though symptoms are absent. Steps to improve health have to be triggered by test results rather than by how one feels. The goal is to bring as many pre and postmeal readings into the normal range as possible. Correct choices for medications and insulin doses make this possible.

Oral Medications That May Help Type 1 Diabetes

Oral medications are used primarily in Type 2 diabetes, but some can help improve control in Type 1 diabetes. For instance, although not FDA approved for use in Type 1 diabetes,[111] some pediatricians find that metformin improves blood sugar control in growing teens with either Type 1 or Type 2 diabetes. Girls between the ages of 11 and 16 and boys between 13 and 18 produce large amounts of growth hormone, which triggers excess glucose production by the liver. Large insulin doses are required to overcome the excess glucose production.

Metformin significantly reduces the liver's glucose production caused by growth hormone but does not appear to interfere with normal growth. The overall effect is better blood sugar control with a rapid reduction in insulin doses over the first month of metformin use. However, teens prone to ketoacidosis are not good candidates for this treatment because ketoacidosis increases the risk of lactic acidosis, a rare side effect of metformin that can be deadly.

Although not FDA approved, Precose or Glyset can be considered in Type 1 diabetes when blood sugars after meals are often high or frequent hypoglycemia is a problem. These medications slow the digestion of carbohydrates and can smooth out blood sugars. Carb boluses may need to be reduced slightly, but once insulin doses are reduced, hypoglycemia is less likely because of the longer time over which carbs are digested. Combining Precose or Glyset with rapid insulins like Humalog or Novolog can work well once carb boluses are lowered. The overnight basal dose also may need to be lowered slightly.

One control issue with Precose and Glyset can be the fasting blood sugar. Fasting blood sugars may be improved when one of these medications is started. However, after a large carb intake in the evening meal, digestion of these carbs may occur after bedtime and cause the next morning's reading to be higher than expected.

Like everyone else, people with Type 1 diabetes may possess genes which promote Type 2 diabetes. As they age, they may develop an apple shape or gain weight, and acquire insulin resistance typical of Type 2 diabetes. This gradual change can be detected by a cholesterol profile which has a low HDL level and high triglycerides, or by the onset of high blood pressure. Oral medications that reduce insulin resistance, such as metformin or one of the glipizides, may help reduce insulin doses.

Weight Gain With Insulin

One drawback to using insulin successfully to control blood sugar is that it can lead to weight gain. When the need for insulin is finally recognized in a person with Type 2, an individual may have gone for months or years with high blood sugar levels. During this time, many calories may have been lost into the urine due to high blood sugars. Often the person adapted to this by eating an extra 500 or 1,000 calories a day without gaining weight.

When blood sugars rise above 180 mg/dl (10 mmol) routinely, weight gain often stops, even if calorie intake is excessive. If the blood sugar is high enough, weight loss may even occur. However, when treatment with insulin is started to bring down the blood sugar level, there is an immediate shift from losing calories in the urine to moving these calories into the cells. Unless the person reduces the calories in the diet as his blood sugars reach normal, a rapid increase in weight will occur.

A good principle for anyone who is overweight is to reduce calories as soon as insulin is started. Be sure to orchestrate your efforts with your physician as you start your new regimen so that your insulin dose will not be based on your past eating habits. A large insulin dose for a reduced calorie meal can cause sudden lows that need not occur.

Basal and bolus doses always have to be closely matched to need to make low blood sugars less likely. If you decide to lose some weight by cutting back on calories and begin to experience low blood sugars, your insulin doses need to be immediately reduced to match the calorie reduction. Otherwise, when hypoglycemia occurs, you will have to eat. If a low does occur, only about 20 grams (80 calories) of quick carb are needed to correct it. If a person avoids overeating in the face of a low blood sugar, it also helps prevent weight gain.

Actually, low blood sugars are unlikely, even if insulin is somewhat excessive, in a person with Type 2 diabetes who has insulin resistance. Fear of having a low may drive some into "protective eating" that is really unnecessary and is sure to drive weight higher. One way to help prevent weight gain with insulin in Type 2 diabetes is to add metformin which reduces the likelihood of weight gain.

Diabetes medications have different effects on weight. Glitazones tend to shift harmful intra-abdominal fat into less harmful fat under the skin. In some people, they also cause fluid retention which adds to weight and may place an additional load on the heart. Glucophage (metformin) generally creates a loss of 2 to 6 lbs in weight. A combination of Glucophage and insulin is usually weight neutral, as is the use of fast insulin releasers. An upcoming therapy, pramlitide (see page ___), may offer additional benefits of weight reduction and improved control after meals.

Special Concerns Related To Medications: Kidney Disease

Although sulfonylureas actually are processed by the liver, much of the active parts of the drugs are eliminated by the kidneys. For this reason, the first generation sulfonylureas are generally avoided if advanced kidney damage is present and creatinine levels are above normal. Furthermore, the insulin level in the blood is increased by these medications, and the action of the insulin is prolonged because it has to wait to be cleared by the kidneys, which are occupied with eliminating remnants of the sulfonylureas.

Second generation sulfonylureas, glimepiride or glyburide, are processed more quickly. Third generation glimepiride (Amaryl) tends to clear faster and is probably the safest sulfonylurea to use if advanced kidney disease is present.

Metformin should never be used when kidney disease is indicated by an elevated creatinine level since it has to be eliminated primarily through the kidneys. Kidney disease is the actual cause of over 80% of the deaths induced by lactic acidosis from metformin.

Special Concerns Relating To Medications: Liver Disease

The use of sulfonylureas is not advised when liver disease exists since these medicines may result in prolonged drug activity and hypoglycemia. Glimepiride (Amaryl) may be an exception to this, as its metabolism does not appear to be affected by liver disease.

The glitazones, Avandia and Actos, may be used but only if the doctor monitors liver enzymes every 3 months for the first year and as needed thereafter for unwanted changes. Because Rezulin, a discontinued drug in this class, caused liver toxicity, these two drugs are required by the FDA to carry warnings that they may cause liver damage. Although this appears to be rare, a glitazone should not be used in the presence of significant liver disease. Metformin also should not be used when significant liver disease exists.

27.7 Common Medication Combinations

Different classes of diabetes medications affect the body differently. Drugs from different classes can control the blood sugar through increasing insulin secretion, sensitizing the body to use insulin better, turning off the liver's production of glucose, and delaying the digestion of carbohydrates. In Type 2 diabetes, it is common to take two or more drugs at the same time. Let's look at how different medications can be combined to enhance their blood sugar lowering capacity.

Metformin And Glitazone

Metformin with Actos or Avandia is more effective at reducing high readings throughout the day than either class alone. Glitazones improve insulin sensitivity, while metformin shuts off the liver's production of glucose, so they lower the blood sugar by different means. The pill Avandamet combines Avandia and metformin for easier use. Fluid retention may occur with use of glitazone.

Sulfonylurea And Metformin

The most common combination is a sulfonylurea for its ability to boost insulin production and metformin for its ability to shut off the liver's glucose production. This combination is so effective it seems to work better together than each drug does individually. These combinations can reduce a fasting blood sugar dramatically and help in weight maintenance. The sulfonylurea can cause low blood sugars, so careful dosing is needed. One pill, called Glucovance, is a combination of glyburide and Glucophage. Another combination pill is Metaglip, made from metformin and glipizide.

Sulfonylurea And Glitazone

Actos or Avandia are often added to a sulfonylurea when the blood sugar isn't being controlled by a maximum dose of sulfonylurea, the person is overweight and insulin resistant. Adding glitazone will not help if insulin resistance is not present. This combination can cause low blood sugars.

Metformin And Alpha-Glucosidase Inhibitor

Use this combination to reduce blood sugars before breakfast and after meals. Studies have shown that Precose and metformin are more effective when taken together in reducing blood sugars after meals than metformin alone. Side effects that may occur are bloating, gas and diarrhea.

Metformin And Rapid Insulin Releaser

Metformin with Prandin or Starlix is also effective at lowering fasting and after meal blood sugars.

Sulfonylurea And Alpha-Glucosidase Inhibitor

For people who have high blood sugars primarily after meals, a combination of Precose or Glyset plus a sulfonylurea is a good combination. Possible side effects include abdominal cramping, gas, diarrhea and low blood sugars.

Rapid-Insulin Releaser and Alpha-glucosidase Inhibitor

This combination taken before a meal is especially helpful for highs after the meals. Prandin or Starlix will stimulate the pancreas to produce insulin to cover the meal, while Precose Glyset slows down digestion of carbs. This combination can cause lows after meals but is less likely to do this than sulfonylureas.

27.8 Common Medication And Insulin Combinations For Type 2

Sulfonylurea And Insulin

If a sulfonylurea by itself is not working around the clock, insulin is often added at night to provide effective control. This combination is called BIDS (bedtime insulin daytime sulfonylurea). You may be prescribed this combination if sulfonylurea and metformin were tried but were not effective to control your blood sugar. One benefit of using a sulfonylurea with insulin is that less insulin is needed, so less weight gain is likely to occur.

Metformin And Insulin

Metformin may be combined with insulin enables a lower dose of insulin to be used to avoid weight gain. Since metformin makes your liver more sensitive to insulin, you need less insulin. Metformin helps you maintain or lose weight. How it does this is not clear, but it may partly suppress the appetite.

Precose And Insulin

These work well together because Precose delays the absorption of carbohydrate and decreases the insulin need so that doses can be reduced. One drawback is an increased risk of low blood sugars after using a rapid insulin.

Actos Or Avandia And Insulin

A glitazone paired with insulin sensitizes the cells to insulin and will usually reduce the amount of insulin that is needed. This can result in better control than when insulin is used alone. The combination can cause low blood sugars. It is wise to start both at low to medium dosages to reduce the risk of side effects. Weight gain can occur, but it is usually from water retention rather than fat.

"The covers of this book are too far apart."
Ambrose Bierce

Wrap Up

Now that you've worked through *Using Insulin*, you have the information and skills to begin to control your blood sugar. You have set yourself the goal of maintaining your blood sugar in your target range 75% of the time and achieving an A1c of 7% or less. Plus, you know good control makes you feel better and reduces the risk of complications in the long run. You've got the knowledge and motivation needed to take control of your diabetes, but what else do you need?

Information is important, but never enough by itself. It has to be supplemented with hands on experience, perseverance, doing the same or similar thing over and over again with better results over time. Setting basal and bolus doses, counting carbs, matching carbs with carb boluses, correcting highs, and recording this information in a useful way are all part of the mix. When a blood sugar control problem appears, the problem pattern needs to be identified so that needed adjustments in insulin, carbs or exercise can be made to improve your blood sugar results.

One thing we can guarantee you will need is patience. Life has a way of changing, and your blood sugar will change with it. Once you finally attain reasonable control, it may last months, years, or only a short time before it's highs and lows all over again. But once you succeed through science or luck, you will have the confidence to try again. You may have no idea why your good control is gone. Just go back, problem solve, trouble shoot, and make changes and keep trying solutions until you again see improvements.

If you draw a blank, get assistance from a trained health professional who can spot details or patterns in your charts that you have missed. Professional experience helps you reach solutions faster. Develop a good relationship with a knowledgeable and supportive health care team to speed your success.

Another aid available in many communities is a support group. Here you'll meet other people with diabetes, their families and friends, local health care providers, researchers, and sales reps from companies that provide diabetes products. This supportive community allows everyone to catch up on the latest breakthroughs in drugs, devices and treatment. People with diabetes give each other advice and help each other accept diabetes and deal with it more effectively. They understand the rewards and difficulties of having diabetes better than people who have not experienced it.

If no support group exists near you, start one. You need no agenda, just the desire to know and share your experience with other people with diabetes and their family and friends.

In finishing this book, you've arrived at the beginning of another adventure in really mastering your diabetes. At times when your control isn't what you want it to be, start over. Set and test your TDD, basals and boluses, review carb counting, change your diet, take on new exercise. Living with diabetes is an ongoing process. Celebrate your successes and grow from your successes and mishaps alike. Keep trying the approaches presented here.

Thank you for being such an engaging and hardworking audience to address. We've learned much from creating this book and hope you learn even more by *Using Insulin*.

Appendix A

How To Count Carbs Using A Gram Scale And Carb Percentages

Few foods, other than table sugar and lollipops, are totally carbohydrate. So the Carb Percentages for a variety of foods are provided on the following pages. These Percentages give the amount of carbohydrate in 1 gram of that particular food. To find out how much carbohydrate you are eating in a particular food, you will need to do a simple calculation:

1. Weigh the food on a gram scale to get its total weight.
2. Find that food's Carb Percentage in one of the Food Groups listed below.
3. On a calculator, multiply the food's weight in grams by its Carb Percentage.
4. The answer is the number of grams of carbohydrate you are eating.

Example

Let's say you place a small apple on a gram scale and find that it weighs 100 grams. You then look up its Carb Percentage and find that it is 0.13. You then simply multiply 100 grams by 0.13 to get the grams of carb you will be eating:

100 grams of apple X .13 = 13 grams of carbohydrate

Additional Information

Carb Percentages give the actual concentration of carbohydrate in foods. For instance, apples are 13% carbohydrate (most of their weight is water), while raisins are 77% carbohydrate by weight, and bagels contain 56% carbohydrate by weight. Both apple juice and regular sodas are 12% carbohydrate, although the carbohydrate in apple juice is higher in fructose, while a regular soda has more of its carbohydrate as sucrose or sugar.

Cranberry juice is even richer in carbohydrate at 16%, while grapefruit juice contains only 9% by weight. A 6-oz. glass of cranberry juice will therefore contain almost twice as much carbohydrate as an identical glass of grapefruit juice. Because it contains more carbohydrate, a glass of cranberry juice will raise the blood sugar about twice as high as the same amount of grapefruit juice. It will also require almost twice as much insulin to cover it.

Carb Percentages For Various Foods

Juices

apple cider	.14	frozen	.09	orange-apricot	.13
apple juice	.12	grapefruit-orange: canned	.10	papaya	.12
apricot	.12	frozen	.11	pineapple: canned	.14
apricot nectar	.15	lemon	.08	frozen	.13
cranberry	.16	lemonade, frozen	.11	prune	.19
grape: bottled	.16	orange: fresh	.11	tomato	.04
grape: frozen	.13	canned, unsweet	.10	V-8	.04
grapefruit: fresh	.09	canned, sweet	.12		
canned	.07	frozen	.11		

Dressings, Sauces, Condiments

bacon bits	.19	olives	.04	soy sauce	.10
BBQ sauce	.13	pickles, sweet	.36	spaghettie sauce	.09
catsup	.25	salad dressings: blue cheese	.07	steak sauce	.09
cheese sauce	.06	ceasar	.04	sweet & sour sauce	.45
chili sauce	.24	diet	.22	tartar sauce	.04
hollandaise sauce	.08	French	.17	tomato paste	.19
horseradish	.10	Italian	.07	Worcestershire sauce	.18
mayonnaise	.02	Russian	.07		
mustard	.04	pickle relish, sweet	.34		

Fruit

apple	.13	dried	.62	pears: fresh	.15
apple sauce	.10	fruit cocktail, in water	.10	canned in water	.09
apricots: fresh	.13	grapes: concord	.14	persimmons: Japanese	.20
canned in water	.10	european	.17	native	.34
canned in juice	.14	green, seedless	.14	pineapple: fresh	.14
dried	.60	grapefruit	.10	canned in water	.10
banana	.20	honeydew	.08	canned in juice	.15
blackberries	.12	kiwi	.15	plums: fresh	.13
blueberries	.14	lemons	.09	canned in water	.12
cantalope	.08	limes	.10	prunes: dehydrated	.91
cherries: fresh, sweet red	.16	mangoes	.17	dried, cooked	.67
fresh, sour red	.14	nectarines	.17	raisins	.77
canned in water	.11	oranges	.12	rasberries, fresh	.14
maraschino	.29	papayas	.10	strawberries, fresh	.08
cranberry sauce, sugar	.36	peaches: fresh	.10	tangerines	.12
dates, dried and pitted	.74	canned in water	.08	watermelon	.06
figs: fresh	.18	canned in juice	.12		

Carb Percentages For Various Foods Cont.

Vegetables

artichoke	.10	cooked	.07	potatoes: baked	.21
asparagus	.04	cauliflower: raw	.05	boiled	.15
avacado	.05	cooked	.04	hash browns	.29
bamboo shoots	.05	celery	.04	French Fries	.34
beans: raw green	.07	chard, raw	.05	chips	.50
cooked green	.05	coleslaw	.12	sweet	.24
beans: kidney, lima, pinto,		corn: canned	.06	pumpkin	.08
red, white, baked	.21	steamed, off cob	.19	radishes	.04
beans sprouts	.06	sweet, creamed	.20	sauerkraut	.04
beets, boiled	.07	cucumber	.03	spinach: raw	.04
beet greens, cooked	.03	eggplant, cooked	.04	cooked	.08
broccoli	.06	lettuce	.03	soybeans	.11
brussel sprouts, cooked	.11	mushrooms	.04	squash: summer, cooked	.03
cabbage: raw	.05	okra	.05	winter, baked	.15
cooked	.04	onions	.07	winter, boiled	.09
Chinese, raw	.03	parsnips	.18	tomatoes	.05
Chinse, cooked	.01	peas	.12	turnips	.05
carrots: raw	.10	peppers	.05		

Cold Cereals, Dry / Combination Dishes / Sandwiches

Cold Cereals, Dry		Combination Dishes		Sandwiches	
All Bran™	.78	beef stew	.06	BLT	.19
Cheerios™	.70	burrito	.24	chicken salad	.24
Corn Chex™	.89	chicken pie	.17	club	.13
Corn Flakes™	.84	chili:with beans	.11	egg salad	.22
Frosted Flakes™	.90	no beans	.06	hot dog with bun	.26
Fruit and Fiber™	.78	con carne	.09	peanut butter and jelly	.50
granola	.68	coleslaw	.14	tuna salad	.24
Grapenuts™	.83	enchilada	.18		
NutriGrain™	.86	fish and chips	.18	**Soups**	
Product 19™	.77	fish sticks	.37	clam chowder	.07
Puffed Wheat™	.77	hot dog	.18	cream of mushroom	.04
Raisin Bran™	.75	lasagna	.16	tomato	.09
Shredded Wheat™	.81	macaroni and cheese	.20	vegetable beef	.04
Special K™	.76	pizza	.28	bean w/ pork	.09
Rice Chex™	.86	potato salad	.13	chicken noodle	.07
Rice Krispies™	.88	spaghetti with meat sauce	.15	chicken w/ rice	.07
Total™	.79	tossed salad	.05		
Wheaties™	.80	tuna casserole	.13		

Carb Percentages For Various Foods Cont.

Desserts and Sweets

apple butter	.46	lollipops	.99	ice cream: plain	.21
banana bread	.47	peanut brittle	.73	cone	.30
brownie	.71	gum drops	.99	bar	.25
brownie with nuts	.50	chocolate syrup	.65	ice milk	.23
cakes: angel food	.60	cookies: animal	.80	jams	.70
chocolate	.55	chocolate chip	.73	jellies	.70
coffee	.52	fig bar	.71	pies: apple	.37
fruit	.57	gingersnap	.80	blueberry	.34
pound	.61	oatmeal & raisin	.72	cherry	.38
sponge	.55	vanilla wafers	.74	lemon meringue	.47
white	.63	danish pastries	.46	pecan	.57
candies: caramel	.76	doughnuts: cake	.52	pumpkin	.23
fudge with nuts	.69	jelly filled	.46	preserves	.70
hard	.96	fruit turnovers	.26	pudding, chocolate	.23
jelly beans	.93	honey	.76	sherbert	.32

Breads and Grains

bagel	.56	couscous	.33	brown	.23
barley, cooked	.28	English muffin	.51	white	.25
biscuits	.45	French toast	.26	rolls	.60
bread: italian	.50	lentils	.19	spaghetti: plain	.26
rye	.47	macaroni: plain	.23	with sauce	.15
wheat	.47	cheese	.20	toast	.70
white	.49	muffins	.45	tortillas: corn	.42
bread crumbs	.74	noodles	.25	flour	.58
bread sticks	.75	pancakes & waffles: dry mix	.70	wheat flour	.76
buns	.50	prepared	.44		
corn starch	.83	rice, cooked	.24		

Alcoholic Beverages / Beverages / Hot Cereals, Cooked

Alcoholic Beverages		Beverages		Hot Cereals, Cooked	
beer: regular	.04	carbonated soda	.12	corn grits	.11
light	.02	chocolate milk	.11	Cream of Wheat™	.14
champagne	.01	eggnog	.08	Farina™	.11
liqueurs	.30	flavored instant coffee	.06	oatmeal	.10
wine: dry	.04	milk	.04	Roman Meal™	.14
sweet	.12	punch	.11	Wheatena™	.12

Carb Percentages For Various Foods Cont.

Snack Foods

almonds	.19	saltines	.70	popcorn, popped, no butter	.78
cashews	.26	marshmallows	.78	with butter	.57
cola	.10	mixed nuts	.18	potato chips	.50
corn chips	.57	onion dip	.10	pretzels	.75
cheese	.58	peanut butter	.17	sunflower seeds, no shell	.19
crackers: graham	.73	peanuts	.20	walnuts	.15
round	.67	pecans	.20		
rye	.50	pistachios	.27		

Dairy

cheese: cottage	.03	ice cream: choc	.28
ricotta	.05	vanilla	.22
cheddar	.01	milk	.05
		yogurt	.08

Sample Smart Cart And Enhanced Logbook

B 16.8 300																								4	
L 14.0 250																								3	Acti-
O																								2	vity
O 11.2 200																								1	
D																									
8.4 150																									
S																									
U 5.6 100																									
G 4.0 70																									
A 2.8 50																									
R 1.8 30																									
mmol 0	BGs:																								
Insulin	4	6 am	8	10	noon	2	4	6	8	10	12	2 am	4												
Carb Bolus H/Nov/R																								TDD	
Basal Lan/L/N/U																									
Correction Bolus																									

Breakfast			**Lunch**			**Dinner**		
Time	Food	Carb Grams	Time	Food	Carb Grams	Time	Food	Carb Grams
Morning Snacks			Afternoon Snacks			Evening Snacks		

Day: _____ Wt: _____ Comments: _____

Date: __/__/__ _____

Smart Charts can be ordered in quantities at (800) 988-4772 or on back page.

Enhanced Logbook		Breakfast		Lunch		Dinner		Night	
		Before	After	Before	After	Before	After	Bedtime	2 a.m.
Sunday ___/___/___ walk/run/bike at _____ am/pm	BG								
	Time								
	Carbs								
	Insulin								
Monday ___/___/___ walk/run/bike at _____ am/pm	BG								
	Time								
	Carbs								
	Insulin								
Tuesday ___/___/___ walk/run/bike at _____ am/pm	BG								
	Time								
	Carbs								
	Insulin								
Wednesday ___/___/___ walk/run/bike at _____ am/pm	BG								
	Time								
	Carbs								
	Insulin								
Thursday ___/___/___ walk/run/bike at _____ am/pm	BG								
	Time								
	Carbs								
	Insulin								
Friday ___/___/___ walk/run/bike at _____ am/pm	BG								
	Time								
	Carbs								
	Insulin								
Saturday ___/___/___ walk/run/bike at _____ am/pm	BG								
	Time								
	Carbs								
	Insulin								
# below target									
# above target									

PATTERNS

My target ranges: Before meals _____ to _____   At bedtime _____ to _____

After meals _____ to _____   At 2 a.m _____ to _____

Your Basal Percentage Affects Your Carb Factor And Correction Factor

The tables on the next three pages are extensions of Table 10.2, the Table of TDDs, Basal and Bolus Doses, that appears on page 118. Table 10.2 works well when someone's basal insulin makes up about 50% of their TDD. However, when the percentage of basal insulin is significantly lower or higher than 50%, the amount of bolus insulin needed to cover carbs and to lower high blood sugars is changed.

The tables that follow provide more accurate estimates for the insulin to carb ratio (Carb Factor) and the Correction Factor when the day's basal insulin makes up 40%, 60%, and 70% of the total daily dose of insulin. For a 40% basal, we use a 450 Rule to estimate the Carb Factor and a 1600 Rule to estimate the Correction Factor. For 60%, we use a 550 Rule and a 2000 Rule, respectively. For 70%, we use a 600 Rule and a 2200 Rule to make the estimates. Overall, these tables allow for more accurate estimates of basal and bolus doses when basal doses differ from 50% of the TDD.

TDDs, Basal And Bolus Doses for 40% Basal

For this TDD =	Day's Basal (40% of TDD)	Carb Bolus 1u covers this many carbs:	Corr. Bolus 1u lowers blood sugar:
16 units	6.4 units	28 grams	100 mg/dl
18 units	7.2 units	25 grams	89 mg/dl
20 units	8.0 units	23 grams	80 mg/dl
22 units	8.8 units	20 grams	73 mg/dl
24 units	9.6 units	19 grams	67 mg/dl
26 units	10.4 units	17 grams	62 mg/dl
28 units	11.2 units	16 grams	57 mg/dl
30 units	12.0 units	15 grams	53 mg/dl
32 units	12.8 units	14 grams	50 mg/dl
36 units	14.4 units	13 grams	44 mg/dl
40 units	16.0 units	11 grams	40 mg/dl
44 units	17.6 units	10 grams	36 mg/dl
48 units	19.2 units	9 grams	33 mg/dl
52 units	20.8 units	9 grams	31 mg/dl
56 units	22.4 units	8 grams	29 mg/dl
60 units	24.0 units	8 grams	27 mg/dl
65 units	26.0 units	7 grams	25 mg/dl
70 units	28.0 units	6 grams	23 mg/dl
75 units	30.0 units	6 grams	21 mg/dl
80 units	32.0 units	6 grams	20 mg/dl
90 units	36.0 units	5 grams	18 mg/dl
100 units	40.0 units	5 grams	16 mg/dl

Approximate basal and bolus doses for someone who receives 40% of their TDD in their basal doses.

© 2003 Diabetes Services, Inc.

TDDs, Basal And Bolus Doses for 60% Basal

For this TDD =	Day's Basal (60% of TDD)	Carb Bolus 1u covers this many carbs:	Corr. Bolus 1u lowers blood sugar:
16 units	9.6 units	34 grams	125 mg/dl
18 units	10.8 units	31 grams	111 mg/dl
20 units	12.0 units	28 grams	100 mg/dl
22 units	13.2 units	23 grams	91 mg/dl
24 units	14.4 units	23 grams	83 mg/dl
26 units	15.6 units	21 grams	77 mg/dl
28 units	16.8 units	20 grams	71 mg/dl
30 units	18.0 units	18 grams	67 mg/dl
32 units	19.2 units	17 grams	63 mg/dl
36 units	21.6 units	15 grams	56 mg/dl
40 units	24.0 units	14 grams	50 mg/dl
44 units	26.4 units	13 grams	45 mg/dl
48 units	28.8 units	11 grams	42 mg/dl
52 units	31.2 units	11 grams	38 mg/dl
56 units	33.6 units	10 grams	36 mg/dl
60 units	36.0 units	9 grams	33 mg/dl
65 units	39.0 units	8 grams	31 mg/dl
70 units	42.0 units	8 grams	29 mg/dl
75 units	45.0 units	7 grams	27 mg/dl
80 units	48.0 units	7 grams	25 mg/dl
90 units	54.0 units	6 grams	22 mg/dl
100 units	60.0 units	6 grams	20 mg/dl

Column labels down the sides: TDD PER DAY · BASAL · CARB FACTOR · CORRECTION FACTOR

Approximate basal and bolus doses for someone who receives 60% of their TDD in their basal doses.

© 2003 Diabetes Services, Inc.

TDDs, Basal And Bolus Doses for 70% Basal

For this TDD =	Day's Basal (70% of TDD)	Carb Bolus 1u covers this many carbs:	Corr. Bolus 1u lowers blood sugar:
16 units	11.2 units	38 grams	138 mg/dl
18 units	12.6 units	33 grams	122 mg/dl
20 units	14.0 units	30 grams	110 mg/dl
22 units	15.4 units	27 grams	100 mg/dl
24 units	16.8 units	25 grams	92 mg/dl
26 units	18.2 units	23 grams	85 mg/dl
28 units	19.6 units	21 grams	79 mg/dl
30 units	21.0 units	20 grams	73 mg/dl
32 units	22.4 units	19 grams	69 mg/dl
36 units	25.2 units	17 grams	61 mg/dl
40 units	28.0 units	15 grams	55 mg/dl
44 units	30.8 units	14 grams	50 mg/dl
48 units	33.6 units	13 grams	46 mg/dl
52 units	36.4 units	12 grams	42 mg/dl
56 units	39.2 units	11 grams	39 mg/dl
60 units	42.0 units	10 grams	37 mg/dl
65 units	45.5 units	9 grams	34 mg/dl
70 units	49.0 units	9 grams	31 mg/dl
75 units	52.5 units	8 grams	29 mg/dl
80 units	56.0 units	8 grams	28 mg/dl
90 units	63.0 units	7 grams	24 mg/dl
100 units	70.0 units	6 grams	22 mg/dl

Leftmost vertical label: TDD — TDD

Vertical label (basal column): BASAL PER DAY

Vertical label (carb column): CARB FACTOR

Vertical label (correction column): CORRECTION FACTOR

Approximate basal and bolus doses for someone who receives 70% of their TDD in their basal doses.

© 2003 Diabetes Services, Inc.

Glossary

A1c

Glycosylated hemoglobin levels reflect blood glucose level during the previous two to three months. A1c is a form of glycosylated hemoglobin commonly used to assess blood glucose control in people with diabetes. Normal A1c levels are generally 4% to 6%. Diabetes treatment typically aims for a target A1c of less than 6.5% or 7%.

Albuminuria

A condition in which high levels of a protein called albumin are found in the urine. Excess albumin in the urine is often a sign of early kidney disease.

Adult diabetes

Now called Type 2 or NIDDM (non-insulin dependent diabetes).

Basal/Bolus Approach To Therapy

Therapy that is based on blood sugar targets, A1c goals, and monitoring at least four times a day. Carbohydrate content of foods, exercise, stress, and other factors are evaluated to determine insulin need. In early Type 1.5 or Type 2, no insulin or one to two injections may be needed. In Type 1 diabetes and in later stages of Type 1.5 and Type 2, insulin is delivered by three or more injections a day or use of an insulin pump with basal and bolus doses calculated from the TDD.

Basal Insulin Dose

Background insulin from a long-acting insulin to match background insulin need. When one or more basal insulin doses are correctly set to deliver about 50% of the TDD, the blood sugar does not rise or fall during periods in which no eating occurs.

Bolus

See Carb Bolus or Correction Bolus.

Beta cells (b-cells)

Cells that make insulin and are found in the Islets of Langerhans within the pancreas.

Blood glucose level

The concentration of glucose in the blood (blood sugar). It is measured in milligrams per deciliter (mg/dl) in the U.S. or in millimoles (mmol) in other countries.

Body mass index (BMI)

A unit of measurement (kg/m^2) that describes weight in relation to height for people 20 to 65 years old.

Brittle diabetes

This is usually seen in Type 1 diabetes where the blood glucose level fluctuates widely from high to low as a result of insulin doses that do not match the lifestyle.

C-peptide

Plasma C-peptide is a by-product of insulin production with a longer half-life than insulin. It measures how much insulin a person is able to make. A level below 0.3 is defined as Type 1 diabetes.

Carbohydrate

One of three main constituents (carbohydrates, fats, and proteins) of foods and the most important for blood sugar control. Carbohydrates are composed mainly of sugars and starches.

Carb Bolus

An injection of a rapid insulin to match carbohydrates in a meal or snack.

Carb counting

Counting the grams of carbohydrate in any food eaten. Matching these grams with appropriate insulin doses is an effective way to maintain a normal blood sugar.

Correction Bolus

An injection of a rapid insulin to bring a high blood sugar back within a person's target for before a meal, after a meal, or at bedtime.

DCCT

The Diabetes Control and Complications Trial (DCCT) was a 9-year study of 1,441 people with Type 1 diabetes. Sponsored by the National Institute of Health, it showed that tight blood sugar control significantly reduces the risk of diabetic retinopathy, neuropathy, and nephropathy.

Dawn Phenomenon

An early morning rise in blood glucose levels, caused largely by the normal release of growth hormone that blocks insulin's effect during the early morning hours.

Diabetic coma

Loss of consciousness due to very high blood sugars. (See ketoacidosis)

Diabetic nephropathy

Kidney disease resulting from diabetes that usually has been poorly controlled for several years. There rarely are symptoms until very late in the disease.

Diabetic neuropathy

Damage to the nervous system most often resulting from high blood sugars. Three different forms of neuropathy can be distinguished: peripheral neuropathy, sensory neuropathy, and autonomic neuropathy. Peripheral neuropathy affects the motor nerves, which can lead to problems with muscle movement and size. Sensory neuropathy impairs the nerves that control touch, sight, and pain perception. Autonomic neuropathy affects the nerves involved in such involuntary functions as digestion. Symptoms such as pain, loss of sensation, loss of reflexes, and/or weakness may occur.

Diabetic retinopathy

Damaged small blood vessels in the eye that can cause vision problems, including blindness.

Exchange lists

Food within any particular list—starch/bread, meat, vegetable, fruit, milk, and fat—may be exchanged with other foods on the same list without changing the nutritional content of the diet.

Fasting plasma glucose (FPG) test

The test is taken after fasting for 8 to 10 hours, typically overnight. A FPG level less than 110 mg/dL is normal; one between 110 and 126 mg/dL indicates impaired glucose tolerance or prediabetes, and one greater than 126 mg/dL supports a diagnosis of diabetes.

Exchange

A serving of food that contains known and relatively constant amounts of carbohydrate, fat, and/or protein. The food is listed in an exchange by portion size determined by weight or measurement. There are exchanges for milk, fruit, meat, fat, bread, and vegetables.

Fat

One of the three main constituents (carbohydrate, fats, and protein) of foods. Fats occur alone as liquids or solids, such as oils and margarines, or they may be a component of other foods. Fats may be of animal or vegetable origin. They have a higher energy content than any other food (9 calories per gram).

Gestational diabetes (GDM)

Elevated blood sugars usually diagnosed during the last half of pregnancy and triggered by insulin resistance. Gestational diabetes increases the risk of perinatal mortality and the development of diabetes in the mother years following the pregnancy. The blood sugar must be tightly controlled throughout the pregnancy to avoid these problems.

Glucagon

A hormone made by the pancreas that raises blood sugar levels. It is injected during severe low blood sugars to raise the blood sugar quickly by releasing glucose stored in the liver.

Glucose

A simple sugar that is found in the blood and is used by the body for energy.

Glycogen

Glycogen is the form in which the liver and muscles store glucose. It may be broken down to active blood glucose during an insulin reaction, a fast, or exercise.

Glycosylated hemoglobin

See A1c.

Gram

A small unit of weight in the metric system. Used in weighing food. One ounce equals 28 grams.

HbA1c

See A1c

Hormone

A chemical substance produced by a gland or tissue and carried by the blood to other tissues or organs, where it stimulates action and causes a specific effect. Insulin and glucagon are hormones.

Hyperglycemia

A higher than normal level of glucose in the blood (high blood sugar).

Hypertension

High blood pressure (excess blood pressure in the blood vessels). Found to aggravate diabetes and diabetic complications.

Hypoglycemia

A lower than normal level of glucose in the blood (low blood sugar), usually less than 60 mg/dl (3.3 mmol) caused by too much insulin, too little food, or extra activity. Symptoms vary from confusion, nervousness, sweating, shakiness, headaches, and drowsiness to moodiness, or numbness in the arms and hands. If left untreated, severe hypoglycemia can cause loss of consciousness or convulsions.

Insulin

A hormone secreted by the beta cells of the Islets of Langerhans in the pancreas. Needed by many cells to use glucose for energy.

IDDM

See Type 1 diabetes.

Insulin reaction

See Hypoglycemia.

Insulin pump

A small, computerized device about the size of a beeper that can be programmed to delivery basal insulin, and give a bolus of insulin for a meal or high blood sugar. It replaces insulin injections. A pump delivers rapid insulin via a plastic catheter to either a teflon infusion set or a small metal needle inserted through the skin. Doses as small as 0.05 unit can be delivered with accuracy.

Insulin resistance syndrome (IRS)

A basic metabolic abnormality underlying Type 2 diabetes. Insulin resistance describes a loss of sensitivity by certain cells to the action of insulin. AKA Metabolic Syndrome and Syndrome X.

Interstitial fluid

A relatively clear fluid between cells in which glucose measurements can be made without drawing blood by puncturing a blood vessel.

Islets of Langerhans

Special groups of pancreatic cells that produce insulin and glucagon.

Ketoacidosis

A very serious condition in which the insulin level is very low in the body, causing an excess release of free fatty acids, and high levels of ketones in the blood and urine. This acidic state takes hours or days to develop, with symptoms of abdominal pain, nausea, and vomiting. It also causes dehydration, electrolyte imbalance, rapid breathing, coma, and possibly death.

Ketones

Acidic by-products of fat metabolism.

Ketosis

An excess of ketones in the blood (and urine) which precedes the acidic state of ketoacidosis.

Nephropathy

See Diabetic nephropathy

Neuropathy

See Diabetic neuropathy

NIDDM

See Type 2 diabetes.

Oral glucose tolerance test (OGTT)

A 3-hour test of plasma glucose after drinking a solution containing 75 or 100 grams of glucose. Values over 200 mg/dL (> 11.1 mmol/L) on two occasions confirm a diagnosis of diabetes.

Pancreas

A gland positioned near the stomach that secretes insulin, glucagon, and many digestive enzymes.

Protein

One of the three main constituents (carbohydrate, fat, and protein) of foods. Proteins are made up of amino acids and are found in foods such as milk, meat, fish, and eggs. Proteins are essential constituents of all living cells and form important structures and enzymes. Proteins (four calories per gram) are burned at a slower rate than fats or carbohydrates.

Proteinuria

Protein in the urine. This may be a sign of kidney damage.

Retina

A very thin light-sensitive layer of nerves and blood vessels at the back of the inner surface of the eyeball.

Type 1 diabetes

Insulin-dependent diabetes mellitus (IDDM). The pancreas makes little or no insulin because the insulin-producing beta cells have been destroyed by several types of antibodies. Usually appears suddenly in people younger than 30. Treatment consists of daily insulin injections or use of an insulin pump, a planned diet, regular exercise, and daily self-monitoring of blood glucose.

Type 1.5 diabetes

Also called LADA. A slower form of Type 1 diabetes in adults in which only one or two types of antibodies attack the beta cells that make insulin.

Type 2 diabetes

Non-insulin-dependent diabetes mellitus (NIDDM). Type 2 diabetes is associated with insulin resistance and impaired beta cell function. It sometimes is controlled by diet, exercise, and daily monitoring of glucose levels, but at other times oral antihyperglycemic agents or insulin injections are needed. Type 2 diabetes accounts for at least 75% of diabetes cases.

References

[1] The Diabetes Control and Complications Trial Research Group: The effect of intensive treatment of diabetes on the development and progression of long-term complications in insulin-dependent diabetes mellitus. *N Engl J Med* 329: 977-986, 1993.

[2] I. Lager et. al.: Reversal of insulin resistance in Type I diabetes after treatment with continuous subcutaneous insulin infusion. *BMJ* 287: 1661-1663, 1983.

[3] J.M. Stephenson et al.: Dawn Phenomenon and Somogyi Effect in IDDM. *Diabetes Care* 12: 245-251, 1989.

[4] A.O. Marcus: Patient selection for insulin pump therapy. *Practical Diabetology* 11: 12-18, 1992.

[5] J.C. Javitt, L.P. Aiello, Y. Chiang, F.L. Ferris, J.K. Canner III, S. Greenfield: Preventive Eye Care in People with Diabetes Is Cost-Saving to the Federal Government: Implications for Health Care Reform. *Diabetes Care* 17(8): 909-917, 1994.

[6] Kroc Collatorative Study Group: Blood glucose control and the evolution of diabetic retinopathy and albuminuria. *N Engl J Med* 311: 365-372, 1994.

[7] D.M. Nathan: Long term complications of diabetes mellitus. *N Engl J Med* 328: 676-685, 1993.

[8] B. Zinman, H. Tildesley, J.L. Chiasson, E. Tsui, T. Strack: Insulin lispro in CSII: results of a double-blind crossover study. *Diabetes* 46: 440-443, 1997.

[9] R.S. Beaser, R.S. Clements, S. Crowell, E. F. Friedlander, E.S. Horton, A.M. Jacobson, R.L. Schneider, D.C. Simonson, and J.I. Wolfsdorf: Upgrading Diabetes Therapy: What every primary physician needs to know. *Novo Diabetes Care*, pg. 5, 1994

[10] I. Lager et. al.: Reversal of insulin resistance in Type I diabetes after treatment with continuous subcutaneous insulin infusion. *BMJ* 287: 1661-1663, 1983.

[11] H. Beck-Nielsen et. al.: Improved in vivo insulin effect during continuous subcutaneous insulin infusion in patients with IDDM. *Diabetes* 33: 832-837, 1984.

[12] J.O. Prochaska, C.C. DiClemente: Transtheoretical therapy toward a more integrative model of change. *Psychotherapy Theory Res Prac* 19(3): 276-287, 1982.

[13] A. Schiffrin and M. Belmonte: Multiple daily self-glucose monitoring: its essential role in long-term glucose control in insulin-dependent diabetic patients treated with pump and multiple subcutaneous injections. *Diabetes Care* 5: 479-484, 1982.

[14] Y. Z. Grasso et al: Autoantibodies to IA-2 and GAD65 in patients with Type 2 diabetes mellitus of varied duration: Prevalence and correlation with clinical features. *Endocrine Practice* 7 (5): 339 - 345, 2001.

[15] T.A. BuchananBuchanan, A.H. Xiang, R.K. Peters, S.L. Kjos, A. Marroquin, J. Goico, C. Ochoa, S. Tan, K. Berkowitz, H.N. Hodis, S.P. Azen: Preservation of pancreatic beta-cell function and prevention of type 2 diabetes by pharmacological treatment of insulin resistance in high-risk hispanic women. *Diabetes* 51: 2796-2803, 2002.

[16] J.L. Chiasson, R.G. Josse, R. Gomis, M. Hanefeld, A. Karasik, M. Laakso, STOP-NIDDM Trail Research Group: Acarbose for prevention of type 2 diabetes mellitus: the STOP-NIDDM randomised trial. *Lancet* 359: 2072-2077, 2002.

[17] W.C. Knowler, E. Barrett-Connor, S.E. Fowler, R.F. Hamman, J.M. Lachin, E.A. Walker, D.M Nathan, Diabetes Prevention Program Research Group: Reduction in the incidence of type 2 diabetes with lifestyle intervention or metformin. *NEJM* 346: 393-403, 2002.

[18] E.S. Ford, W.H. Giles, W.H. Dietz: Prevalence of the metabolic syndrome among US adults: findings from the third National Health and Nutrition Examination Survey. *JAMA* 287: 356-359, 2002.

[19] S.M. Hafner, S. Lehto, T. Ronnemaa, K. Pyorala, M. Laakso: Mortality from coronary heart disease in subjects with type 2 diabetes and in nondiabetic subjects with and without prior myocardial infarction. *N Engl J Med* 339: 229-234, 1998.

[20] Executive Summary: Third Report of the National Cholesterol Education Program (NECP) Espert Panel on Detection, Evaluation, and Treatment of High Blood Cholesterol in Adults (Adult Treatment Panel III). NIH, Nov. 19, 2002.

[21] J. R. Downs, M. Clearfield, S. Weis, E. Whitney, D.R. Shapiro, P.A. Beere, A. Langendorfer, E.A. Stein, W. Kruyer, A.M Gotto Jr.: Primary prevention of acute coronary events with lovastatin in men and women with average cholesterol levels: results of AFCAPS/TexCAPS. Air Force/Texas Coronary Atherosclerosis Prevention Study. *JAMA* 279 (20): 1615-1622, 1998.

[22] M.R. Law, N.J. Wald, A.R. Rudnicka: Quantifying effect of statins on low density lipoprotein cholesterol, ischaemic heart disease, and stroke: systematic review and meta-analysis. *BMJ* 326(7404): 1423, 2003.

[23] J. Gerontol et. al.: Reduction of new coronary events and new atherothrombotic brain infarction in older persons with diabetes mellitus, prior myocardial infarction, and serum low-density lipoprotein cholesterol >/=125 mg/dl treated with statins. *A Biol Sci Med Sci* 57(11): M747-50, 2002.

[24] M. Cucherat, M. Lievre, F. Gueyffier: Clinical benefits of cholesterol lowering treatments. Meta-analysis of randomized therapeutic trials. *Presse Med* 29(17): 965-76, 2000.

[25] Seventh Report of the Joint National Committee on Prevention, Detection, Evaluation, and Treatment of High Blood Pressure (JNC7). NIH, May 14, 2003.

[26] E. Cabrera-Rode, et al: Slowly progressing type 1 diabetes: persistence of islet cell autoantibodies is related to glibenclamide treatment. *Autoimmunity* 35(7): 469-474, 2002.

[27] D.R. Matthews, C.A. Cull, I.M. Stratton, R.R. Holman, R.C. Turner; UK Prospective Diabetes Study (UKPDS) Group: Sulphonylurea failure in non-insulin-dependent diabetic patients over six years. *Diabet Med* 15(4): 297-303, 1998.

[28] T. Kobayashi, et al: Multicenter intervention trial of slowly progressive IDDM with small dose of insulin (The Tokyo Study). *Diabetes* 45: 622-626, 1996.

[29] H.E. Lebovitz: Types of diabetes and their implications regarding heart and vascular disease. In **Medical Management of Diabetes and Heart Disease**, New York, Marcel Dekker, pg. 9-33, 2002.

[30] C.G Fonarow, A. Gawlinski: Rationale and design of the Cardiac Hospitalization Atherosclerosis Management Program at the Univ. of California Los Angeles. *Am J Cardiol* 85(3A): 10A-17A, 2000.

[31] P. Gaede et. al.: Multifactorial intervention and cardiovascular disease in patients with type 2 diabetes. *N Engl J Med* 348(5): 383-393, 2003.

[32] P. Valensi, I. Moura, M. Le Magoarou, J. Paries, G. Perret, J.R. Attali: Short-term effects of continuous subcutaneous insulin infusion treatment on insulin secretion in non-insulin-dependent overweight patients with poor glycaemic control despite maximal oral anti-diabetic treatment. *Diabetes Metab* 23: 51-57, 1997.

[33] H. Ilkova, B. Glaser, A. Tunckale, N. Bagriacik, and E. Cerasi: Induction of long-term glycemic control in newly diagnosed type 2 diabetic patients by transient intensive insulin treatment. *Diabetes Care* 20: 1353-1356, 1997.

[34] S. Park and S.B. Choi: Induction of long-term normoglycemia without medication in Korean type 2 diabetes patients after continuous subcutaneous insulin infusion therapy. *Diabetes Metab Res Rev* 19: 124-130, 2002

[35] S. Skovlund, N. Van Der Ven, F. Pouwer, F. Snoek: Appraisal of insulin therapy among Type 2 diabetes patients with and without previous experience of insulin treatment. *Diabetes* 52(Sup 1): Abstract 1818-P, 2003.

[36] D. Luery and D. Chayer: Physician's reaction to inhaled insulin, a new insulin delivery system. *Diabetes* 52(Sup 1): Abstract 456-P, 2003.

[37] P. Hollander, S. Schwartz, R. Sievers, P. Strange, B. An, W. Lyness: Insulin plus metformin vs. triple oral therapy following failure of a combination of 2 OADs: Efficacy and costs of therapy. *Diabetes* 52(Sup 1): Abstract 521-P, 2003.

[38] D.S. Bell and F. Ovalle: How long can insulin therapy be avoided in the patient with type 2 diabetes mellitus by use of a combination of metformin and a sulfonylurea? *Endocr Pract* 6: 335-336, 2000.

[39] N. Perrotti, D. Santoro, S. Genovese, et. al.: Effect of digestible carbohydrates on glucose control in insulin-dependent diabetic patients. *Diabetes Care* 7: 354-359, 1984.

[40] G. Boden and F. Jadali: Effects of lipid on basal carbohydrate metabolism in normal men. *Diabetes* 40: 686-692, 1991.

[41] D.M. Mott, S. Lilloija, and C. Bogardus: Overnutrition induced decrease in insulin action for glucose storage: in vivo and in vitro in man. *Metabolism* 35: 160-165, 1986.

[42] J.A. Marshall, S. Hoag, S. Shetterly and R.F. Hamman: Dietary fat predicts conversion from impaired glucose tolerance to NIDDM. *Diabetes Care* 17: 50-56, 1994.

[43] E. Ferrannini, E.J. Barrett, S. Bevilacqua, R.A. DeFronzo: Effect of fatty acids on glucose production and utilization in man. *J Clin Invest* 1983; 72: 1737-1747.

[44] G.M. Reaven: Banting Lecture 1988: Role of insulin resistance in human disease. *Diabetes* 37: 1595-1607, 1988.

[45] P. Halfon, J. Belkhadir and G. Slama: Correlation between amount of carbohydrate in mixed meals and insulin delivery by artificial pancreas in seven IDDM subjects. *Diabetes Care* 12: 427-429, 1989.

[46] F.Q. Nuttall, A.D. Mooradian, M.C. Gannon et al.: Effect of protein ingestion on the glucose and insulin response to a standardized oral glucose load. *Diabetes Care* 7: 465-470, 1984.

[47] D.J.A. Jenkins, T.M.S. Wolever and A.L. Jenkins: Starchy foods and glycemic index. *Diabetes Care* 11: 149-59, 1988.

[48] D.J.A. Jenkins, T.M.S. Wolever, et al.: Glycemic index of foods: a physiologic basis for carbohydrate exchange. *Amer J Clin Nutr* 34: 362-66, 1981.

[49] T.M.S. Wolever, L Katzman-Relle et al.: Glycemic index of 102 complex carbohydrate foods in patients with diabetes. *Nutr Res* 14: 651-69, 1994.

[50] J.A. Ahern, P.M. Gatcomb, N.A. Held, W.A. Petit, W.V. Tamborlane: Exaggerated hyperglycemia after pizza meal in well-controlled diabetes. *Diabetes Care* 16: 578-580, 1993.

[51] G. Perriello, P. De Feo, E. Torlone, et. al.: The Dawn Phenomenon in Type I (insulin-dependent) diabetes mellitus; magnitude, frequency, variability, and dependency on glucose counterregulation and insulin sensitivity. *Diabetologia* 42: 21-28, 1991.

[52] C. Binder, T. Lauritzen, O. Faber, S. Pramming: Insulin pharmacokinetics. *Diabetes Care* 7: 188-199, 1984.

[53] P.M. Jehle, C. Micheler, D.R. Jehle, D. Breitig, B.O. Boehm: Inadequate suspension of neutral protamine Hagendorn (NPH) insulin in pens. *Lancet* 354: 1604-1607, 1999.

[54] K Hermansen, S. Madsbad, H. Perrild, A. Kristensen, M. Axelsen: Comparison of the soluble basal insulin analog insulin detemir with NPH insulin: a randomized open crossover trial in type 1 diabetic subjects on basal-bolus therapy. *Diabetes Care* 24(2): 296-301, 2001.

[55] G. Perriello, E. Torlone, S. Di Santo, C. Fanelli, P. De Feo, F. Santeusanio, P. Brunetti, G.B. Bolli: Effect of storage of insulin on pharmacokinetics and pharmacodynamics of insulin mixtures injected subcutaneously in subjects with type 1 (insulin-dependent) diabetes mellitus. *Diabetologia* 31(11): 811-815, 1988.

[56] J. Beyer, U. Krause, A. Dobronz, B. Fuchs, J.R. Delver, R. Wagner: Assessment of insulin needs in insulin-dependent diabetics and healthy volunteers under fasting conditions. *Horm Metab Res* Suppl 24: 71-77, 1990.

[57] The 500 Rule for covering carbs with Humalog or Novolog was modified from the 450 table developed for Regular insulin by J. Walsh and R. Roberts in the *Insulin Pump Therapy Handbook*, page 19, 1992.

[58] B. Zinman: The physiologic replacement of insulin. An elusive goal. *NEJM* 321: 363-370, 1989.

[59] P. Davidson, H. Hebblewhite, R. Steed, B. Bode: A deductive framework to aid in understanding CSII parameters: carbohydrate-to-insulin ratio (CIR) and correction factor (CF). *Diabetes* 52 (Suppl 1): Abstract 443-P, 2003.

[60] Published in **Pumping Insulin** by J. Walsh and R. Roberts, page 62, 1989, after Dr. Paul Davidson of Atlanta brought up the idea of his 1500 Rule in a discussion with him at the 1988 ADA meeting.

[61] P.S. Denker, D.R. Leonard, P.E. DiMarco, P.A Maleski: An easy sliding scale formula. *Diabetes Care* 18(2): 278, 1995

[62] The 1500 Rule worked well for Regular but provided correction boluses that were too large with Humalog. We modified it to an 1800 Rule for Humalog in the third edition of **Pumping Insulin**, page 116, 2000.

[63] The Unused Bolus Rule was developed in 1984 by John Walsh while teaching a weekly diabetes intensive management workshop at Kaiser. It was first published as the Insulin-Used Rule in the first edition of **Pumping Insulin**, page 70, 1989.

[64] D.J. Menzies, P.A. Dorsainvil, B.A. Cunha, D.H. Johnson: Severe and persistent hypoglycemia due to gatifloxacin interaction with oral hypoglycemic agents. *Am J Med* 113(3): 232-4, 2002.

[65] J.M. Stephenson and G. Schernthaner: Dawn Phenomenon and Somogyi Effect in IDDM. *Diabetes Care* 12: 245-251, 1989.

[66] D. Cox, L. Gonder-Frederick, W. Polonsky, D. Schlundt, B. Kovatchev, W. Clark: Recent hypoglycemia influences the probability of subsequent hypoglycemia in Type I patients. *Diabetes* 42: Abstr 399, 1993.

[67] T.L. Levien, D.E. Baker, J.R. White Jr, R.K. Campbell: Insulin glargine: a new basal insulin. *Ann Pharmacother* 36(6): 1019-1027, 2002.

[68] V. Bhatia and J.I. Wolfsdorf: Severe hypoglycemia in youth with insulin-dependent diabetes mellitus: frequency and causative factors. *Pediatrics* 88(6): 1187-1193, 1991.

[69] S.N. Davis, S. Fowler, and F. Costa: Hypoglycemic Counterregulatory responses differ between men and women with Type 1 diabetes. *Diabetes* 49: 65-72, 2000.

[70] A. Avogaro, P. Beltramello, L. Gnudi, A. Maran, A. Valerio, M. Miola, N. Marin, C. Crepaldi, L. Confortin, F. Costa, I. MacDonald and A. Tiengo: Alcohol intake impairs glucose counterregulation during acute insulin-induced hypoglycemia in IDDM patients. *Diabetes* 42: 1626-1634, 1993.

[71] E.W. ter Braak, et. al.: Clinical characteristics of type 1 patients with and without severe hypoglycemia. *Diabetes Care* 23(10): 1467-1471, 2000.

[72] J. Anderson, S. Symanowski, and R. Brunelle: Safety of [Lys(B28), Pro(B29)] human insulin analog in long-term clinical trials. *Diabetes* 43(1): abstract 192, 1994.

[73] T. Veneman, A. Mitrakou, M. Mokan, P. Cryer and J. Gerich: Induction of hypoglycemia unawareness by asymptomatic nocturnal hypoglycemia. *Diabetes* 42: 1233-1237, 1993.

[74] C.G. Fanelli, L. Epifano, A.M. Rambotti, S. Pampanelli, A. Di Vincenzo, F. Modarelli, M. Lepore, B Annibale, M. Ciofetta, F. Bottini, F. Porcellati, L. Scionti, F. Santeusanio, P. Brunetti and G.B. Bolli: Meticulous prevention of hypoglycemia normalizes the glycemic thresholds and magnitude of most of neuroendocrine responses to, symptoms of, and cognitive function during hypoglycemia in intensively treated patients with short-term IDDM. *Diabetes* 42: 1683-1688, 1993.

[75] K. E. Powell et al.: Physical activity and chronic disease. *Am J Clin Nutr* 49: 999-1006, 1989.

[76] M. Tanasescu et. al.: Physical activity in relation to cardiovascular disease and total mortality among men with Type 2 diabetes. *Circulation* 107(19): 2392-2394, 2003.

[77] G. Zoppini, M. Carlini, M. Muggeo: Self-reported exercise and quality of life in young type 1 diabetic subjects. *Diabetes Nutr Metab* 16(1): 77-80, 2003.

[78] K.J. Cruickshanks, R.Klein, S.E. Moss, and B.E.K. Klein: Physical activity and proliferative retinopathy in people diagnosed with diabetes before age 30 yr. *Diabetes Care* 15: 1267-1272, 1992.

[79] K.J. Cruickshanks and B.E.K. Klein: Physical activity and the progression of diabetic retinopathy. *Diabetes* 43 (1): abstract 84, 1994.

80 A. Festa, C.H. Schnack, A.D. Assie, P. Haber and G. Schernthaner: Abnormal pulmonary function in Type I diabetes is related to metabolic long-term control, but not to urinary albumin excretion rate. *Diabetes* 43 (1): abstract 610, 1994.

81 P. Felig and J. Wahren: Role of insulin and glucagon in the regulation of hepatic glucose production during exercise. *Diabetes* 28(1): 71-75, 1979.

82 J. Wahren: Glucose turnover during exercise in healthy man and in patients with Diabetes Mellitus. *Diabetes* 28(1): 82-88, 1979.

83 E.B. Marliss and M. Vranic: Intense exercise has unique effects on both insulin release and its role in glucoregulation: implications for diabetes. *Diabetes* 51 (Suppl 1): S271-283, 2002.

84 R.J. Sigal et. al.: Hyperinsulinemia prevents prolonged hyperglycemia after intense exercise in insulin-dependent diabetic subjects. *J Clin Endocrinol Metab* 79(4): 1049-1057, 1994.

85 American Diabetes Association Position Statement: Gestational Diabetes Mellitus. *Diabetes Care* 25 (suppl 1): S94-96, 2002.

86 P. White: Pregnancy complicating diabetes. *Am J Med* 7: 609-616, 1949.

87 J. Pedersen: Fetal mortality in diabetics in relation to management during the latter part of pregnancy. *Acta Endocrinol* 15: 282-294, 1954

88 J. Pedersen and E. Brandstrup: Fetal mortality in pregnant diabetics: strict control of diabetes with conservative obstetric management. *Lancet* I: 607a-612, 1956.

89 J. Pedersen, L. Molsted-Pedersen and B. Andersen: Assessors of fetal perinatal mortality in diabetic pregnancy. *Diabetes* 23: 302-305, 1974.

90 K. Fuhrmann, H. Reiher, K. Semmler, F. Fischer, M. Fisher and E. Glockner: Prevention of congenital malformations in infants of insulin-dependent diabetic mothers. *Diabetes Care* 6: 219-223, 1983.

91 J.L. Kitzmiller, L.A. Gavin, G.D. Gin, L. Jovanovic-Peterson, E.K. Main and W.D. Zigrang: Preconception care of diabetes: Glycemic control prevents congenital anomalies. *JAMA* 265: 731-736, 1991.

92 B. Rosenn, M. Miodovnik, C.A. Combs, J. Khoury and T.A. Siddiqi: Preconception management of insulin-dependent diabetes: Improvement of pregnancy outcome. *Obstet Gynecol* 77: 846-849, 1991.

93 J.M. Steel, F.D. Johnstone, D.A. Hepburn and A. Smith: Can prepregnancy care of diabetic women reduce the risk of abnormal babies? *Br Med J* 301: 1070-1074, 1990.

94 M. Miodovnik, C. Skillman, J.C. Holroyde, J.B. Butler, J.S. Wendel and T. A. Siddiqi: Elevated maternal glycohemoglobin in early pregnancy and spontaneous abortion among insulin-dependent diabetic women. *Am J Obstet Gynecol* 153: 439-442.

95 J.L. Mills, J.L. Simpson, S.G. Driscoll, L. Jovanovic-Peterson, M. Van Allen, J.H. Aarons, B. Metzger, et.al.: The National Institute of Child Health and Human Development: Diabetes in Early Pregnancy Study: Incidence of spontaneous abortion among normal women and insulin-dependent diabetic women whose pregnancies were identified within 21 days of conception. *N Engl J Med* 319: 1617-1623, 1988.

96 L. Jovanovic-Peterson, M. Druzin and C.M. Peterson: Effect of euglycemia on the outcome of pregnancy in insulin-dependent diabetic women as compared with normal control subjects. *Am J Med* 71: 921-927, 1981.

97 C.A. Combs, B. Wheeler, E. Gunderson, L. Gavin, and J.L. Kitsmiller: Significance of microproteinuria in the first trimester of pregnancies complicated by diabetes. *Diabetes* 39: 36A, 1990.

98 S. Bo et al: Clinical characteristics and outcome of pregnancy in women with gestational hyperglycaemia with or without antibodies to beta-cell antigens. *Diab Med* 20 (1): 64-68, 2003.

99 I. Ostlund and U. Hanson: Occurrence of gestational diabetes mellitus and the value of different screening indicators for the oral glucose tolerance test. *Acta Obstet Gynecol Scand* 82 (2): 103-108, 2003.

[100] J.S. Sheffield, E.L. Butler-Koster, B.M. Casey, D.D. McIntire, K.J. Leveno: Maternal diabetes and infant malformations. *Obstet Gynecol* 100 (5 Pt 1): 925-930, 2002.

[101] L. Jovanovic-Peterson and C.M. Peterson: Dietary manipulation as a primary treatment strategy for pregnancies complicated by diabetes. *J Am Coll Nutr* 9: 320-325, 1990.

[102] B. Rosenn, M. Miodovnik, C.A. Combs, J. Khoury and T.A. Siddiqi: Preconception management of insulin-dependent diabetes: Improvement of pregnancy outcome. *Obstet Gynecol* 77: 846-849, 1991.

[103] L. Jovanovic, R.H. Knopp, Z. Brown, M.R. Conley, E. Park, J.L. Mills, B.E. Metzger, J.H. Aarons, L.B. Holmes, J.L. Simpson: Declining insulin requirement in the late first trimester of diabetic pregnancy. *Diabetes Care* 24(7): 1130-1136, 2001.

[104] E.A. Masson, J.E. Patmore, P.D. Brash, M. Baxter, G. Caldwell, I.W. Gallen, P.A. Price, P.A. Vice, J.D. Walker, S.W. Lindow: Pregnancy outcome in Type 1 diabetes mellitus treated with insulin lispro (Humalog). *Diabet Med* 20(1): 46-50, 2003.

[105] S.K. Garg, J.P. Frias, S. Anil, P.A. Gottlieb, T. MacKenzie, W.E Jackson: Insulin lispro therapy in pregnancies complicated by type 1 diabetes: glycemic control and maternal and fetal outcomes. *Endocr Pract* 9(3): 187-93, 2003.

[106] Bhattacharyya A, Brown S, Hughes S, Vice PA: Insulin lispro and regular insulin in pregnancy. *QJM* 94(5): 255-60, 2001.

[107] L. Jovanovic, S. Ilic, D.J. Pettitt, K. Hugo, M. Gutierrez, R.R. Bowsher, E.J. Bastyr 3rd: Metabolic and immunologic effects of insulin lispro in gestational diabetes. *Diabetes Care* 22(9): 1422-7, 1999.

[108] L. Jovanovic-Peterson, W. Bevier, and C.M. Peterson: The Santa Barbara County Health Care Services program: birth weight change concomitant with screening for and treatment of glucose-intolerance of pregnancy: a potential cost-effective intervention? *Amer J Perinatol* 14: 221-228, 1997.

[109] O. Langer, D.L. Conway, M.D. Berkus, E.M. Xenakis, O.N. Gonzales: A comparison of glyburide and insulin in women with gestational diabetes mellitus. *N Engl J Med* 343(16): 1134-1138, 2000.

[110] W. Berger, F. Caduff, M. Pasquel, A. Rump: The relatively frequent incidence of severe sulfonylurea-induced hypoglycemia in the last 25 years in Switzerland. Results of 2 surveys in Switzerland in 1969 and 1984. *Schweiz Med Wochenschr* 116(5): 145-51, 1986.

[111] R.C. Turner, C.A. Cull, R.R. Holman: U.K. Prospective Diabetes Study. *Diabetes Care* 19: 182-183, 1996.

[112] E. Haupt and U. Panten: Value of biguanide in therapy of diabetes mellitus. *Med Klin* 92 (8): 472-9, 505, 1997.

[113] J. Mamputu, N. Wiernsperger, G. Renier: Antiatherogenic properties of metformin: the experimental evidence. *Diabetes Metab* 29(4 Pt 2): 71-76, 2003.

[114] J.R. Daniel, K.O. Hagmeyer: Metformin and insulin: is there a role for combination therapy? *Ann Pharmacother* 31(4): 474-80, 1997.

[115] S. Sarnblad, M. Kroon, J. Aman: Metformin as additional therapy in adolescents with poorly controlled type 1 diabetes: randomised placebo-controlled trial with aspects on insulin sensitivity. *Eur J Endocrinol* 149(4): 323-9, 2003.

Index

Order Using Insulin

Please send me _____ copies of **Using Insulin** at $23.95 each. (CA residents add 7.75% sales tax ($1.86) or $25.81 each.) I understand that I may return this book for a full refund within 30 days for any reason. Please call for discounts on quantity orders.

Name _____

Addr _____

City _____ State _____ Zip _____

Phone ( ) _____ – _____

_____ copies of **Using Insulin** at $23.95 each ($25.81 in CA) $_____

_____ copies of **Pumping Insulin** at $23.95 each ($25.81 in CA) $_____

_____ *My Other CheckBooks* (Pocket Pancreas & 4 mos. Smart Charts) at $12.95 $_____

_____ *Smart Charts* (refill for 4 mos.) at $8.95 $_____

_____ *Smart Charts* (refill for 12 mos.) at $21.45 $_____

                        Shipping cost: $_____

            ❑ Priority Mail $4.50 (+ $1.25 for each add item) $_____

            ❑ Bookrate $3.25 (+ $0.50 for each add item) $_____

                                 Total $_____

Payment: ❑ Check   ❑ Visa   ❑ Mastercard   ❑ American Express   ❑ Discover

Card #: _____   Expires: _____ / _____

Signature: _____

By Mail:
Torrey Pines Press   **By Phone:**   (800) 988-4772
1030 West Upas St.   **By Fax:**   (619) 497-0900
San Diego, CA 92103   **Online:**   www.diabetesnet.com/ishop/